Praises for the UCAT Study Guide

"This study guide is definitely different from other UCAT resources. It is very specific in guiding you on how you should improve based on your individual weaknesses. Practising UCAT questions alongside this guide really helps to narrow down which sections I should focus on at any given time throughout my preparation. It also allows me to be specific in HOW I should improve, rather than aimlessly doing a bunch of questions"
- Tiana, scored 2870

"The strategy laid out in this guide helped me achieve a score in the 9th decile having only achieved one in the 4th decile last year"
- Danny, scored 2940

"All you need is this guide and some practice questions"
- Dana, scored 2850

"The study guide gave a really good basis and 'plan for action' for my UCAT revision and massively helped me achieve a score I couldn't have dreamt of when I first started practising!"
- Sarah, scored 2870

"People who are beginners and want to jump straight to constructive studying, this book is highly recommended. The schedule and recommended book list it provided will save you time groping around in the dark"
- Han-Ting, scored 2740

"A good guide with respect to assessing which areas you need to work on the most. Helps you create a structured study plan which otherwise I would not have done"
- Jack, scored 2830

"Great platform to help further your understanding of the Aptitude test. Helps improve strategy and focus your practise to outcome"
- Hafsah, scored 2720

"This was helpful in understanding the UCAT strategically and helped me improve my score a lot"
- Monica, scored 2540

"For those who do not know where to begin with UCAT revision, like me, this guide is absolutely perfect"
- Ishan, scored 2900

"Would've been lost without it! Really helped structure my preparation"
- Gabriella, scored 2560

"The study guide helped me immensely with preparation techniques and helped me gain more confidence in my abilities as the test approached"
- Natacha, scored 2850

"I really liked it and found all the advice really helpful, especially for the abstract reasoning section. I also liked how it helped me organise my revision and prioritise what to spend the most time on."
- Bethanh, scored 3200

"This guide helped me to effectively identify my weakest section of the UCAT and improve upon it. I think this had the biggest positive impact on my total score because it meant that I was no longer aimlessly doing questions but instead targeted focused revision"
- Serena, scored 2710

"This guide completely changed how I approached the UCAT"
- Mason, scored 2820

"Helped me to refine my practice, give me confidence, and calm my anxiety and got me 2930 and Band 1."
- John, scored 2930

"An incredible book with thorough and clear explanations of the individual subtests and tips on improving. This is not like any other book - Mike goes in depth about strategies that enabled me to recognise my weaknesses and turn them around into strengths. I am beyond grateful for this book, a hund-

red percent worth the money and beyond. Thank you!"
- Hassan, scored 2940

"Really helpful advice and tips to help improve your scores in each subset of the UCAT. I was struggling with QR and DM and the strategies to improve have been really beneficial. I also love all the extra advice you can get from the website and the 30-day challenge too. It's really helped keep me on track and focus on my weak spots"
- Mohammed, scored 3240

"I love this book and the blog also. It's literally all you need to be prepared for the UCAT, it's also easy to read and understand."
- Derek, scored 2810

"I ordered this book after looking at the reviews and recommendations from YouTube channels. This book is simply amazing - it's so easy and quick to read/follow. It provides so many techniques, bonus chapters and tips! I would definitely recommend purchasing this book, as it's helped me improve greatly"
- Nadir, scored 2950

"This is a zero to hero guide on how to prepare for the UCAT. Highly recommend"
- Manisha, scored 2560

"Michael has done a great job! It gives a good systematic approach to all the UCAT components and really helps in building up technique and resilience"
- Mohammed, scored 2760

"It's great getting exam prep advice from someone who has been in the same shoes. Very helpful in preparing for the exam"
- Becky, scored 2480

UCAT STUDY GUIDE

HOW TO SCORE IN THE TOP PERCENTILE

*250 exam tips, strategies and preparation tactics
from top scoring candidates*

Michael O. Carter

www.themedicblog.co.uk

Printed in the United Kingdom

First Printing, 2019

Published by THE UKCAT BLOG LIMITED
Proofread & edited by Nia Edwards

This book is dedicated to all the subscribers and followers of the MEDIC BLOG, old and new, thank you for the gift of your support. I only hope this UCAT study guide can begin to repay you for all the feedback and support that you've given me.

Here's to you and your continued success

Contributors, Thank you!

If you find anything amazing in this book, it's thanks to the brilliant minds who acted as teachers, critics, contributors and proofreaders. If you find anything ridiculous in this book it's because I didn't heed their advice or made a mistake.

Though indebted to hundreds of people, I wish to thank here the many UCAT candidates who have graced the pages of this book and shared what worked for them through this guide, listed in no particular order with their corresponding UCAT scores:

Marc Adams (3100)

Amelia Engle (2820)

Evan Fox (2640)

Ed Engle (2780)

Chris Gladwell (2690)

Sophie Lee (2530)

Sophia Belsky (2750)

Kevin Godin (2800)

Noah Close (2830)

Justin Beck (2930)

Sophia Amoruso (2570)

Eric Juarez (3170)

Olu Ogunyemi (3150)

Joe Gazzaaley (2950)

Dilion Loper (2550)

Jon Costner (2930)

Monica Betts (2620)

Samet Yagci (2690)

Mike Fussman (2530)

Emily Clapp (2790)

Hage Ziad (2830)

Malcolm Godin (2745)

Robin Brown (2840)

Sajid Khan (2950)

Margaret Ching (2810)

Tony Kumar (2910)

Esther Meiji (3230)

Peter Dorsey (2490)

Jimmy Nguyen (3240)

Shaul Tsor (2560)

Mo Salim (2945)

Ana Neves (2670)

Damini Wild (2850)

Glenn Fadiman (2810)

Mohamed Omar (2590)

Ivan Parcel (2530)

Alex Booke (3240)

Connor Braaten (2730)

Regina Ono (3240)

Paulo Martins (2560)

Lamia Jarrah (2705)

Ian Recker (2550)

Ibrahim Ayo (2715)

Ron Ermel (2590)

Rishi Raj (2640)

Priyanka Simas (2630)

Vi Rethin (2550)

Barnes Tyler (2580)

Nikesh Farmah (2720)

Aaron Krasner (2810)

Carl Blanco (2600)

Shyam Patel (2610)

Orlando Riveira (2920)

Duan Plavak (2710)

Raghav Bhara (3020)

Doug Fieselman (2460)

Tom Knight (2470)

Margaret King (2860)

Shawn Ross (2440)

Aarif Nughal (2590)

Contents

SITUATIONAL JUDGEMENT 389

BEST FROM THE BLOG 396

UCAT CHECKLIST 418

MY STORY AND WHY YOU NEED THIS BOOK

My Story and Why You Need this Book

'K ing's College, University of London - unsuccessful'. There it was. My UCAS homepage was relentless in its confirmation that, as of February 2010, I received rejections from all four medical schools I applied to. I sat at the desk in my bedroom in a weird semi-conscious state thinking it was the end of the world. Later, I wandered online trying to consider alternative options, I remember I was so utterly dispirited that I was unable to bring myself to share the news with my family. So what now? I had applied the previous October with confidence that I would get at least one offer. I had straight "A" predictions for my A-levels (Chemistry, Physics and Maths) and amazing work experience at my local hospital to support my application. I had accumulated 5 month's work experience as a volunteer in the Diabetes Clinic at Darrent Valley Hospital in Dartford, I was well briefed on NHS current affairs and had been given so much valuable guidance from healthcare professions and medical students. Yet I had failed to convert all the support into a single offer! I despaired at the thought of going through the long application process again. But worst of all was the fear gnawing away at me that I would never be a doctor!

"Making your mark on the world is hard. If it were easy, everybody would do it. But it's not. It takes patience, it takes commitment, and it comes with plenty of failures along the way. The real test is not whether you avoid this failure because you won't. It's whether you let it harden or shame you into inaction, or whether you learn from it; whether you choose to persevere" - **Barack Obama, US President from 2009 – 2017**

After a few days of pathetic wallowing, I decided to put it behind me. I came across the quote by Barack Obama and decided, that moment, to persevere! My ambition did not change, final A-level exams were fast approaching so I had to refocus quickly if I was going to give myself a fighting chance of reapplying. At least the shock of rejection had not depleted my motivation to work; I was desperate to prove the universities wrong by achieving my predicted grades. It took a lot of hard work and determination, but I did it! I achieved 3 A's in Physics, Chemistry and Maths, and decided I was going to take a gap year and reapply.

Once my A-levels were out of the way, I felt free to explore why I had failed to secure a place. All my medical school choices rejected me at application review due to my below the par score in the University Clinical Aptitude Test (UCAT), formerly known as the United Kingdom Clinical Aptitude Test - UKCAT. I discovered that the year I first applied there were over 80,000 applications for medicine, that was one place for every 10 applicants! To fall at just one hurdle meant immediate rejection. I soon realised that I was so naive to have been so confident of an offer. While my application was strong in some parts I had let myself down with my UCAT score. I was so determined to beat the odds that I practised harder for the exam the second time.

Before my second attempt at the UCAT, I signed up for a two-day crash course in London and spent an additional six weeks practising questions. The fate-deciding two hours in front of a computer screen eventually came around and surprisingly it was not as terrifying as the previous year. I did score a higher average of 640 but I was a little bit disappointed; it was not as high as I was hoping. However, I still applied, hoping my A-level grades and proven commitment would tilt things in my favour, but unfortunately it did not. I was still rejected by all my choices! To be fair, I had been invited to two interviews but was not able to convert them into an offer, so what now? In all honesty, I gave up. I decided to take on my 5th choice and study Pharmacology at the University of Manchester.

Pharmacology was amazing, learning about different medications, their sources, chemical properties, biological effects and therapeutic uses was great. I particularly enjoyed exploring drug interactions in biological systems, how chemical formulation interacts with living cells and tissue. In third year there was a lot of focus on clinical trials, including understanding how animals were used in research and the critical role they play in scientific understanding of biomedical systems. This research is leading to successful drug therapies and cures for diseases from Hypertension, to Spinal cord injuries. However, I soon realised that a career in Pharmacology might not be for me. I remember it like yesterday, it was at the Stopford building, the main lecture building for life science related courses - I had to inject a live rat with saline solution during an animal handling exercise (do not worry, saline is a harmless mixture of salt and water which is used to train students on proper animal handling techniques).

"Are you nervous?" my supervisor asked as I was stalling.

"I'm good. Just trying to figure out the logistics" I replied.

I was trying to adopt the handling technique that had been taught in-order to reduce animal stress and decrease the likelihood of getting bitten. Rodents were popular research subjects because their genetic, biological and behaviour characteristics closely resemble those of humans, and many symptoms of human conditions can be replicated in rodents. Most of the rodents used in our clinical practice were inbred so that, other than sex differences, they are almost identical genetically. This helps make the results of the trials more uniform; according to the National Human Genome Research Institute as a minimum requirement, mice used in experiments must be of the same purebred species. Many Manchester students might not be aware that on the top floor of this Stopford building is a huge 'secret' research facility with high level security. Before you can even access this floor as a student you are required to pass some nationally recognised test and fill in a non-disclosure agreement (NDA). This was where all our clinical practices were being carried out and it gave me first hand exposure to life as a clinical research scientist (my back-up career choice since medicine wasn't working out). Nonetheless, I took a deep breath, grabbed the rodent, it squirmed a bit - I dropped it!

"Do you need a hand, mate?" my supervisor asked impatiently

"I'm good, was just caught by surprise, going to give it another try" I replied

At that moment I suddenly became self-aware and began to notice the queue of students behind me. They were waiting their turn with cringing looks coupled with excitement, kind of the look trainee doctors have when witnessing a baby being delivered during medical training. I also realised it had been 10 whole minutes and I was no closer to successfully handling the rodent and injecting it with saline.

"5 minutes to go before it's the end of your turn" the supervisor reminded.

It was now or never, I said to myself. I took another deep breath and went for it. After two more tries and about thirty seconds to spare, I successfully handled the rat, holding it with my left hand and injecting the solution with my right without a single bite, I remember a few mates bragging they did it in one go but I was just glad I passed. I heard a rumour that a girl on the course got bitten and fainted. She dropped the rat and they had to lock down the entire practice area to prevent the rodent from escaping; not sure how true that story is but it gave me the confidence I needed to know that things could have gone a lot worse.

*"Every failure brings with it a seed of an equivalent lesson" - **Napoleon Hill***

Overall, I did enjoy clinical practice but with time, I realised it was not what I want to do for the rest of my life. It is hard to put into words why I felt this way, and over the years I have never really figured it out - all I can say is that it doesn't give me the fulfilment I normally get when I'm passionate about something. For me, the theoretical side of Pharmacology was more appealing. This gradually rekindled my passion to become a doctor and in the summer before my final year I decided to apply to graduate-entry medicine. This would be my third time applying! I was determined not to fail again, I took the time to reflect on my previous attempts at the exam and work out where I could improve. Upon reflection, I came up with a preparation plan that would accomplish FOUR things:

- Effectively identify weak areas in the UCAT and improve my reasoning skills in a short amount of time.

- Learn exam strategies and techniques to improve performance in each section.

- Effectively practice questions to increase familiarity with the exam as well as potential traps laid out by examiners.

- Include a feedback loop and performance indicators to regularly assess progress over time and adapt preparation accordingly.

After seven weeks of studying and adopting this new strategy, the UCAT finally came around and this time I could feel my hands sweating. I eventually managed to keep my cool and kept going over the 'study notes' I had put together from my revision.

"Michael O. Carter" the test supervisor yells with a strong Mancunian accent across the test centre waiting room.

"Yes?" I nervously replied

"Computer number 16 is now available for you to take your test", she continued.

I got up and walked towards the screen. All I could think of at that moment, as I was walking over, was that my dream to become a doctor came down to this test. I had three A's at A level under my belt and was on track to get at least a 2.1 in Pharmacology - I strongly believed a good UCAT score would tilt things in my favour.

I sat down, logged in and the test began.

Arguably it was the longest two hours of my life but eventually, it was over. I walked out and waited for my results in the waiting room.

A few minutes later, "Michael O. Carter!" supervisor yelled again.

"Here is your score report. Good work!" she praised before handing me a piece of paper.

I stared down at it I couldn't believe my eyes, I did it! I had exceeded my target score with an average of 710 in each section (Total of 2840), my entire approach to preparing for the exam paid off. I went from an average of 600 to 710 by strategically adapting my preparation.

Over the ensuing weeks I began getting a lot of questions from family friends planning to apply to Medicine and Dentistry the following year; my mum had pretty much told her friends I was going to be a doctor (when in fact I had not even applied at this point). I was so busy balancing my studies, part-time job and volunteer experience that I thought it would be easier to create a blog that would address all their questions instead of replying individually. The general idea of the blog was to share the tips and techniques that worked for me when I took the test. After a few months, to my surprise, the blog started getting a bit of traffic, I remember it reaching 1,000 monthly visits after 5 months. I couldn't believe it! The result inspired me to include more advice and tips for preparing for the exam. Today, the blog is visited by over 15,000 students each month during the exam period and the numbers continue to rise. The testimonials and feedback continue to inspire me to update the website and this guide.

A year after launch, I would occasionally get emails from readers seeking more specific advice on how to prepare for the exam. Some of the most common questions included:

- Where do I start with my UCAT revision?

- What amount of preparation time should I give each section?

- What is the minimum UCAT score I need to achieve?

- Is 1 month enough time to prepare for the exam?

- How did you save time with the onscreen calculator?

- How did you attempt practice questions?

- How many mocks would you recommend doing before the test?

- Can I improve my verbal reasoning skills in 1 month?

- How did you keep motivated with your UCAT preparation?

Little did I know where questions like this would take me. It was these types of questions that birthed this study guide.

"An expert is a person who has made all the mistakes that can be made in a narrow field" - **Niels Bohr, Nobel Prize Winner**

The main mistake I made the first two times I took the test was that I practiced loads of questions but had no clear strategy. Besides attempting questions and learning from their solutions - I thought I was improving but in actual fact I was only familiarising myself with the questions in the exam. In hindsight, it is no surprise my score didn't improve much the second time. I was, essentially, just getting used to the type of questions in the exam - this is what I believe is the most common mistake made by most candidates when preparing for the UCAT. There is a long list of books and courses that focus on practice questions rather than preparation or exam strategies. I would argue that strategy, for overall preparation and attempting the individual subtests, is just as important because the UCAT doesn't contain any curriculum content, rather your cognitive and reasoning abilities are being tested. Therefore, it is more effective to place equal emphasis on strategies for each subtest rather than 'improving familiarity' with the test. The third time I took the exam, I incorporated just that, and with an effective feedback loop I not only familiarized myself with the exam, but also significantly improved my reasoning skills and thus, my overall score.

This book covers over 250 tips, strategies and preparation tactics, I encourage you find the ones that work for you and master them before your big day. Here is the step-by-step process you will follow to achieve UCAT success:

1. Set: Introduces concepts for setting a target score by understanding how universities use the UCAT. For example, what is the minimum score needed to be invited for an interview? This section explores all the key factors to determine a target practice score.

2. Identify: Explains an effective step-by-step approach for discovering weak areas in the exam and shortcomings in reasoning skills.

3. Prioritise: Introduces a new approach for determining the order of dealing with the UCAT subtests. It explains which subtest to spend the most time preparing for, and by how much.

4. Improve: Recommends proven strategies to boost performance in each section by recognising the underlying reasons for incorrect answers. These include SWOT, 5-why technique, categorising weaknesses and more.

5. Practice: Introduces key rules for attempting practice questions and boosting productivity. Learn techniques for boosting productivity and studying efficacy.

6. Assess: Introduces new concepts, such as key performance indicators (KPIs), to evaluate progress over time. Spot patterns more effectively by following the strategies recommended in this step.

I should note that this entire book is designed to be very specific in guiding you on how to improve based on your individual weaknesses and jumpstart you into constructive studying. As a result, I've included a comprehensive **30-day UCAT study schedule** to help provide assistance in managing your revision time. It applies the key concepts in this book and includes daily exercises to help ensure you stay motivated and on track.

Last but not the least, I will share **exam strategies for each section** from pattern finding techniques for the abstract reasoning to speed reading techniques for the verbal reasoning subtest. I will cover everything that worked for me and the advice from many of the top scorers that contributed to this guide. I encourage you to try them and find what works for you. Many of the times past readers take out or build on elements to create their own strategies. This guide has been designed to act the foundation on which you mould your own approach to the exam.

I've also created a **private Facebook UCAT Study Group** for readers to join. It provides an opportunity to learn from other students taking the exam in the same year. Share advice and gain new perspectives as you prepare for the exam. Visit the blog for access to the UCAT Facebook group at www.themedicblog.co.uk/ucat-facebook-group

I'm about to show you step-by-step how to achieve a UCAT score in the top percentile. I remember looking on forums a while back and reading posts from successful applicants claiming that they did not really prepare for the exam, they only familiarised themselves with the questions. They further stated that preparation will not significantly improve an applicant's score! I am living proof that those claims are utter rubbish! It is **POSSIBLE** to significantly increase your UCAT score and I'm going to show you how I did it. Some exercises in this book may require you to write things down. To help you with this, you can download the study aids and templates mentioned and utilised throughout from the MEDIC BLOG store at www.themedicblog.co.uk/store. I've also included bonus materials to help keep you motivated.

It is truly an honour sharing this strategy with you, it was a huge game changer for me and I hope it does the same for you.

Take a deep breath and let me guide you on your journey to UCAT success. I am and will continue to be a humble tutor to you all.

Mike

How to use this book – Read this First

The first edition of the study guide was first published on May 8th, 2016. I did my best to cover all of the bases when it debuted, but there were a lot of gaps. Though I included everything that worked for me, I would occasionally get emails from candidates asking for more advice because some of the techniques provided didn't work for them. It was hard to provide advice beyond the scope of my experience.

Not anymore. Things have changed. There have been over 120,000 visitors on the blog since then, hundreds of candidates have shared their successes and failures with me via e-mail. For this edition I've reached out and included tips, strategies and techniques from other top scoring candidates, most of which scored higher than me in the test.

I remember during my research I had about two notebooks worth of strategies and tips compiled from other successful candidates. Once my research was out the way, the hardest part was organising the content in a logical way so that it can make sense to readers. It took an extra 3 months to sort it all out - I'll forever be grateful to sticky post-it notes. I had gone through four packs and had them all stuck on the wall of my room. After a while, some of the post-it's would loose stickability and fall off, I would freak out and cellotape them back up on the wall. My girlfriend thought I had gone mad, she would occasionally call me Rick (from the Rick and Morty tv show). For instance, I would be in the middle of a conversation with her and out of the blue I'd get a great idea, run over to the post-it wall, write my idea on a sticky note and place it. It used to annoy her because I would do it almost every day during the course of organising the contents of this book. One moment we are talking about taking a trip to Edinburgh for her birthday, the next thing you know I'm completely ignoring her and filling in a sticky note...oops. Nonetheless, one of these random idea surges was creating this chapter. Before diving into the contents of this guide, I want to share my advice on how to use it. The book is comprised of five sections, namely:

→ UCAT preparation guide

→ 30-day UCAT study schedule

→ 200+ exam strategies

→ Best from the blog

→ UCAT checklist

Preparing for the exam takes a long time so it's unrealistic to expect readers to spend every day studying for the UCAT. I took this into consideration and created a set of rules to help you get the most from the guide.

Rule #1: Read preparation guide cover-to-cover before starting 30-day schedule

Before starting the 30-day study schedule I provide a comprehensive UCAT preparation guide. Rather than regurgitating information that can be found on the official UCAT site I provide step-by-step advice from how to practice questions to what to do if you don't see any improvement. These were some of the most common questions from my readers, and I've included more detailed advice in this guide. I would recommend reading this chapter cover to cover, take notes and implement them during preparation.

Rule #2: Follow the 30-day study schedule at your own pace

The 30-day study schedule I have included in this book is broken down day-by-day, designed to help structure your revision and instil a sense of urgency when preparing for the exam. It has been designed to ensure you work up to 3 -5 hours per day. I do not expect you to follow it religiously, feel free to follow it at your own pace, I expect you to fall behind due to other commitments so it may take you longer to complete. The key thing is that it is used as a guide to structure your revision.

Rule #3: Skip strategies Intelligently and liberally - Do not read cover to cover

There are over 200 strategies in this guide - so treat it as a choose-your-own-strategies buffet. I want you to skip anything that doesn't grab you right away, take a mental note of them and return to it later. Perhaps, fold the top corner of the page or highlight the headline. This book should be fun to read. My goal is for each reader to find 80% of the content helpful, try 25% of the strategies, and use 10% in the exam. I expect you to discard plenty so don't get bogged down on reading the book cover to cover. For instance, you might realise on Day 15 of the study schedule that you struggle with 'according to the passage' questions in verbal reasoning. Rather than continuing with the schedule look into the verbal strategies for these types of questions and test one of them to improve your accuracy. If it works great! If it doesn't try another one.

Rule #4: Start with weakest subtest

All that said, I would advise you to initially refer to the strategies that improve the subtest that you have identified as your weakest. Then gradually work your way up to your strongest section. Whilst it is important to practice ALL sections of the UCAT, ensure you allocate an appropriate amount of time to practising weak areas.

Rule #5: Have a designated notebook for UCAT practice

Most students spend roughly 4 - 8 weeks preparing for the exam, which is a very long time. I recommend having a designated UCAT notebook to review regularly and help consolidate study. The notes you write should be more like hieroglyphics than your usual course notes. You should aim to write notes that trigger understanding and exam approach. I give more detailed advice on how to create effective UCAT study notes on the blog at www.themedicblog.co.uk/how-to-make-effective-ucat-study-notes.

Rule #6: Construct your attack plan as you go

Your attack plan is an outline of the techniques and strategies you intend to use on test day based on trial and error. It should give a critical breakdown of the techniques you intend to adopt based on what works in improving your accuracy and pace during practice. I give more detailed advice on how to construct an effective UCAT attack plan for each subtest on the blog at www.themedicblog.co.uk/how-to-construct-a-ucat-game-plan.

Rule #7: Reward yourself

Stepping away from distractions long enough to get some serious studying done can be difficult. That's why you should always be thinking of ways to reward yourself for studying that are specific and appealing to your situation. I'm living proof that establishing a reward system works, I use it all the time to help myself complete long-term tasks - like writing this book. For example, whenever I finished a chapter, I would take a few days off or spend a weekend away from university. Recently I went to Berlin with my best friend and it was great for unwinding, I was recharged after the break, and my work turnover increased. I encourage you to have a reward system in place when you reach a goal or milestone. You can implement it on a weekly basis when you complete all your study goals or perhaps daily when you've completed all your study tasks for the day. Trust me! It makes a difference. Perhaps you could give an episode of the Rick and Morty show a try as a reward.

We are about to go through what you need; these are resources I recommend you have in place before studying with the guide.

What You Will Need

This guide serves as a launching point for further reading. Many of the links provided will direct you to pages on the blog, I highly recommend you explore them to help support learning. I also recommend having a few resources in place before we start. Here is a list of the materials you will need before you begin the UCAT study guide:

- **UCAT Notebook:** Any notebook will do, but I recommend a small one to encourage you make shorter and more efficient study notes.
- **Official UCAT website:** The official exam website has helpful resources and practice questions to help prepare for the exam. This is where we will begin our preparation!
- **UCAT Practice book:** There are many UCAT books with thousands of practice questions, visit the blog for the latest recommendations at www.themedicblog.co.uk/ucat-books/. I do not recommend buying all of them, look at reviews and pick the most suitable.
- **Online UCAT Course:** The UCAT is a computer-based exam so investing in an online course may prove invaluable. The best courses offer additional tutorials and mock tests, so make sure to pick the most suitable one. Check out the latest recommendations on the blog: visit www.themedicblog.co.uk/online-ucat-courses/.

- **UCAT Facebook Study Group:** Includes additional tips and advice from other successful candidates. Visit www.themedicblog.co.uk/ucat-facebook-group to get link and private code to join.

I must stress that it is not mandatory to invest in a practice book or online course, but it will give you a massive advantage over other candidates as you will gain more familiarity with the spectrum of questions in the exam. A survey conducted by the exam board showed that use of these third-party materials correlated with higher scores in the exam.

UCAT PREPARATION GUIDE

PROVEN STEP-BY-STEP GUIDE TO PREPARE FOR THE UCAT TEST

UCAT Preparation Guide - Overview

t took three attempts at the UCAT before finally scoring in the top 10%. I made every possible mistake that one could make. However, during my third attempt at the test I designed a preparation plan that would accomplish FOUR key things:

- Effectively identify weak areas and improve my reasoning skills
- Learn exam strategies and techniques to improve performance in each section.
- Effectively practice questions to increase familiarity with the exam as well as potential traps laid out by examiners.
- Include a feedback loop and performance indicators to regularly assess progress over time and adapt preparation accordingly.

These goals were accomplished by splitting my preparation into 6 steps, they are as follows:

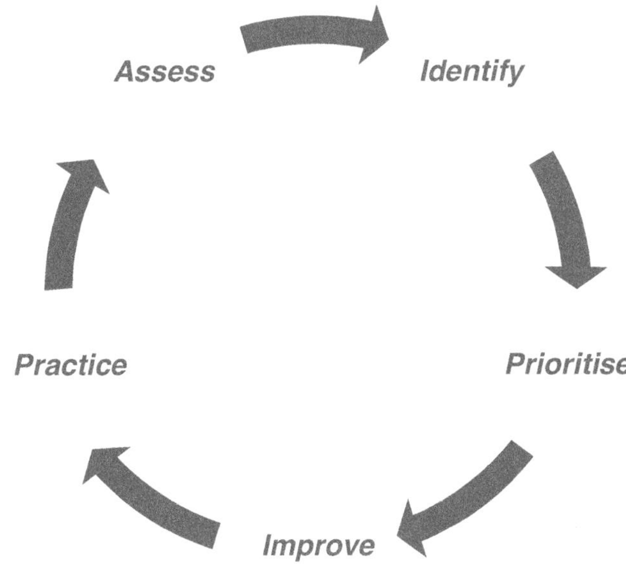

Set

This must be completed before we begin the next step in preparing for the exam, it involves setting a target practice score that will act as a benchmark throughout your entire preparation. When you attempt any mock or practice test, it will be compared to this target score. The idea is that you have a way to assess progress over time. Your target score should reflect your chosen University's requirement for the UCAT. I have not included this in the cyclic process because we will not repeat this step throughout preparation.

Identify

This is the second step during preparation, it involves identifying your weakness and strengths in the exam. It is important to identify this early on as it will dictate how you prepare for the exam. Although it is important to practice all sections of the UCAT you should aim to spend a majority of time working on your weak areas, hence the necessity of this step.

Prioritise

This is the third step and it involves prioritising the subtests and question-types in the exam. One of the most common mistakes candidates make is that they assume that their lowest score during practice is their weakest, which isn't necessarily the case. Using the results from the identify stage, prioritise the subtests and have a rough plan for the amount of time you will spend on its section.

Improve

Learn tips, techniques and strategies to improve your score in each section. Spend more time on your weakest subtest and question-types. Pay attention to accuracy and speed in each subtest. Select a hand full of strategies that work well and hone them before the live test.

Practice

This is the fifth step and it involves practising questions. Spend the initial stages attempting questions untimed to improve accuracy then increase the speed by attempting questions under exam conditions. During which you should implement the strategies shared in this book to improve your accuracy and speed in each subtest

Assess

The final step involves creating a feedback loop, this is usually in the form of full mocks or practice tests, which must be under timed conditions. You want to replicate the same environment as the exam and assess a number of key performance indicators (KPIs) that will influence your score. These are Error rate and Speed. Keep a close eye on these two metrics. Assess them thoroughly and regularly. They can be calculated with straightforward maths, which we will dive into later in the book.

After Step 6, repeat the entire cycle again starting with the identify stage. Use the results from assessment (step 6) to recognise new areas to work on. Repeat cycle until your skill and test results are at a level you are pleased with. The idea is that as you move from one cycle to another you begin to narrow your preparation, giving priority to the weakest subtest (as seen below).

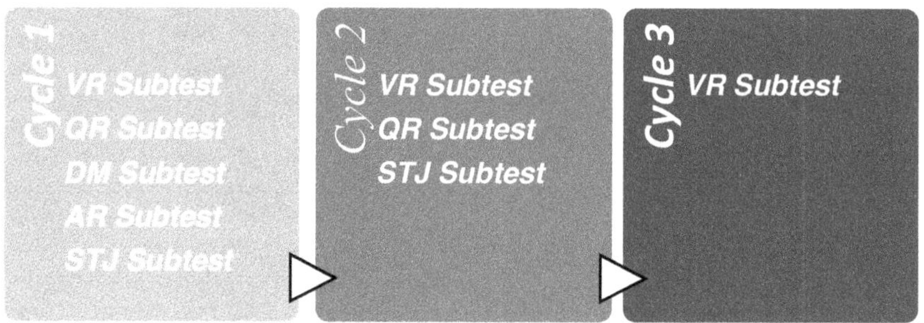

In the example above, the student has identified their weakest section as the verbal reasoning subtest. Hence why it is included in all three cycles. Furthermore, this cyclic approach can also be used when digging into each subtest to practice specific question-types (see below an example digging into the verbal reasoning subtest).

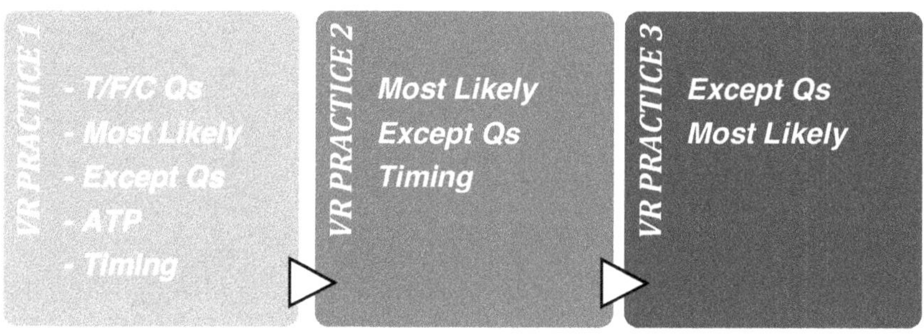

By the third cycle, the student had improved on all main question-types in the VR subtest besides in the 'Except Questions' and 'Most Likely questions' so they remain priority in the third cycle of the strategy. Within each subtest you must find your weakness and drill into them, understand the underlying cause for mistakes and learn strategies to fix them (as seen in diagram below).

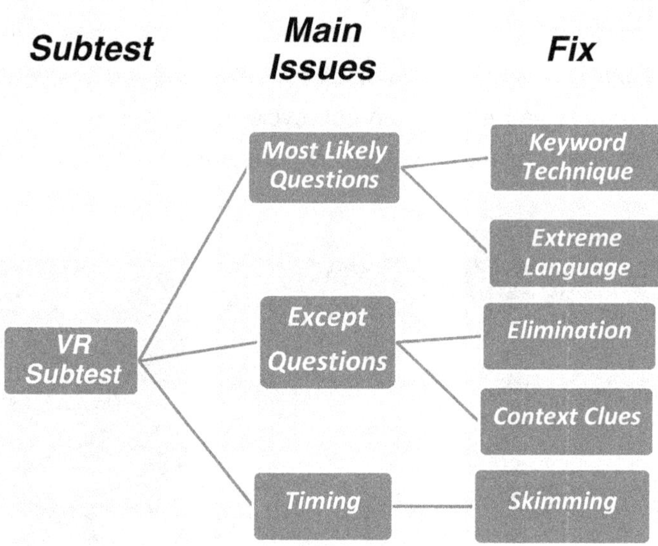

Step 1: Set

Setting Your Target Practice Score

A few years ago, I received an email from someone named Jade, a medicine applicant and regular reader of the blog. I get a lot of emails from readers but this one had an eye-catching subject line.

Subject: I got 690 is that good enough?

Hi Michael, I did my UCAT yesterday and got 2760 as an overall score (VR -590, QR -760, DM -680, AR-730 and Band 2). I've been following your blog and the advice has been great so far and was really helpful in preparing for my UCAT. Can you please advise if 2760 is a good enough score to apply to Medicine?

Kind Regards

- Jade

I regularly get similar questions like this from readers and I usually find myself replying by asking the same question every time:

Hi Jade, Thank you for the email. Glad you found the blog helpful. With regards to your question, how does your first choice assess the UCAT?
- Mike

The most common response from readers is that they have no clue, whilst some are not sure. In Jade's case, she mentioned her choice stated on their website they did not have a minimum requirement and rank applicants based on their overall application where their UCAT score is taken into account.

Universities use the UCAT differently, some have a cut-off where a score good enough for admittance into one university might not be good enough for another. Whilst others rely more on a ranking approach, where the UCAT is one of many components taken into consideration to rank applicants. Nonetheless, it is of great importance to understand how your choice assesses the UCAT because it helps understand if your score is good enough, even though, in some cases your choice may not have a minimum requirement. All universities part of the UCAT consortium assess the exam in some way; it is by understanding this 'assessment' you can set a target practice score, i.e. your goal during your UCAT preparation. To help further explain this, let's take a quick look at the exam and its format.

UCAT Format

The UCAT is a computer-administered exam lasting 2 hours. The test consists of five parts: Verbal Reasoning, Quantitative Reasoning, Abstract Reasoning, Decision Making and Situational Judgement.

Subtest	Time Allowed	Number of Questions	Time Per Question
Verbal Reasoning	21 minutes	44	30 seconds
Decision Making	31 minutes	29	64 seconds
Quantitative Reasoning	24 minutes	36	40 seconds
Abstract Reasoning	13 minutes	55	15 seconds
Situational Judgement	26 minutes	69	22 seconds

Each of the five parts of the UCAT is in a multiple-choice format and is timed separately, they are as follows:

Verbal reasoning subtest: According to the official UCAT site "the verbal section tests the ability to read and think carefully". You are given 21 minutes to complete 44 questions. Some questions assess critical reasoning skills, where you are required to make inferences and draw conclusions. Others might be an incomplete statement or a question, with four response options where you are required to pick the best or most suitable answer from the options provided. For other questions, your task is to read each passage carefully and then decide whether the statement provided is True, False or Can't Tell.

Quantitative Reasoning: According to the official site "tests the ability to solve numerical problems". You are given 24 minutes to complete 36 questions. The problems are at GCSE level and include texts, tables, charts and graphs, where you are required to extract relevant information. A simple on-screen calculator is made available to use in this section.

Abstract Reasoning: According to the official site "the abstract reasoning tests the ability to spot patterns amongst abstract shapes, where distracting patterns may lead to incorrect conclusions". The test measures the ability to critically evaluate, generate hypotheses and change track if necessary. You are given 13 minutes to complete 55 questions. The subtest includes 4 different types of questions, which we will cover in more detail later in the book.

Decision Making: According to the official site "tests the ability to apply logic to reach a decision or conclusion, evaluate arguments and analyse statistical information". This is a relatively new subtest where some questions will have 4 answer options with one correct answer, others may give you a statement options where you are required to place a 'yes' or 'no' next to each statement. You are given 31 minutes to complete 29 questions and will be provided with an onscreen calculator for the subtest.

Situational Judgement: According to the official site "tests your capacity to understand real world situations and identify critical factors and appropriate behaviour in dealing with them". You will be given 26 minutes to complete 69 questions, there are two types of questions in this subtest, we will cover them in detail later in the book.

UCAT Marking

The UCAT is marked based on the number of correct responses you give on the test. The test doesn't use negative marking. That means your score does not go down if you give a wrong answer, but instead you just fail to gain on that particular question. The number of correct responses in each subtest (except for the Situational Judgement subtest) is scaled into a mark ranging from 300 to 900. The total score for the entire test therefore ranges from 1200 to 3600.

Unlike the other subtests, you receive a band score in the Situational Judgement section. The bands reflect the degree to which your answers match the same answers determined by a panel of medical experts and are assessed from Band 1 to Band 4.

Band 1 means that most of your answers were the same as the panel of medical experts; Band 4 means very few of your answers matched. Your goal is to match the answers of the panel.

Band 1 – Very Good
Band 2 – Good
Band 3 – OK
Band 4 – Poor

The key thing to take from this is that the UCAT does not have a specific pass mark, and universities have different opinions on what they consider to be a good score.

How Universities use the UCAT

In order to set a target score you must first understand how your choices use the UCAT. Each university part of the consortium independently decides the importance of the test. There is significant variation in how the various universities use the exam during their selection process. There are categorically two main approaches used by universities and they are as follows:

Approach #1 - Cut-off system

This is when a university sets a universal cut-off, it is the lowest possible score, or band score, a candidate must achieve to be considered for the next stage in the application process. Typically, a UCAT cut-off is based on the overall score achieved in the exam. However, there are universities that have a minimum requirement for each individual subtest. At the time of writing this book, St George's, University of London required applicants to have a minimum of 500 in each section of the UCAT.

Many universities who adopt this approach tend to review and set their cut-off scores annually once the testing cycle is over and applications are submitted. So, there is no way of knowing the UCAT cut-off for the year you apply. A bit frustrating, I know, but not to worry. With some digging, which I will share later in this chapter, you can get a rough idea on the score needed to be considered and therefore increase the likelihood of being invited for an interview.

Nowadays, there is an increasing number of universities considering the band score in the situational judgement subtest and setting a banding cut-off. Whilst some universities do not take the STJ section into consideration, there are some that place a significant amount of emphasis on it. At the time of writing this guide, universities such as Keele, Leicester and Nottingham did not further consider candidates with a band 4 in the STJ section. More popularly, the STJ band score can be used for 'borderline cases' – this is when a university has two candidates who achieve the same score, and they can only invite one to interview or make one an offer, then they might look at the Situational Judgement as a final tool in making their selection.

Approach #2 - Ranking system

Universities that do not have a UCAT cut-off tend to use a ranking or scoring system to shortlist applicants. This is usually when applicants are awarded points based on the outcome of their UCAT score as well as the overall application. Students that achieve high scores receive more points than students with lower scores. Most scoring systems take into account other parts of an application such as academics, personal statement and reference, which are awarded points to create a total score which is ranked against other competing applicants.

At the time of writing, Hull York medical school for example, used a point-based ranking system taking into consideration applicants' total UCAT score and GCSEs. Other medical and dental schools such as University of Edinburgh, Queen Mary University of London and University of Warwick are some of the popular choices known to adopt this scoring approach as well. Each university has their own approach to using the points-based system and consider different factors of one's entire application. I recommend considering these types of universities if you do not perform particularly well in the UCAT, as other elements of your application may help boost total points earned.

When I applied for Medicine back in 2015, I looked into every medical school in the UK that required the UCAT and created the table below. The table gives an overview of the approach respective universities used to assess the UCAT the year I applied. I encourage you to do the same and research into how all the medical or dental schools in assess the exam. You may need to refer back to this, depending on the outcome of your UCAT Score.

University	Assessment Type
University of Aberdeen	Ranking
Barts	Cut-off
University of Birmingham	Ranking
Cardiff University	Ranking
University of Central Lancashire	Ranking
University of Dundee	Ranking
University of Durham	Ranking
University of East Anglia	Ranking
University of Edinburgh	Ranking
University of Exeter	Cut-off
University of Glasgow	Ranking
Hull York Medical School	Cut-off
Keele University	Ranking
King's College,	Ranking
University of Leicester	Ranking
University of Liverpool	Ranking
University of Manchester	Cut-off
University of Newcastle	Cut-off
University of Nottingham	Ranking
Plymouth University	Ranking
Queen's Mary, University of	Cut-off
University of Sheffield	Cut-off
University of Southampton	Cut-off
University of St Andrews	Ranking
St George's, University of London	Cut-off
University of Warwick	Cut-off

Please note the table above refers to when I applied back in 2015, the universities above might have changed their approach in assessing the exam or may no longer be part of UCAT Consortium. For the latest list of universities part of the UCAT test consortium, visit the blog at www.themedicblog.co.uk/ucat-universities.

43

Assessing how Universities use UCAT

For a majority of universities, you should be able to find information regarding how they use the UCAT on their website. However, there are some cases where the information might not be so easy to find. Just like in Jade's case, her first choice did not provide much information on their website, only that they "do not use a UCAT cut-off". Unfortunately, this is not sufficient to help determine whether Jade's UCAT score is good enough for applying.

Another popular case is when a university uses a cut-off but it is determined after the testing cycle, once applications are submitted. I remember stumbling upon these issues myself when I applied to Medicine. However, there are some resources you can use to assess whether your score is good enough and set a target score before taking the test; they are as follows:

Resource #1 - Official UCAT University Guide

The UCAT university guide is a document released by the exam board every year that provides an overview of how each university part of the consortium uses the UCAT during their admission process. The document tries to provide up-to-date information directly copied from the university's website.

The document includes a retrieval date i.e. the date that the information was cited. To reduce the likelihood for any omissions, inaccuracies or changes, the document also includes links to the respective websites where it was cited for you to check again. There is always a chance a university may make some changes, so I encourage going through the links provided. You can find a download link to the latest version of the university guide on the blog at www.themedicblog.co.uk/how-universities-use-the-ucat. I recommend going through the document with the following points in mind during your research:

- Is there a minimum UCAT requirement?
- If there is no cut-off, how are applicants ranked?
- How much emphasis is put on the other parts of an application?
- Is the situational Judgement taken into consideration? If so, at what stage?

Resource #2 - Admissions Office

Every medical and dental school has an admissions team responsible for managing admission for their respective courses. They are very helpful and can provide valuable information not included on their website. However, they may at times not give much information regarding how they assess the UCAT the year you are applying. However, you are more likely to get information about previous application cycles. I remember when I applied the third time I was so 'desperate' that I called the respective admission teams to get more insight into their application process. If the tutor on the phone did not know the answer to my question, I followed up with an email. In some cases, I called again to follow up when I got no answer. Below are a few questions that worked really well:

- Did you have a cut-off last year?
- How is the cut-off determined?
- What was the cut-off last year?
- How much emphasis was put on the exam last year?
- Did you use a ranking system last year?
- How was the exam assessed last year?
- What would you say is a good score?
- How did you rank applicants last year?
- I understand you use a point-based system to rank applicants, how are the points determined?
- How many students applied last year and how many did you invite for interview?
- How many places do you have on your course?

I discovered that I got more information asking direct questions like "what was the UCAT score cut-off last year?" than questions like "what UCAT score do I need?". I noticed admission tutors responded better to questions that showed I've done a bit of research before calling. For example, "I understand you use a point-based system to rank applicants, how are the points determined?". When you begin to look into how universities assess the UCAT, I strongly recommend you record your findings as you may need to refer back to it from time to time. I recorded mine on an excel spreadsheet and found this very convenient for referring back to when I had to shortlist my choices.

Now let's take a deeper dive at some of the questions that worked really well. I want to explain their significance and how you can use the information to set a target score:

Question 1: Did you use a UCAT cut-off system last year?

For universities that do not provide much information on their websites, I found this question extremely helpful. The last thing you want is to be applying to a university with an achieved score below their UCAT cut-off. This question is great because it is closed and the tutor only has two options to respond - Yes or No. If they respond with Yes, record it on a table, as seen below, that they use a 'cut-off'. If NO, record it as 'ranking' If there was a cut-off for the previous year, a good follow-up question would be something like "What was the cut-off last year?" and record the response. Always seek to ask additional questions that will help mould out a rough estimate for the score you need. If the tutor doesn't seem sure or has no clue, politely ask for their name and email address and then immediately send an email to follow up. Highly unlikely, but if for whatever reason they refuse to provide an answer, I recommend calling back and rephrasing your question, something like "What was the minimum score for candidates you invited for interview last year?", or perhaps, "What is a good score?". Below is a list of universities that used a cut-off the year I applied, ranked from lowest to highest. Please note that some of the cut-off scores are estimates based on calls with the admissions office or information from their website. Also note that this may most likely not be the same for the year you apply.

University	Cur-off Score
Barts	2400
Hull York	2400
Exeter	2500
Southampton	2500
St Georges	2590
Sheffield	2600
Warwick	2690
Newcastle / Durham	2718
Manchester	2810
King's College	2920

Question 2: Did you use a ranking system last year?

This is another great closed question for universities that may award points. Great follow up questions include "Which components of an application is ranked/scored?" or "Which component holds the most weight on the total score?". The key thing you want to know is how points are awarded and which component is the most important factor. Universities that use a ranking system where they factor other parts of your application may be a better consideration if you do not perform particularly well in the UCAT. However, some ranking universities place a lot of emphasis on the UCAT. At the time of writing this book, King's College University of London mentioned the exam as the most important factor when shortlisting applicants - these types of universities might be better applying to if you don't have particularly strong academics but have achieved a high score. At the same time, there are universities that do not put much emphasis on the exam, like the University of Aberdeen that used a score ranking system where the UCAT accounted for 40% and academics accounted for 60%.

Question 3: Did you consider the band score in Situational Judgement last year?

The Situational Judgement is the final subtest of the UCAT. Unlike the other sections, you do not receive a score out of 900. Instead, you are assessed from Band 1 (Very Good) to Band 4 (Poor). The section measures your ability to understand real world situations and identify critical factors and appropriate behaviour in dealing with them. Some universities such as Keele, Nottingham and Liverpool consider this section of the exam and automatically reject candidates with a band 4 score. Whilst others such as Warwick and Southampton do not even consider this section at the time of writing this guide. Even If you achieve a high UCAT score but end up with a band 3 or 4 in the STJ section, I wouldn't advise applying to a university that considers the STJ section, chances are, you'll get rejected.

Question 4: How many students applied last year and how many places do you have on your course?

To help measure the 'competitiveness' of a course, I asked the above question to create an **Applicants to Places** ratio. The ratio is a measure of how competitive a course is based on how many students apply versus the number of places on the course. It is calculated using the formula below:

$$Application: Places Ratio = \frac{Total\,Number\,of\,Applicants}{Total\,number\,of\,places}$$

Let's take another look at the universities that used a cut-off when I applied and rank them according to 'competitiveness' using this ratio.

	Cut-off	No of Applications	Places	Application: Places Ratio
St George's	2590	1000	135	7.4
Manchester	2810	3000	380	7.9
Bart's	2400	2369	260	9.1
Newcastle	2718	3000	327	9.2
Sheffield	2600	2500	237	10.5
Kings	2920	3500	330	10.6
Hull York	2400	1400	130	10.8
Exeter	2500	1700	130	13.1
Southampton	2500	4000	276	14.5
Warwick	2690	3000	164	18.3

From the table above, we can deduce that for St George's, about 7 people were applying for every place, for Manchester that about 8 people were applying for every place, Bart's about 9 people were applying for every place and so on.

Let's assume I achieved a score of 2600 when I took the test, then the following cut-off universities would be the ones I would consider:

University	Cut-off	Applications: Places
Barts	2400	9.1
Hull York	2400	10.8
Exeter	2500	13.1
Southampton	2500	14.5
St Georges	2590	7.4
Sheffield	2600	10.5

At first glance, you might be thinking that applying to Barts or Hull York would be the best option as they have the lowest cut-off scores, but when you consider the application to places ratio this might not be the case. Let's take another look at Hull York for example, it is far more competitive than applying to St Georges and Sheffield. Therefore, all things considered, Hull York might not be a great choice despite the low UCAT requirement.

The Application:Places ratio approach is flawed in some parts as it doesn't tell you about the real nature of the competitive selection process at each university. Nonetheless, I strongly recommend that you choose a medical or dental school based largely on its course structure, its teaching style and whether you have a strong chance of getting in. Working out the Application:Places ratio can be an additional factor to help indicate your chances of getting selected for an interview.

Last but not least

Once you understand how universities use the UCAT, use results from your research to set a target score. Your UCAT target score is the minimum score you need to achieve to apply to your ideal choices, not factoring other parts of your application. It is the minimum score needed to increase the likelihood of being invited for an interview or being offered a place. I appreciate you want to score as high as possible in the exam but setting a minimum target score beforehand helps with assessing your performance as you prepare for the exam.

Target Score = UCAT Cut-off For #1 Choice

If your first choice uses a UCAT cut-off, you may want to set your target practice score as this minimum. For universities that use a ranking system or are not clear about how they use the exam, I recommend giving them a call to get a rough estimate. If that proves futile, use the official UCAT results data released each year. The exam board uses a statistical approach called *decile* or *percentile* to report the overall performance of candidates each year. A decile is any of the nine values that divide the results into ten equal parts where each decile represents 10% of the total candidates based on their overall test performance. The 1st decile represents a score at the 10th percentile; the 2nd decile represents a score at the 20th percentile, and so on. This statistical approach is descriptive and gives a good overview of candidate's performance in the UCAT each year. The highest scoring applicants will be in the 9th decile, while the lowest scoring candidates will be in the 1st decile. Universities analyse the official results and compare them with their applicant pool. When setting my target score in 2015, I used the decile rank from the previous year i.e. the 2014 UCAT results, to set a minimum target practice score for universities that used a ranking approach.

Decile	2014 Results (Out of 3600)
1st	2210
2nd	2330
3rd	2410
4th	2470
5th	2540
6th	2600
7th	2660
8th	2740
9th	2840

The total score for each decile indicates the score a candidate can achieve to be classified in that decile. For example, in 2014, a candidate that scored 2330 in the exam would be in 2nd decile or 20th percentile, which means they scored better than 20% of all the candidates that took the exam in 2014. The overall UCAT performance is released by the exam board after each testing cycle and can be found on the official website. You can find the latest deciles and mean scores on the blog: www.themedicblog.co.uk/ucat-mean-scores-deciles/.

Use the UCAT results from the previous year to set a target score if your first choice isn't clear how they assess the exam. In some cases, where your first choice does provide information on how they rank applicants, I suggest using their formulae to set a target. The decile/percentile approach should only be used if your first choice does not provide much information or if it is suggested that the UCAT is the main component when ranking candidates.

Based on my research in 2015, I decided to set a minimum practice target score of 2600 which was the 6th decile rank in 2014. After looking into my ideal 4 choices I set my ideal target score to 2800 (i.e. 700 in each section).

Ideal Score – 2800

(Based on Researching Ideal Choices)

Minimum Score - 2600

(Based on Researching Previous year results)

Generally, scores in the 6th decile, i.e. the top 40%, are typically considered to be good UCAT scores. However, this doesn't mean that if you achieve below this you will not get a place into medicine or dentistry, you may just need to consider universities that do not rely so heavily on the exam. As a rule of thumb, you can set your target score as the 6th decile rank from the previous year. This will help with gauging your performance during practice in cases where it's not clear what you need to achieve to be invited for an interview. It is possible that the cut-off for your first choice might be below the 6th decile for the previous year. If this is the case, I recommend setting the decile score as the ideal and the university's cut-off as the minimum target score. Before we move into the second step, have an ideal and minimum UCAT target score set. You will refer back to these scores as you prepare for the exam.

Now let's identify your weakest areas and create an attack plan to improve both skill and familiarity with the exam.

Step 2: Identify

Identifying Your Weakest Areas

Whilst it is important to practice all sections of the UCAT, the subtest you identify as weakest will ultimately define how you tailor your preparation. Identifying and focusing on weak areas is a bullet-proof way to significantly increase your total score. However, with so many resources available, it can be confusing and difficult to know where to start. In this chapter I'll show you step-by-step, how to identify your weakest section and recognise the element(s) you struggle with the most. The TWO main mistakes most candidates make during this step are firstly, they assume the subtest they score the lowest in, is their weakest and secondly, once they have falsely identified this weakness, they would attempt more practice questions rather than doing more targeted study that involves analysing question-types and shortcomings in skill. For instance, let's assume a candidate discovered that the abstract reasoning section was their weakness. Rather than practice more abstract questions they could deep dive into the subtest to improve - the abstract section has 4 different question-types. Depending on their shortcomings, a more effective approach would be identifying which question-type the candidate struggles with the most and the practicing more of this specific type. Another approach could be honing their technique for spotting patterns. Both approaches are far more effective in improving one's overall abstract score than attempting practice questions.

So, before we begin to identify your weakest section, you will need to fully understand the tasks, question-types and skills being tested in each section to effectively recognise the key areas you may need to work on.

Verbal Reasoning - Task, Questions & Skills

The verbal reasoning section assesses your ability to read and think carefully about the information presented in passages, and to determine whether specific conclusions can be drawn from them. You are not expected to use prior or external knowledge - for example, if the passage states that London is the capital of France, you must use this to answer the questions and apply information only provided in the passage. The verbal subtest includes five main types of questions, they include:

True/False/Can't Tell Questions - These are questions where you are given a statement and must decide if, based on the passage, it is true, false or you can't tell.

Incomplete Statements - This question-type isn't written as a question, instead you must pick an appropriate option that would best finish the statement provided.

According to the Passage - These questions usually start with the phrase 'According to the passage', where you must pick the most appropriate answer solely based on information provided in the passage.

Except Questions - These are questions where you are required to select the answer that is an exception to the options provided. You must weigh up the evidence and draw conclusions from the passage in-order to select the correct answer.

Most likely Questions - These are questions where you have to pick the answer that is most likely true or false. You also have to weigh up evidence provided from the passage and draw conclusions in order to deal with this question-type.

For examples of each type of verbal reasoning question visit the blog at www.themedicblog.co.uk/ucat-verbal-reasoning-subtest. Each type of verbal question requires you to think carefully about the passage to answer all 44 items. There are three skills being tested in the verbal section and they are as follows:

Comprehension - This is your ability in understanding and interpreting of what is being read. If you find yourself getting a majority of questions wrong because you misunderstood the passage, then this is probably a weakness. We will cover tips and strategies to boost comprehension later in the guide.

Critical Thinking - Some questions may require you to read between the lines, i.e. make inferences and draw conclusions from various parts of the passage. If you find this difficult then you may need to work on this skill. I must admit this was a weakness of mine. We will cover tips for improving critical thinking when preparing for the subtest.

You have 21 minutes to answer 44 questions, that's about 30 seconds per question! If, during practice, you find yourself not finishing the section in time then this probably is a weakness. We will take a look at time-saving strategies and tips for improving both reading and processing speed.

Decision Making - Task, Questions & Skills

The Decision-Making subtest tests your ability to apply logic to reach a decision or conclusion, evaluate arguments and analyse statistical information. The question-types are not as straightforward as the verbal section; instead candidates can expect questions broken down into the type of skill being tested, and they include:

Deductive Reasoning - This is your process of reasoning from one or more statements to reach a logically certain conclusion. In the test, you will be presented with items that are in the form of syllogism or logical puzzles.

- **Syllogism** - These are questions where a conclusion is drawn from two given or assumed propositions (premises); a common or middle term is present in the two premises, but not in the conclusion, which may be invalid. E.g. all dogs are animals; all animals have four legs; therefore, all dogs have four legs. If you are getting these types of questions wrong, then this is an area for improvement.
- **Logical Puzzles** - The UCAT also includes puzzles where statements are provided, and you have to piece together what is happening. This involves clear and logical thinking.

Evaluating Arguments - The Decision-Making section also includes questions that assess your ability to evaluate arguments. These types of questions usually account for 35% of the real test. They are in the form of two question types:

- **Recognising assumptions** - These types of questions are typically standalone statements where you'll be will have four answer options.
- **Interpreting information and drawing a conclusion** - These types of questions typically involve a graph, chart or table where you will be given

5 statements and be required to respond to each statement by placing a 'yes' or 'no' answer next to each statement.

Statistical Reasoning - These are questions that require some degree of mathematical skills; they test the ability to assess probability and deal with statistical information. There are two subtypes:

- **Venn Diagrams** - A venn diagram is a diagram that shows all possible logical relations between a finite collection of different sets. You should be aware of this from GCSE's, the UCAT has incorporated this into the DM subtest.

- **Probability** - This is the other type of statistical reasoning question. Probability is about estimating how likely (probable) something is to happen. The DM section includes probability questions that require candidates to select a response from four options.

For examples of each type of decision-making question visit the blog at www.themedicblog.co.uk/ucat-decision-making-subtest. You have 31 minutes to complete 29 items, that's just over 1 minute per question. It might seem like a lot of time compared to the verbal section but bear in mind you have to read statements and constantly re-evaluate the options provided, which can take some time.

Quantitative Reasoning - Task, Questions & Skills

The quantitative reasoning subtest assesses your ability to use numerical skills to solve problems, by extracting relevant information from text, tables and other numerical presentations. The subtest draws on your ability in evaluating and deducing data to solve problems. The subtest assumes you have familiarity with core Maths concepts at secondary school level. You'll be expected to draw on problem-solving and data analysis skills in this subtest. Key areas include:

- Percentages, ratios and fractions
- Proportionality: inverse and direct
- Rate - Speed, distance and time calculations
- Working with money

- Areas and volumes
- Graphs and charts

For examples of quantitative reasoning question-types visit the blog at: www.themedicblog.co.uk/ucat-quantitative-reasoning-subtest. Remember, Questions can come in any form covering key areas such as percentages, proportions, rates and averages to name a few. You have 24 minutes to answer 36 questions, that's on average about 40 sections per response, so decisions have to be made quickly and accurately, some questions may take longer, and others may be quicker to answer. The key is to have an efficient method to get to the right answer.

Abstract Reasoning - Task, Questions & Skills

The abstract reasoning section assesses your ability to identify patterns or rules that apply amongst abstract shapes. There are four different types of questions in this section, they include:

Type 1 - You are presented with two sets of shapes labelled "Set A" and "Set B" are then given a test shape and asked to decide whether the test shape belongs to Set A, Set B, or Neither.

Type 2 - You are presented with a series of shapes then asked to select the next shape in the series.

Type 3 - You are presented with a statement, involving a group of shapes, then asked to determine which shape completes the statement.

Type 4 - You are presented with two sets of shapes labelled "Set A" and "Set B". Then asked to select which of the four response options belongs to Set A or Set B.

For examples of each type of decision-making question visit the blog at: www.themedicblog.co.uk/ucat-abstract-reasoning-subtest. You have 13 minutes to answer 55 questions, that's on average about 15 seconds per item which may not seem like enough time but with enough practice you can develop an efficient method to get to the right answer.

Situational Judgement - Task, Questions & Skills

The situational judgement subtest measures your capacity to understand real world situations and how to identify critical factors and appropriate behaviour in dealing with them. Unlike the other subtests, you do not receive a score out of 900. Instead you are given a band score (from 1 to 4), where band 1 is the highest. There are two types of questions tested, they include:

Appropriateness Questions - This usually accounts for most of the items. This is where you are given a scenario and presented with an action. You will need to rate how appropriate this action is in the context of the scenario. You are given four answer choices to choose from, they include:

- A very appropriate thing to do
- Appropriate, but not ideal
- Inappropriate, but not awful
- A very inappropriate thing to do

Other questions are drag-and-drop where you will be presented a few actions to a scenario and asked to choose the most appropriate and least appropriate actions.

Importance Questions - This is where after each scenario you are presented with an action. You must rate how important it is to carry out that action in the context of the scenario. Those actions which are considered essential should be awarded high importance. If an action is inconsequential, or even detrimental, then it will be of lower importance, you are given four answer choices to choose from, they include:

- Very important
- Important
- Of minor importance
- Not important at all

For examples of each type of situational judgement question visit the blog at: www.themedicblog.co.uk/ucat-situational-judgement-subtest. You have 26 minutes to complete 69 questions in this section, that's on average about 22 seconds per item.

> **Please note:** *The UCAT includes a 1-minute instruction section preceding each subtest. Now that you are aware of the question-types within each subtest let's begin to identify your weaknesses and strengths.*

Attempting the Official UCAT Questions

There are so many commercial resources available that advise on how to pass the UCAT. The problem is that the UCAT does not work with any of them, so you potentially run the risk of spending a lot of money on irrelevant or dated material. However, a survey conducted by the UCAT does prove that using these unofficial books, courses or seminars are associated with higher overall performance. The only official resources are on the UCAT website, we will use these resources to identify your true weakness.

The preparation tools provided on the UCAT website are extremely helpful. The exam board covers a variety of topics ranging from test strategies to candidate advice as well as tips for preparing for the test. I recommended you go through all the resources available on their website. The first exercise in identifying your weakest skill involves using the official practice tests and question banks. During my first attempt at the UCAT, I did the official practice tests at the end of my preparation; I thought it would give me a rough idea of what my score would be in the actual exam. In hindsight, this was a bad idea because I achieved a poor score and it was too late to improve my skills. I discovered that this is a common mistake made by many applicants. The practice tests and question banks are the only official resources available, so I recommend taking advantage of them early on. They are updated every year to reflect the same level of difficulty candidates will encounter in the exam. The first step in identifying your weakness is attempting the official practice questions and tests.

The first exercise in identifying your strengths and weakness involves attempting the official question banks (not to be confused with the official practice tests) for each subtest untimed. You will need a pen and notebook to make notes as you attempt questions.

Exercise 1: Attempt Official UCAT Questions Banks Untimed

The UCAT provides practice questions for each subtest: Verbal reasoning, Decision Making, Quantitative Reasoning, Abstract Reasoning and Situational Judgement. Attempt each set of practice questions untimed. The aim of this is to familiarize yourself with each section of the exam; do not practice any questions beforehand nor worry about time management. If it takes you a whole day to go through the entire set of practice questions that's fine. It's not a race, attempt each set and take notes of the question-types you found difficult.

Use the Official Question Banks to familiarise yourself with the exam. Do no prior practice beforehand nor worry about time management. The whole point is to familiarize yourself with the exam.

Verbal Reasoning Question Banks

Go through the question banks provided untimed and review your answers at the end. I recommend taking note of question-types you find difficult and learn from the solutions afterwards. After you have completed the verbal question banks and reviewed answers, try to reflect on the entire test and think about what you struggled with the most. Do not get too caught up in specifics for now, try to identify which of the skills being tested you could improve on, using the points below for assistance:

Comprehension

- Misunderstanding or misinterpreting information from the passage
- Guessing answer options at random
- Making assumptions
- Poor retention: cannot remember the topic for each paragraph

Critical Thinking

- Drawing false conclusion
- Making wrong inference
- Unable to draw conclusion from multiple sources of information
- Unable to eliminate answer options effectively

Speed (or Pace)

- Reading text one word at a time
- Vocalising while reading (subvocalization)
- Fixating on a word or sentence
- Regressing: regularly going back to re-read the passage
- Running out of time in subtest

When I attempted the verbal question bank I struggled on pacing and critical thinking. I was also a slow reader, without realising it I would constantly regress and at times vocalise. This significantly reduced my reading speed and level of comprehension. Identifying this early on enabled me to adopt strategies to improve and ultimately increase my verbal score in the UCAT. Try to spot which element you struggle with the most and write it down. We will go over this list later on.

Decision Making Question Banks

Go through the question banks provided untimed and review your answers at the end. I recommend taking note of question-types you find difficult and learn from the solutions afterwards. After you have completed the Decision-making question banks and reviewed the answers, reflect on the entire test and think about which skill you struggled with the most:

Deductive Reasoning

- Struggle on puzzle problems
- Not recognising links between different information
- Making wrong assumptions

Evaluating Arguments

- Misinterpreting Graphs and Charts
- Misinterpreting information from problems in text

Statistical Reasoning

- Poor grasp of venn diagram concepts
- Poor grasp of key probability concepts

Speed (or Pace)

- Spending too much time on a question
- Not using onscreen calculator
- Reading text one word at a time

- Hyper Regressing: Going back to re-read words or sentences regularly

Quantitative Reasoning Question Banks

Go through the question banks provided untimed and review your answers at the end. I recommend taking note of topics you find difficult and learn from the solutions afterwards. You may notice you feel rusty on some topics. Take note of them. Also pay attention to the format of questions, for example, items presented in the form of tables, charts or graphs, were you able to rapidly identify relevant variables? If not, then you may want to take note of this as well. The list below provides assistance to help identify areas for improvement:

Numerical Skills

- Slow to perform simple numerical operations
- Uncomfortable dealing with fractions and decimals
- Rusty at converting and changing percentages, ratios and fractions
- Rusty at calculating speed, distance and time
- Rusty at converting units
- Unable to calculate interest e.g. compound interest
- Poor at Interpreting graphs and charts

Speed

- Spending too much time on an item
- Not using the onscreen calculator when appropriate
- Reading one text at a time
- Hyper-regressing
- Obsessing over exact answer
- Not estimating and rounding when appropriate

Abstract Reasoning Question Banks

Go through the question banks provided untimed and review your answers at the end. I recommend taking note of which of the 4 question types you find difficult and learn from the solutions afterwards. The abstract reasoning sections test your relationship-finding skills and pace. You rarely notice pattern similarity instantly. With enough practice you will improve, the more questions you practice, the easier you'll find the subtest. Do not get dispirited if you struggle with it. We will cover pattern finding strategies later in this guide, but for now, work at your own pace, try to think of your own best approach to answering questions and use the following list of ideas to focus on the commonality within each set:

- Shape of components
- Number of corners on each component
- Type of edges on each component
- Colour of each component
- Number of components
- Orientation of components
- Consistent (or consistently evolving) position of one component relative to the others
- Size of components

The above suggestions are a good starting point. By applying this list of possibilities to each set, you can improve generating hypothesis and spot the patterns quicker. The list below provides assistance to help identify areas for improvement:

Abstract Skills (Pattern or Relationship finding skills)

- Slow or unable to spot basic or complex patterns
- Unable to spot conditional patterns
- Not wary of red herrings or distractors
- Unable to take a step back and look at whole picture

Speed (or Pace)

- Spending too much time on an item
- Slow at changing tactic when initial thesis for relationship fails
- Poor at eliminating answer options
- Fixating on a shape or pattern
- Not using the flagging function
- Not utilising keyboard shortcuts

Situational Judgement Question Banks

The Situational Judgement section (STJ) is different from the other subtests; technically there is no right or wrong answer when you think about how it is marked. My advice would be to take note of which of the two question-types you struggle with the most and carefully monitor pace, you should notice a pattern. After you have attempted the STJ practice questions and reviewed the answers, learn from the answer rationale provided by the UCAT. I'll show you how I was able to improve my Situational Judgement band score later in this book, for now only review answers and learn from them. Use the list below to help identify areas for improvement:

Key Issues and concepts

- Integrity
- Teamwork
- Safety and Quality
- Maintaining trust
- Duties of a doctor

Speed

- Spending too much time on an item
- Poor at eliminating answer options
- Not using the flagging function
- Not utilising keyboard shortcuts

> *Review your notes for each subtest before moving to the next exercise, proposing solutions of your own and try to implement them for the next exercise. There is no need to do any further practice or refer to any other resource at this time.*

Exercise 2: Attempt the official UCAT practice tests under exam conditions

The exam board provides three practice tests (A, B and C), you will attempt all three tests under timed conditions. There is no need to dive into books or courses at this stage. You have familiarised yourself with the exam by going through the practice questions in the question banks, now you must mimic the testing conditions and identify where your natural capabilities lie.

Each test is about 2 hours long, so I recommend doing one practice test a day and reviewing your answers afterwards on the same day. For example, if you take Practice Test A on Day 1, review your answers afterwards, then attempt Practice Test B on Day 2 and so on. I recommend this approach because the test is really exhausting. When you are attempting a practice test, treat it like the real exam, try to mimic the same environment. Make sure you are in a quiet place and be sure you won't be disturbed the entire 2 hours you are taking the test. The whole point of this is to give you first-hand experience of the time limitations in each section of the exam and identify the part of the exams you find difficult with no practice.

> *Once you have gone through the question banks and familiarised yourself with the exam, attempt all three official practice tests under timed conditions with no prior studying. This is the most effective way to identify where your natural capabilities lie.*

Exercise 3: Review your practice test scores

Once you have completed a practice test, you will be taken to a review screen - this screen shows your score in each section. Spend time reviewing all the questions in each section, don't just go through the items you got wrong, **work through every solution in comparison to your own and identify differences in approach and thought process**. There is an "explain answer" button for each question on the top left-hand corner; by clicking on this you will obtain an explanation for the correct answer. Make sure that you fully understand them and take note of the question-types you got wrong, and the one's you guessed. For instance, you might realise that you didn't do well on logical puzzles in the Decision-Making subtest but quite well on the venn diagram questions. This suggests you will need to practice more logical puzzles to boost your overall Decision-Making score.

***Advice from Mike:** You want to reflect on your use of time in each subtest as well, did you finish each section in time? If not, why? Did you rush towards the end in a specific section? Before learning any of the strategies recommended in this guide, try to propose solutions of your own and try to implement them in the remaining practice tests.*

To summarise, make sure after each practice test to do the following:

- Understand the explained answers for ALL items (you might have fluked a few).
- Identify the question-types in each section you find most difficult.
- Identify the question-types that are your strongest

- Reflect on your use of time.

Exercise 4: Calculate Practice Test Scores

After you've completed a practice test, you will notice that the final review screen doesn't give a score out of 900 in each section. Instead, you are provided with the total number of incorrect responses in each section. You can simply calculate the number of correct responses achieved by subtracting the number of incorrect responses from the total number of items in each subtest. For example, if the review screen states you achieved 11 incorrect responses in the verbal reasoning section then you scored 33 out of 44. Record the number of correct responses for each section and put into the format of the table below.

	Practice Test A	Practice Test B	Practice Test C	Average Score
Verbal Reasoning (out of 44)				
Decision Making (out of 29)				
Quantitative Reasoning (out of 36)				
Abstract Reasoning (out of 55)				

Please note that the Situational Judgement scores are not included in our calculation. This is due to the fact that your score in this section will not count towards your overall test score out of 3600. Instead you'll be given a band score from 1 to 4. Once you've recorded your scores as seen above, the next step is to convert the average score in each section into an approximate UCAT score out of 900 using the conversion table on the blog. Visit the blog at **www.themedicblog.co.uk/ucat-conversion-table/**.

Please be aware that the conversion table is for approximation purposes only. Scores on the UCAT are given in 10-point intervals, so actual scores will vary slightly. It is designed to err on the side of caution, so in most cases, a similar performance on the exam would result in a slightly higher score. Using the conversion table, record your average score in each subtest out of 900 as seen in the table:

	Average score (out of 900)
Verbal Reasoning	
Decision Making	
Quantitative Reasoning	
Abstract Reasoning	

Exercise 5: Use UCAT Results to Identify 'True 'Weakness

As you are now aware, the UCAT uses a statistical approach called deciles to report the overall performance of candidates each year. The score for each decile indicates the minimum score a candidate can achieve to be classified in that decile. For example, in 2015 (the year I took the exam), a candidate that achieved 2540 would be in the 5th decile and a candidate score at 2840 would be in the 9th decile. The term percentile can also be used instead of decile, which means out of 100. For instance, a score in the 1st decile represents a score at the 10th percentile; the 2nd decile represents a score at the 20th percentile, and so on.

Advice from Mike: Your practice test scores will most likely be very low at this stage – don't be discouraged as this is expected.

The data provided by the UCAT is valuable because you can compare your practice test scores to the candidates scores in the previous cycle. Take a look at Gary's practice test results, a 2018 medicine applicant:

	Average score (out of 900)
Verbal Reasoning	580
Decision Making	600
Quantitative Reasoning	624
Abstract Reasoning	610

You are probably at this point thinking that Gary's weakest section is verbal reasoning because it is his lowest score. However, when compared to the official UCAT results from the previous year (2017 test statistics), it reveals a whole different picture, see below:

	Average score (out of 900)	2017 UCAT Average (previous year)
Verbal Reasoning	580	570
Decision Making	600	647
Quantitative Reasoning	624	695
Abstract Reasoning	610	629

The table above compares his practice score with the previous year averages in each section. When compared to last year's result, Gary scored above average in verbal reasoning and below average in all other sections. Using basic statistics, which we will dive into in the next chapter, we can conclude that Gary's strongest section is the verbal reasoning subtest. The key thing to take from this is that **your lowest score isn't necessarily your weakest section**. This is one of the most common mistakes made by candidates when preparing for the exam; they assume their lowest score is their weakest and spend more time trying to improve this 'false weakness'.

Compare your practice test results with the previous year average. If your average in a subtest is below last year's average consider it weak, if it's above, consider it strong. Once you have completed all five exercises, you

If you have scored below the previous year averages in all four subtests, not to worry, it's expected. I will run through how to spot your true weakness and prioritise each subtest in the next chapter. For those that have scored above the average in all sections, well done! Regardless, you still need to identify your true weakness. The next part of the strategy will help with prioritising each subtest and determining the amount of time to prepare for each one.

Step 3: Prioritise

Prioritising the UCAT Subtests

One afternoon during my final year at university, I was sitting in the middle of my Neuropharmacology lecture when my phone's vibration went crazy. I was included in a trend on The Student Room Forum where a candidate wanted to know the amount of practice time he should spend on each section of the exam. The trend was read by thousands of students and lead to a lot of replies to the post. After my lecture, I had a look at the responses, there were a few good tips from other students but a lot of really bad ones. The bad advices stemmed from two main misconceptions:

- Spend a majority of time on the subtest you score in the lowest
- You only need 3 - 4 weeks to prepare, practice as many questions as possible within that time and you'll be fine

They are common mistakes candidates make when prioritising the UCAT subtests. Firstly, candidates assume that the section where they achieve the lowest score is their weakest subtest. Secondly, candidates can at times fall into the trap of spending too much time on sections of the exam they find most comfortable, sometimes without even realising it. These two problems create the necessity of this step, to help prioritise each section and manage time appropriately.

Bad Advice #1 - Spend a majority of time on the subtest you score the lowest

This is really bad advice, determining the order of dealing with the UCAT subtests is important because it mostly defines the amount of practice time you will allocate to each section. I recommend spending the majority of time focusing on your weakest section; it is the most effective way to significantly increase your total UCAT score. However, your lowest score isn't necessarily your weakest; it is common for candidates to assume their lowest score is their weakest. Let's take another look Gary's practice results, the family friend I taught my preparation strategy back in 2016.

	Gary's Average Practice Score (out of 900)
Verbal Reasoning	580
Decision Making	600
Quantitative Reasoning	624
Abstract Reasoning	610

You immediately assume his weakest section is the verbal section because it's his lowest score. However, when compared to the previous year, he scored above average and it is in fact his strongest section. I use Gary's practice result to explain this concept because it's a great example and extreme case, where the highest scoring section is in fact the weakest and lowest scoring subtest is the strongest.

	Gary's Practice Score (out of 900)	2017 UCAT Averages
Verbal Reasoning	580	570
Decision Making	600	647
Quantitative Reasoning	624	695
Abstract Reasoning	610	629

When I took the official practice tests in 2015, I compared my score to the 2014 averages, the table below shows how my practice score averages compared:

	My Average Practice Score (out of 900)	2014 UKCAT Averages (out of 900)
Verbal Reasoning	527	571
Quantitative Reasoning	640	684
Abstract Reasoning	680	636
Decision Analysis*	585	614

Please note that the Decision Analysis subtest no longer features in the UCAT test, it has been replaced with the Decision-Making Subtest.

As you can see my average UCAT practice score in the verbal, quantitative and decision analysis sections were below average. The only section I scored above average was in abstract reasoning. From this, I concluded my strongest section was abstract reasoning. The next part was identifying the order of weakness with respect to the previous year.

Determining the order to deal with each Subtest

Exercise 1: Calculate Percentage Difference

In some cases, it might not be as easy to spot your weakest or strongest section. For example, candidates that score below average on all four sections or even above average in all sections. Calculating the percentage difference between your score and the official averages gives a good indication of the extent of your skill, which we will use to identify your true weakness and rank the subtests in order. Find the formulae for calculating percentage difference below:

$$P.D = \frac{Practice\ score - Last\ Year\ Score}{Last\ Year\ Score} \times 100$$

Use the formulae above to calculate the percentage difference for each subtest.

Example: My average practice score in Verbal Reasoning (VR) = 527; Last year Candidat VR Average = 571

$$P.D = \frac{527 - 571}{571} \times 100$$

Percentage difference = **-7.7%**

In other words, I scored **7.7% below last year's average.**

The table below shows the percentage difference of my practice score and the UCAT averages in 2014 to give an indication the extent of my skill.

Essentially, the UCAT section with the largest percentage difference below the previous average is considered the weakest section and the section with the largest percentage difference above average is considered strongest. This technique is great because if you achieve below (or above) the average UCAT scores in all sections, you can still identify the true weakness and rank the subtests accordingly. Take a look below at my UCAT performance after calculating the percentage difference for each section:

	Average Practice Score (out of 900)	2014 Averages (out of 900)	Percentage difference
Verbal Reasoning	527	571	-7.7 %
Quantitative Reasoning	640	684	-6.4%
Abstract Reasoning	680	636	+6.9%
Decision Analysis	585	614	-4.7%

As you can see from the table, I scored 7.7% below the previous year in Verbal Reasoning, which suggests that the subtest is my weakest section. Quantitative Reasoning came in second at 6.9% below previous average, Decision Analysis as my third weakest (or second strongest) subtest at 4.7% below the average and Abstract Reasoning was my strongest subtest at 6.9% above average.

Calculate the percentage difference of your practice score and the previous UCAT averages for each subtest. You can find the latest averages at the official UCAT website or on the blog at www.themedicblog.co.uk/ucat-mean-scores-deciles/.

Exercise 2: Create A Priority Table (Optional)

I believe calculating the percentage difference between your practice score and the previous year's results is an effective way to prioritise the subtests. Once you've worked out the differences for each subtest, create a priority table showing the order of priority and the minimum number of hours you plan to spend practising. The figure below shows my priority table when preparing for the UCAT back in 2015.

Subtest	Strength	Priority
Verbal Reasoning	Weakest	1st
Quantitative Reasoning	2nd Weakest	2nd
Decision Analysis*	2nd Strongest	3rd
Abstract Reasoning	Strongest	4th

The table shows my weakest (highest priority) to strongest (least priority). I arranged the subtests in order of priority based on the results from calculating the percentage difference. I strongly recommend spending the majority of your time improving your weakest subtest i.e. the UCAT section with the largest percentage difference below average. Studies have shown that more time spent on strong areas improves overall test mark by an average of 10 to 15 percent, while more time spent on weakest areas can improve overall test score by 20 to 35 percent. That equates to an extra 180 points in each UCAT subtest by simply focusing on weak areas.

Bad advice #2 - You only need 3-4 weeks to prepare, practice as many questions as possible within that time and you'll be fine.

This is more bad advice that provides no structure to preparation and doesn't take into account that every candidate is different. The following exercises will help you to determine how long to prepare for the UCAT and the amount of time to spend on each section.

Determining How Long to Prepare for The Test

Exercise 3: Determine how long to prepare for the test

Most students take the UCAT at the end of the Summer, in either August or September. This is probably due to the fact that summer is a busy time.

Many students will either be working or enjoying a break from their studies. Some students might be travelling, for part or all of the summer. Depending on your personal plans, there are any number of factors that could impact your decision on how long to prepare for the test.

My advice would be to consider all the factors that might affect your preparation or performance on test day and schedule your test appointment appropriately. Since you can choose any available test appointment, there is no reason not to choose the appointment that will give you the greatest advantage. Not taking into account other external factors that might influence preparation, I suggest determining how long you prepare for the exam based on how easy you find the official practice test in Step 2, if you found it ok then 3-4 weeks should be enough time to prepare. However, if you found it extremely difficult you may need longer. For those that struggle the most I personally think 6 - 8 weeks is more than enough time to prepare. For more advice on this visit www.themedicblog.co.uk/how-long-to-prepare-for-ucat.

Advice from Mike: Remember quality over quantity, try not to get too caught up on the length of your preparation, what's more important is the quality.

Exercise 4: Determine the amount of practice time for each section

The strategy below helps give structure to preparation and provides a minimum number of hours candidates must commit to each section. In order to calculate the recommended hours, follow these steps:

- Calculate the number of days until actual test days (e.g. 30 days).
- Calculate the average number of hours per day you can realistically spend preparing for the exam (e.g. 3 hours per day, so that's 90 hours over 30 days).
- Dedicate 45% of the Total Time to your weakest section (e.g. 45% of 90 hours is 40.5 hours).
- Dedicate about 28% of the total time to the 2nd weakest section (e.g. 28% of 90 hours is 25 hours).
- Dedicate 18% of the total time to your 2nd strongest section (e.g. 18% of 90 hours is 16 hours).
- Dedicate 9% of the total time to your strongest section (9% of 90 hours

is 8 hours).

This calculation is based on my personal experience and feedback from other high scoring candidates. Nonetheless, it should be used as a rule of thumb and act as a rough guide to help balance your time, you can modify or personalize as you see fit. I spent roughly 41 hours preparing for the Verbal Reasoning subtest and was able to improve my score significantly. By essentially spending 5 times more hours on my weakest section than my strongest section I saw a significant boost in overall score.

Subtest	Strength	Priority	Minimum Time Allocated to Each Section
Verbal Reasoning	Weakest	1st	40.5 hours
Quantitative Reasoning	2nd Weakest	2nd	25 hours
Decision Analysis*	2nd Strongest	3rd	16 hours
Abstract Reasoning	Strongest	4th	8 hours

Once you've identified your true weakness and prioritised the UCAT sections accordingly, the next part of the strategy involves improving your skills, we will look at the fundamentals in improving your performance in the exam. Take a moment to breathe. When you're ready, let's begin.

Step 4: Improve

Improving Your UCAT Score

Despite what some candidates might believe, you can significantly improve your performance in the UCAT. I'm living proof that it's possible, I went from scoring an average of 600 to 710 by simply changing my approach to preparing for the exam. Like any other test you've taken in your life, the right preparation is key. Instead of just practising thousands of questions and learning from worked solutions, I focused on improving my overall approach, learning tactics to compensate weakness and moulding an attack plan for each section based on my skills. There have been hundreds of testimonials from students that have adopted this approach and the numbers continue to rise.

One of the most important pieces of advice I can give for the UCAT is to move away from the mindset of "what do I need to get the correct answer to this question?" and towards the mindset of "How, given the 15 seconds I have to answer, can I maximise the chance of selecting the correct answer to this question?" That's an entirely different mindset as it is strategy-dependant.

Reviewing UCAT practice tests correctly is the key to getting better quickly, you must **critically evaluate your skills and determine an optimal strategy for each subtest.** I would go as far as to say that if you do not have a strategy for how you intend to attack each subtest, chances are you are setting yourself up for a low score. Top students are able to critically review practice to the point they switch from merely practice to actually teaching themselves.

Reconsidering How You React to Mistakes

I want you to think back to how you reacted to the mistakes made when reviewing answers to the official UCAT question bank and practice tests (in step 2: Identify). Getting questions wrong must have been anywhere from mildly disappointing to absolutely infuriating. For many students, discovering that they have answered a UCAT question incorrectly can trigger any or all of the following impulses:

- Focusing on what you did well and ignoring what you did wrong.
- Disregarding questions you got wrong because they were just "careless mistakes".
- Reviewing mistakes but not critically evaluating the reason you answered incorrectly.
- Accepting the fact that you got things wrong and ignoring to review test all together.

All of the above impulses are unhelpful. The UCAT is like any other skill: you have to see what you are doing wrong in order to improve, but more importantly you have to understand the underlying reason. Sports like tennis are great because players get instant feedback: if they mess up a shot (i.e. it doesn't stay in play or goes the wrong direction), they adjust their next swing, right? In tennis, practice and reinforcement occurs at the same time. It's a little harder to get the mix of practice and feedback right on the UCAT, but nonetheless it is crucial to improve in the exam. In this chapter I share multiple strategies to critically review your mistakes so you can improve your performance in each subtest. I recommend giving them all a try and sticking with the most effective technique(s) for you.

Strategy: Categorise Each Incorrect Response

It is important that you review incorrect responses effectively. A helpful way to do this is by sorting them into categories. Many times, incorrect responses can be sorted into these general categories:

- Skipped (picked randomly or didn't apply logic or strategic process)
- Guessed (guessed through strategy or logic e.g. elimination, eyeballing, estimation, etc)
- Knew (thought you knew but was wrong)

Seeing how many questions you skipped, how many you guessed, and how many you were certain were correct can help to focus your studying. For instance, if the majority of the questions you answered incorrectly in the

VR section were ones you 'knew', it is possible that your reading strategy is ineffective. Alternatively, you might be answering incorrectly due to the time pressure. The table below shows this strategy being used to categorise incorrect responses in the VR section. As you can see from the table, the student answered a total of 13 questions incorrectly, out of which they randomly answered 3 items, guessed 6 and were certain they knew 4.

Skipped	Guessed	Knew
Qs 21, Qs 24, Qs 3	Qs 4, Qs 7, Qs 8, Qs 12, Qs 15, Qs 35	Qs 17, Qs 19, Qs 23, Qs 28

Once you've sorted the questions into these general categories, make sure to review them all, think about your approach and thought process. Once completed, **review the remaining questions answered correctly**. Compare questions that you guessed incorrectly with the ones you guessed correctly. Was it just blind luck? Or is there a difference between the way you approached the guessed questions you got correctly? Is there a particular skill-set or question hindering your performance?

Strategy: Understand the Reason for Incorrect Response

Sort the questions by the fundamental reason you answered them wrong. I find that nearly all incorrect answers in the UCAT falls into four categories:

- **Timing:** You were pressed for time and rushed to answer the question, either due to length or complexity of the question.
- **Comprehension:** Picked the wrong option due to misunderstanding the question or task, either by being tricked by the question or misinterpreting information provided.

- **Procedural or Content:** You don't know how to work out the answer or do not know the material being covered.
- **Error in Judgement:** You made a careless or stupid mistake.

The cross grid below shows this strategy being used to understand the reason for the incorrect responses categorised in VR practice example shared earlier. As you can see from the grid, the student answered a total of 13 questions incorrectly. Out of which, 3 were due to timing issues, 2 were due to poor comprehension (or grasp), 5 were due to lack of knowledge on content and 3 were due to careless mistakes.

	SKIPPED	GUESSED	KNEW
TIMING	Qs 3	Qs 4	Qs 19
GRASP		Qs 35	Qs 28
CONTENT	Qs 24	Qs 7, Qs 8	Qs 17, Qs 23
ERROR	Qs 21	Qs 12, Qs 15	

Now, that you have a structured approach to recognising the most common mistakes that result in selecting wrong answers, you will need to take things one-step further with self-evaluation. Here are some examples of common reasons you answer incorrectly, and how you can take your analysis one-step further:

Timing: The question was too complex, so didn't have enough time to finish.
One step further: What specific shortcut do I need to learn, and how will I adopt it to save time?

Content: I knew the content, but I didn't know how to approach this question.

One step further: How do I solve the question, and is there a general rule that I need to know for the future?

Guessing: I was stuck between two answer choices, and I guessed wrong.
One step further: Why could I not eliminate one of the last answer choices? Knowing the correct answer now, how I can eliminate it? Does this suggest a strategy I can use for the future?

Error in Judgement: I misread what the question was asking or solved for the wrong thing
One step further: Why did I misread the question? What should I do in the future to avoid this?

Advice from Mike: Be ruthless about understanding your mistakes. Adopt a no-mistake-left-behind policy. Letting one slip through can mean you make the same mistake in the real UCAT.

Strategy: The Five Why's Technique

Here's another useful strategy when reviewing your responses: **ask yourself "Why?" five times.** By doing this you'll dig deeper and deeper to understand what the underlying cause is, and how to fix it. Here's an example. Let's say you answered an 'incomplete statement' question wrong in VR section. Here are the things to consider using the 5 why approach:

Starting point: I scored poorly on 'Incomplete Statement' question during VR practice.

- Why? – Because I picked the wrong answer choice, out of the two I had left.
- Why? - Because the wrong answer choice had a phrase that was in the passage, I got tricked.
- Why? - I didn't fully understand the passage when I was reading it.
- Why? - I read the passage too quickly.
- Why? - I was scared about running out of time.

You can see how a single question can take you down a rabbit hole of additional questions that can give you a ton of insight about where you went wrong. This technique is great because you have a lot of opportunities to improve on core skill such as how you read passages, how you eliminate answer choices and how you process each type of question.

Advice from Mike: *Always reflect and dig deeper when reviewing practice test results and consider/plan future approaches and processes.*

Strategy: The SWOT Method

The SWOT method is another framework for identifying and analysing the internal and external factors that can have an impact on your UCAT performance. The framework is credited to Albert Humphrey, who tested the approach in the 60s and early 70s. It is now adopted by organisations of all types as an aid to making business decisions. However, it is a great tool for tuning preparation, and we can apply the framework to assess UCAT practice. It can be used at the start of your UCAT preparation to evaluate practice test results, and full mock completed under testing conditions. The framework provides powerful support for decision-making because it enables you to uncover opportunities for exam success that weren't initially recognised. As its name states, SWOT examines four elements:

Strengths (S): The skills or concepts which you find easiest and are confident in answering most questions correctly.

Weaknesses (W): These are concepts or skills you are not very confident about. For example, you may find probability as a weak area in DM. But learning the concepts and doing some problem practice could potentially convert this weakness into a strength.

Opportunities (O): These are the questions in which with more practice they could turn to strengths. These are those areas where you use guesswork at times but still get them right most of the time.

Threats (T): These are the questions in which you always score fewer marks despite understanding concepts and applying learned techniques to improve. This is the danger zone. You just cannot seem to get these concepts and always score a low mark.

A SWOT matrix is often used to organize items identified under each of these four elements. It is usually a square divided into four quadrants, with each quadrant representing one of the specific elements. You identify and list specific strengths in the first quadrant, weaknesses in the next, then opportunities and, lastly, threats (see below). The matrix allows you to effectively grasp your strengths, improve weakness, explore opportunities and overcome threats when you prepare for the exam. I've worked with students who just love drilling their strong points because it's comfortable. Unfortunately, this **is a waste of time** - you have to confront your demons and consistently pick at what you are weak at, which is uncomfortable and difficult – but necessary.

STRENGTHS	WEAKNESSES
True, False or Cant tell	Except Questions Inference Questions
OPPORTUNITIES	**THREATS**
Comprehension Flagging	Timing Author Questions

How to use a SWOT matrix during UCAT preparation: After you have attempted a mock or practice test, write out which question-type you were able to answer correct and easily; these are your *strengths*. Such questions where you could absolutely not answer, are your *weaknesses* or *threats*. Questions that you could answer correctly, but were not very sure on, are your *opportunities* because with a little hard work they could turn into strengths. You can also split strategies and/or skills into the four quadrants as well.

Difference between Threats and Weaknesses: Weaknesses are areas that that require a lot of work to improve, you are confident that with enough practice you can significantly improve. However, threats on the other hand are more complicated, you have practised and done as much as you can to improve but your efforts seem a bit futile. Weaknesses can turn into either strengths or threats, just as threats can turn into weaknesses and strengths.

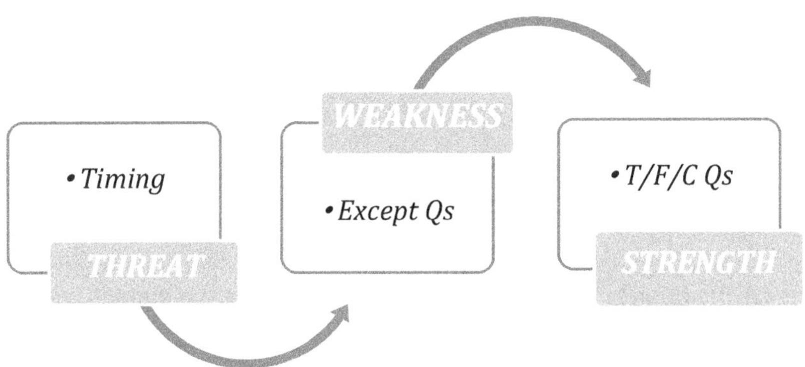

The above diagram shows an assessment of the verbal reasoning question-types into Threats, Weaknesses and Strengths. The goal during UCAT preparation is to **turn as many question-types and skills into strengths**. It's impossible to convert all of the skills required for each subtest into strengths, however you can learn tips to compensate for shortcomings. This thus proves the need to learn tips, techniques and strategies to compensate or improve troubling areas for each subtest.

> *Focusing on your weaknesses is critical because you have a limited amount of time to study, and you need to spend that precious time on the areas that will have the most impact on your overall UCAT score.*

Step 5: Practice

Practising UCAT Questions

The saying goes 'practice makes perfect', but only when there is a goal in mind. Take tennis, for example, which requires a higher-order skill. To play good tennis you must be able to run, hit a forehand and a backhand as well as watch your opponent. But mastery of these separate skills is not sufficient. You must be able to combine them into a fluent interplay of actions that result in scoring a point. By merely reading a book about critical thinking you do not develop your critical thinking skills. That only happens when you practice intensively in a way that is specific, determined and concentrated.

Many candidates preparing for the test, without realising, skip the earlier steps in this guide and dive straight into practice. This leaves them at risk of only familiarizing themselves with the questions and not improving their test skills. I found myself in this situation the first time I took the test. I remember spending the majority of my revision practising questions without having a real goal or attack plan, to make things worse, I subconsciously practised mostly abstract questions because I found it the most comfortable. In hindsight, this created a false sense of assurance which was later shattered when I took the actual test. Through the study group, I came to realise that this is a common mistake; in this chapter, we will look at how to practice questions during UCAT revision. I share key rules you must adopt during practice and provide examples to explain each one:

Rule #1: Use Multiple Resources

There will be exceptions, but in general, I recommend using multiple resources during UCAT practice to effectively improve your testing skills. Unfortunately, the official resources are not comprehensive enough, and the type of preparation required cannot come from using them alone. You need to view UCAT concepts from multiple angles and perspectives in order to develop a truly 'three dimensional' technique for each question-type in the exam. I would recommend the official resources initially, then moving onto practice books and/or some sort of online resource as a minimum.

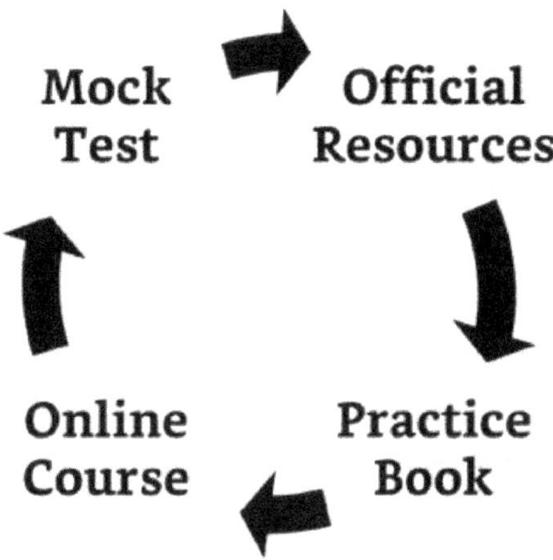

Official UCAT Resources

The official practice questions are the most reliable way to identify weak areas in the exam, they are updated every year to reflect the same level of difficulty candidates will encounter in the exam. One negative is that the total number of practice questions is limited, so you will probably have to supplement it with other resources. I strongly advise using them to identify key areas that need focus during preparation (See Step 2).

Advice from Mike: Once sufficient time has passed, I recommend re-attempting the official UCAT questions and comparing the results to previous performance.

UCAT Practice Book

Practice books are arguably the most popular resources used to prepare for the exam, with the most popular books including thousands of questions that replicate the breadth and depth that can be expected in the UCAT. The major drawback with practice books is that they do not mimic the testing environment since the UCAT is a computer-administered test. Nonetheless, they are extremely beneficial to practice individual questions and further familiarize yourself with the different questions in the exam. Every year I ask the study group to recommend the best practice books and I share them on the blog, visit the link www.themedicblog.co.uk/best-ucat-books for the latest recommendations. If you are unsure which book from the list to get I provide tips on how to pick the right practice book for you and choose my picks for the best book for each subtest

Online UCAT Course/Online UCAT Practice Questions (Strongly Recommend)

Online courses can be a great resource, they provide thousands of practice questions and replicate the test environment as well, this is huge benefit, and why I strongly recommend investing in one. The best courses include additional learning materials and tutorials to further aid with preparation. When using this type of resource, it can be beneficial to keep an eye on your pace in each subtest, be sure time yourself and become familiar with the time limitations and pressures in the exam. Every year I review the most popular online UCAT courses and shortlist the best ones, visit the link www.themedicblog.co.uk/online-ucat-courses for my recommendations of the year.

Advice from Mike: Monitor your pace during practice with an online course, aim to complete each subtest within the set time. That way, you can hone time-saving strategies to avoid running out of time in each section.

UCAT Crash Courses and Tuition

Crash courses or tuitions can be an asset and give you an edge over other candidates because you are learning directly from experienced professionals. It is important to realise that no crash course is good enough that is has helped every single student that as enrolled on them and no crash course is so bad that it has failed every student who has used them. That being said, the key to increasing your chances of success is by finding a course that ideally suits your style of studying. The major benefit of enrolling in a crash course or tuition is that you get real-time advice and strategies to improve your skills, where you are put through a series of exercises to help identify and improve your score. The major drawback is that they are expensive, there is always the risk that you may spend thousands and not benefit anything. I recommend never spending more than you are willing to lose and seek to get a recommendation from past candidates or friends that have taken the UCAT course or tuition you are considering. If you do not know anyone, ask on the Facebook study group or forums, but beware of spammers who may try to give a false review to persuade you to buy their course. Put zero faith in the reviews on the courses website or anyone who is affiliated with the course (i.e. gets paid per referral), only trust the words of people you know personally when it comes to recommendations.

Rule #2: Give Priority to Weakest Areas

Whilst it is important to practice all sections of the UCAT, you must practice more of your weakest areas. As a rule of thumb, your **weakest areas must account for at least 50% of the total questions attempted during revision**. By doing this, you not only become more comfortable but are able to effectively drill down and find patterns to your weaknesses. This might be a content issue - like problems with venn problems, or a specific grammar rule. Or it might be a personal habit of yours, like misreading the passage or eliminating the wrong answer. When I was studying for the UCAT the third time, I discovered I consistently misread inference questions because I was reading too far into what the author was saying. From this insight, I began drilling those specific types of questions until I had developed my own strategy for solving them. Some days, my verbal reasoning practice would consist only of inference questions. I recommend you do the same and work on your weakest areas at three levels, they include: *Subtest*, *Question-type* and *Concept*.

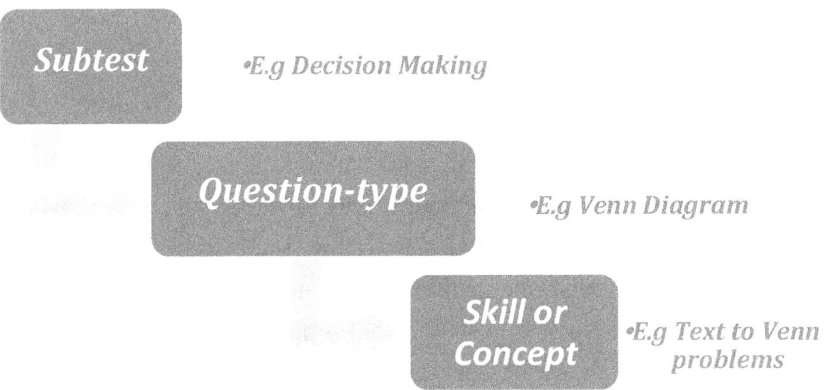

Weakest subtest

Start by identifying the weakest subtest, this is not necessarily the subtest with the lowest score (see step 2). Use resources such as books to practice more questions and look more closely at the subtest. Work on techniques and strategies to improve accuracy. It might be that the QR subtest is your weakest section, practice more questions to figure out the underlying reason for incorrect responses and work on fixing this.

Advice from Mike: Make sure to follow the exercises in step 2 of the preparation plan to effectively identify your weakest subtest.

Weakest Question-type

Take things further by analysing the questions types within your weakest subtest, I provide a breakdown of each subtest (see step 2) to aid your analysis. Aim to identify patterns and fix the question-type(s) with the highest error rate. Finding out the fundamental reason why you answer these question-types won't be easy and will require more practice of the question-type in consideration. You may have to use non-UCAT questions to get more exposure. For example, it might be that for the QR subtest you are rusty in converting percentages, I would recommend using old Maths textbooks or online resources like BBC Bitesize to practice more questions. YouTube videos could help learn shortcuts or Maths tricks to convert from percentages to decimals (or vice versa) that may prove helpful in saving time in the exam.

Advice from Mike: Fixing your weakest points might require creative ways to practice. Feel free to use non-UCAT materials that may seem beyond the scope of the exam. Do not shy away from using apps, old textbooks, YouTube videos or looking up exam tips for other similar aptitude tests.

Weakest Skill or Concept

There are exceptions, but in general, skills can take a long time to improve. It is **more effective to learn techniques and strategies to compensate shortcomings**. For instance, if you are a slow reader develop a reading strategy, slow at a particular Maths operation? Learn some Maths shortcuts. Can't find pattern relationships in AR? Adopt a mnemonic. It can take a lot of practice to find the right set of exam strategies that work for you. You may even find yourself combining multiple strategies to develop your own unique approach.

Advice from Mike: *Use the exam strategies in this guide as a starting point. You can add or take out elements that do not work for you and possibly create an entirely unique approach to fix your weakest skills.*

Rule #3: Work on Accuracy first then Pace

It's extremely beneficial to practice individual questions untimed before leaping into timed practice. That way, you can look more closely at how a question is supposed to be answered and hone your strategies to improve accuracy. The idea is to understand and hopefully formulate an approach to each question-type in a subtest. For instance, venn diagrams feature quite a bit in the Decision-Making section, so you could set a quiz with just venn diagram questions, complete it with no time constraints, and try find ways to simplify these questions (or even shortcuts in the question) to work quicker.

It's also worth pointing out that when you go through the answers as you're marking your quizzes, read the explanations very carefully. Make sure you understand why you got certain questions wrong (i.e. what mistakes you're making during your thought process while attempting the question). The opposite is just as, if not more important; you must make sure you know how you achieved the right answers too (i.e. you didn't just luck out!).

UCAT examiners are a bit sneaky; they sprinkle the test with complex questions to exploit one's urge to answer every question in-depth and lure test-takers into a "sticky" situation where they are wasting time. These complex questions can be confusing, long, or both! The thing you must remember is, **every question in the UCAT is worth equal marks**. Those who are able to identify these "complex" questions and skip them until later will maximise their marks on the easy questions. It's definitely worth putting some time into learning how to identify these questions and getting used to spending very little time on them in preference to the straightforward ones.

89

Generally speaking, **untimed practice should aim to improve accuracy, while timed practice should aim to improve speed**. When learning strategies start with the ones that work on your accuracy, once that has improved, turn your efforts to time-saving strategies to step up your pace.

Advice from Mike: There will be exceptions, but in general, always work on one thing at a time. For example, work on accuracy in VR before moving on to improving VR speed.

Reviewing untimed Practice

In the early part of the UCAT prep schedule, you are mostly only doing untimed questions (see 30-day UCAT study schedule). With untimed questions, it's very tempting to jump ahead to the answer choices right away (often before you are done reasoning through the problem) to see if you got the right answer. Here's the thing about the real UCAT test you are studying for: there's no answers in the back. **You have to learn how to do the best thinking you can do on your own**. Untimed prep is all about learning how to reason through these questions under the best conditions possible before you add time pressure later in your prep. If you short-change yourself by jumping to the answer too quickly, often you'll find you guessed the wrong answer. Now you'll never know if you could have reasoned through the problem successfully and learned something from it in the process. Here is what you should instead of that:

Step 1 – Pick some problems and start doing them: Decide on a block of 10 to 30 questions that you are going do in a row without looking at the answers. Sit down and start doing them.

Some questions are going to be pretty easy. You'll be close to 100% sure not only that the answer you chose is right, but also that the other answer choices are wrong for a some reason that you can readily identify. Don't do anything special to mark these questions. Just do them, eliminating the wrong answer choices and circling the one you think is correct, then move on.

Step 2 – Mark hard problems: When you get to harder questions, reason them out as best as you can. Eliminate any and all answer choices that you are sure are incorrect. Then really think hard and pick the one you think is best. Now, mark the question so you can come back to it later. What we would do is circle the question number at the top left of the question so it's easy to find again.

Step 3 – Specially mark problems that have you totally stumped: Often there will be one problem that you just can't decide at all which of two or three remaining answer choices are best. Do your best, but move on when it becomes absolutely clear you aren't making progress on your own (still pick an answer just like you would on the real test). Mark these problems with a star around the question number.

Step 4 – Before checking the answers, take one more pass at any questions that had you totally stumped: Sometimes a second look after can help you see something you didn't see the first time, and suddenly the problem becomes easier. For this reason, take a quick second try at starred problems (and maybe some of the harder circled ones) before you check the answers.

Step 5 – Check the answers and review incorrect answers: If any are wrong, review those questions until you understand absolutely why the correct answer is better than the one you picked. It might take a lot of thinking, but usually if you look at a question long enough, you will see why your answer choice was wrong and the correct answer choice was right.

Step 6 – Review circled and starred questions you got right: Now, quickly review the circled (hard) and starred (very hard) questions you got right. You want to make sure you understand exactly why you got any questions right, meaning you should be able to identify exactly why the answer you picked is right and exactly why the other answer choices are wrong. Having the right answer doesn't guarantee that you understood it. You always want to understand each and every UCAT problem that you encounter.

Step 7 – Keep notes in your log: You always want to keep a log of problems that you had difficulty with. Keep 3 separate lists of the specific question type for each problem you got wrong, circled, or starred. You do this so that later in your UCAT prep you can see patterns as to which questions types are giving you the most difficulty. Make sure to learn how to identify questions by type (See Step 2 of the preparation guide).

Reviewing timed Practice

After you begin to feel more comfortable solving the questions untimed, which can take a while. Then, and only then, are you ready to tackle timing. How long it takes to get there varies from person to person. Reviewing timed UCAT practice is a slightly different game. Here, you do a whole section within the time limit before doing any kind of review. Almost everyone likes to look straight at the answers after finishing a section. This is a huge mistake! Do this and you will be missing out on valuable opportunity to reason through the hard problems untimed before learning the answer. Here is the proper way to review a timed UCAT practice:

Step 1 – Pick a subtest and do it within the time limit: Pick one of the 5 subtests and do them under timed conditions. Alternatively, you can choose to do a specific question-type under timed conditions.

Step 2 – Mark hard problems with a circle: Same as you did with untimed questions, mark any question you aren't sure about with a circle around the question number.

Step 3 – Specially mark problems that have you totally stumped with a star: Again, same as before, mark the ones that have you no clue with a star. Still pick an answer and move on.

Step 4 – Before checking the answers, redo all circled and starred questions UNTIMED: Here's the key move: before you see if you got questions right, go back and redo all the circled (hard) and starred (very hard) questions untimed. This way your brain gets another chance to learn how to do them right without the time pressure. This actually helps develop speed on future questions. Think about it: when you do a question under time pressure you often have to give up on that one and move on before you've really had a chance to reason it out fully. For example, on QR, you are generally well advised to move on if an individual question is taking more than 40 seconds to answer. Because you didn't see your way through to the correct answer, you really won't get much of a benefit from that question unless you go back and do it right untimed. By doing it right untimed there is a better chance that next time your brain will know how to do a similar question within the proper amount of time.

Step 5 – Check the answers and review incorrect answers and correct answers for difficult problems: This part is the same as for untimed problems. Again, the key is to make sure understand each and every difficult problem (and any easy ones you got wrong for some reason. Extra tip: look carefully at what tripped you up every time you make a careless mistake. Often you can see a pattern and just knowing that will make you more alert when you encounter that again).

Step 6 – Keep detailed notes in your log so you can attack weaknesses: This part is a little different for timed tests. Here you want to keep a separate log of problems that you got wrong under time pressure and any you got wrong even when you did them untimed after. Pay special attention to the problems that you got wrong untimed. These are problems that you might be having substantive issues with and may require extra attention. You should also do this for problems that you had difficulty with under time pressure, but with these, place extra emphasis on learning how to build speed. Consider going through more practice questions and drilling the question-type being considered and build speed.

Advice from Mike: Once you introduce the timing element of the exam, I fully expect you won't be getting an average of 80% correct anymore. For the rest of your prep, your primary goal is to slowly close the gap between your untimed & timed scores until you're hitting about the same level of accuracy on timed exams that you had achieved in untimed conditions. If your accuracy falls through the floor when you introduce timing (for example, if you fall from 80% to 50% or worse), then you have some serious timing issues. My recommendation is to hold off on doing timed practice. Instead, do a full subtest untimed and see how long it takes, then begin to cut down your time. Say a full VR subtest is taking you 40 minutes to complete untimed. Now, try to shave a little bit of time off the subtest each time you practice. Continue cutting a minute or two until you get down to 21 minutes. If at any point your accuracy drops severely again, pause and practice at that time constraint for a while until the accuracy comes back. For example, say you manage to get your timing in VR down from 40 minutes to 32 minutes whilst maintaining an 80% accuracy average, but then went down to 50% average at 30 minutes. Continue to practice at 30 minutes until you've fixed the issue and your accuracy goes back up.

Rule #4: Set timed Mini-tests not Full Mocks

A good way to evaluate your progress is by attempting practice tests regularly. After sufficient practice with a newly developed approach or strategy, put it to the test. I recommend **setting multiple mini-tests before doing a full practice test (mock).**

A mini-test is a **timed practice test specific to only one subtest**. It can be either full (i.e. same number of questions in the exam) or partial (i.e. about half the number of questions expected in the exam) – see table below. Mini-tests act as quick evaluation tests that can be carried out whenever you want to **test a technique or assess your progress in a specific subtest**. You can set a mix of different question-types or the same type of question depending on your goal. Use the time per questions table on page 102 to calculate timing. E.g. 20 questions VR mini-test will be 10 minutes.

	Full mini- test	**Partial Mini test**
Verbal Reasoning	44	20 - 22
Decision Making	29	15
Decision Making	36	18 - 20
Abstract Reasoning	55	25
Situational Judgement	69	30 -35

Mini-tests are not to be confused with a mock, a fully timed 2-hour UCAT paper that includes all 5 subtests and mimics the testing conditions. These are great for assessing overall performance which we will cover in the next step of the strategy, but during practice you will need quicker and specific feedback, thus the need for mini-tests.

Advice from Mike: *Whether you are testing a specific technique or trying to spot patterns answering a specific question-type, mini-tests are a great way for testing newly learned skills under exam conditions. Set Mini-tests during specific practice and set full mock during general assessment. We will cover this in the next step.*

Step 6: Assess

Assessing Your Performance

Pressure can do funny things to candidates. For some, it can lead to nerves, anxiety, frustration and sloppy mistakes, culminating in a poor performance. For others, pressure allows them to concentrate more, work harder and perform better. It takes time and practice to perform well under pressure. Mock exams are a great opportunity for students to figure out and practise what works best for them under exam pressure. By completing a fully timed mock under exam conditions, you get a real feel of the exam, and in addition recognise areas that may need more attention. These may be new issues that come to light due to working under strict exam conditions.

After you begin to feel more comfortable practising each subtest timed, attempt a full mock exam under strict exam conditions. Treat it like the real test, make sure it is computer-based (visit www.themedicblog.co.uk/online-ucat-course for my recommendations) and that you are not interrupted of 2 hours. No breaks will be permitted in the real test so do not take any breaks until you finish the mock. The idea is that you mimic the testing conditions and become desensitised to external factors that can influence your performance. I remember when preparing for the UCAT I had completed a total of 5 mocks before test day. With each mock I became more comfortable with the exam and my overall confidence increased.

Advice from Mike: Get more accustomed to sitting for a long period of time answering test questions and pacing yourself. The more you practice, the more comfortable you will feel when you actually sit down to take the test.

Most importantly, mocks act as **feedback mechanisms** to help direct future studying. Results help recognise areas that you've mastered and spot weak areas that may need more attention. If framed right, mocks can allow you to conduct an elaborative interrogation on tips, techniques and strategies used to improve both accuracy and speed. In this chapter, we will look at how to effectively review mock tests and share strategies to help spot trends and patterns in performance. In addition, I share tactics to help with choosing and discarding strategies to adopt in the real exam.

Advice from Mike: I recommend taking at least 4 mocks before your actual test and spacing them out equally - I did 5 mocks in 5 weeks, i.e. a mock test every week leading to my exam.

Reviewing UCAT Mock Test Performance

This is slightly different from reviewing timed practice covered in step 5. Instead of attempting a specific subtest or question-type, you do an entire 2-hour paper under exam conditions before review:

Step 1 – Pick a mock and do it within the time limit: The mock must include all five subtests, I strongly advise to do test in a computer-based environment. Use one of the recommended online courses mentioned on the blog (visit www.themedicblog.co.uk/online-ucat-course).

Step 2 – Flag problems that you are not 100% sure: When you get to harder questions, reason them out as best as you can. Eliminate answer choices that you are sure are incorrect. Then really think hard and pick the one you think is best. Flag the question so you can come back to it later for review.

Step 3 – Flag and quickly jot questions that you have no conceptual understanding: Often there will be questions that you just have no clue on how to answer. Do your best but move on (still pick an answer though). Quickly jot down the question on a piece of paper to interrogate later.

Step 4 – Check the answers and review all answers: This part is the same as for timed practice. Again, the key is to make sure understand each and every question, especially the ones you got wrong. Remember to look carefully at what tripped you up and the underlying cause for your mistake.

Step 5 – Keep detailed notes in your log: Again, keep a log of problems that you got wrong. These are problems that you might be having substantive issues with and may require extra attention. Place extra emphasis on strategies to help fix the issues you come across.

Elaborative Interrogation: Spotting Patterns and Trends

Asking yourself a number of what and why questions when reviewing mocks, will encourage you to produce explanations for the mistakes and get to the bottom of any issue that may arise. If you can key in on the specific content of the types of problems that you are having trouble with, then you can work on developing an effective strategy for attacking those types of problems. This is otherwise known as elaborative interrogation, it is a specific method where you ask yourself questions about how and why things work, and then produce the answers to these questions. The specific questions that you ask yourself will depend, in part, on the area you are addressing during prep (e.g., why does x happen? What caused x? What is the result of x? And so on). When reviewing UCAT mocks ask yourself two questions:

What am I missing? (see some examples below)

- Are you missing a specific question type? (e.g. according to passage, venn etc.)
- Are you missing questions with a logical element?
- Are you missing questions with heavy conditional elements?
- Are you missing questions with numbers and percentages?
- Are you missing questions that require a specific skill?

Why am I missing this question(s)? (see some examples below)

- Are you having timing issues and only missing questions when you are rushing at the end of the section? (focus on timing)
- Are you misreading? (focus on attention to detail)
- Are you misunderstanding the stimuli? (focus on attention to detail)
- Did you get frustrated? (focus on mental/emotional strength & stamina)
- Did you lose focus? (focus on mental/emotional strength & stamina)
- Is there a more effective way that you could've attacked the problem? (focus on approach)
- Did you misunderstand and/or mis-diagram the relationship between elements in the stimuli? (focus on attention to detail/conditional reasoning/formal logic)

- Did you narrow the answer choices down to the correct answer choice and the answer choice that you incorrectly selected? Why did you choose the incorrect answer choice? Why was it attractive? Are you choosing the same types of incorrect answers over and over?

Many candidates make similar errors time and time again because they don't realize what they are having trouble with and why they are making mistakes. Carefully consider your weak areas, and aggressively work to develop those skills. If you realise that you are struggling with True, False and Can't tell questions, carefully skim through a UCAT practice book or online course locating "T/F/C" questions. One-by-one work through ONLY these questions untimed. Review after each question. Don't move on until you are comfortable that you thoroughly understand that question - develop a methodical approach to a question type, then drill until that approach is ingrained in your mind and becomes almost reflexive. I have provided a few strategies below to help with elaborative interrogation, try each one but pick the one(s) that works best for you:

Strategy: Developing the Pareto Lens

Three years ago, I was recommended a book by an old friend from sixth form, who had quit his job at the time to start a photography business. James was very passionate about capturing moments, his attention to detail when describing cameras and lens would have a regular person like myself muddled. His obsession with cameras matched his love of anime (Japanese animation). Don't get him started on 'Attack on Titans', a popular Japanese manga series he relentlessly recommended that I watched for years before eventually gave in, and now I'm a huge fan myself. Nonetheless, despite how well-versed he was in photography, he admitted that he had been struggling to manage his time running his business until reading a book titled the 4-hour work week by Tim Ferriss. I was struggling with balancing my time with managing the blog and he recommended this book. He was able to convince me to watch a Japanese animation I never thought in a million years I would watch, so thought I'd give his book recommendation a chance and I must admit it changed my life forever.

The book covers a wide range of principles around building wealth whilst freeing up time. There is a particular principle that can be applied to preparing for the UCAT, and it is called the 'Pareto Law', popularly known as the '80/20 Principle'. It states that 80% of an output results from 20% of the input. The principle is named after Vilfredo Pareto, an economist, who in 1906 noticed that 80% of the land in Italy was owned by 20% of the population. The mathematical formula he used to demonstrate this distribution also applied to almost everything. Eighty percent of Pareto's garden peas were produced by 20% of the pea pods he had planted, for example. This distribution became popular because it occurred over and over again in numerous scenarios, and it is still widely applied worldwide by companies, economists and governments, for example:

- About 20% of the world's population controls about 80% of the world's income.
- You would wear about 20% of the clothes in your wardrobe about 80% of the time.
- About 20% of a business's customers account for 80% of complaints.
- About 20% of your studying will lead to 80% of the outcome of your result.

The list is infinitely long and diverse. Imagine applying this to your UCAT prep, structuring your entire attack plan through the lens of a single question:

What 20% of new strategies caused 80% of my desired UCAT result?

That's an entirely different mindset that will give your UCAT preparation a significant edge over other competing students. Let's dig abit further:

- What 20% of exam strategies caused 80% of my desired VR results?
- What 20% of exam techniques caused 80% of my desired DM results?
- What 20% of mental maths shortcuts caused 80% of my desired QR results?
- What 20% of exam tactics caused 80% of my desired AR results?
- What 20% of exam tactics caused 80% of my desired AR results?

It's important to note that this 80/20 principle isn't a law for nature, it isn't as clean cut, but simply a principle of distribution. Sometimes, people will get 90% of results from 15% of their efforts. Or, they'll get 65% of results from 25% of efforts. But even then, the underlying logic of the principle — the minority of input responsible for the majority of results — applies. So as long as you are able to identify an area where such a distribution exists, there's room to apply the principle and design a more effective study plan.

In other words, **seek and focus on the 20% of work that will result to 80% of your desired UCAT outcome.** This will vary with every candidate.

Strategy: Using Exam KPIs

A key performance indicator (KPI) is a type of measurement that evaluates progression over time. It is widely used by businesses to monitor and analyse factors deemed crucial to the success of an organization. We can adopt this concept to assess our performance against a set of targets. By setting KPIs it enables you make smarter decisions about the direction of your revision by applying elaborative interrogation. Often success in an exam like the UCAT is simply the repeated, periodic achievement of micro study goals. Accordingly, choosing the right KPIs relies upon a good understanding of what is important to pass the exam.

Measuring and monitoring your performance is critical but focusing on the wrong performance indicators can be detrimental. Poorly structured KPIs, or KPIs that are too difficult to monitor on a regular basis are no good. To be useful, KPIs must be monitored and be actioned on immediately, let's look at the two most important KPIs during UCAT preparation and how to calculate them:

Error Rate

Error rate refers to the frequency at which you answer questions incorrectly within a specific subtest. It is measured as a percentage and can be calculated using the formula below:

$$\text{E.R} = \frac{Total\ number\ of\ incorrect\ responses}{Total\ questons\ attempted} \times 100$$

This metric is a good way to monitor accuracy over time as you attempt mock tests. I recommend calculating your error rate for each subtest after every mock test, as seen in the table below. That way, you can spot accuracy patterns in each subtest over time.

Subtests	Error Rate (%)		
	Mock 1	Mock 2	Mock 3
Verbal Reasoning			
Quantitative Reasoning			
Abstract Reasoning			
Decision Making			
Situational Judgement			

What to do if Error Rate isn't improving: I recommend diving deeper into the subtests with the highest error rates. Look more closely at question-types and work on strategies to improve accuracy. Challenge your reasoning and carefully consider the underlying cause, then aggressively work to develop a strategy to combat it. After sufficient practice, set multiple mini-tests (See Step 5: Practice) before doing another mock test.

Speed

Speed is a measure of how quickly you complete a subtest within its time limitations. This is an important KPI that must be monitored during every timed exercise. I strongly recommend reflecting on your use of time in each section after attempting mini-tests and mocks.

UKCAT Subtests			
Subtest	Time Allowed	Number of Questions	Time Per Question
Verbal Reasoning	21 minutes	44	30 seconds
Quantitative Reasoning	24 minutes	36	38 seconds
Abstract Reasoning	13 minutes	55	15 seconds
Decision Making	31 minutes	29	64 seconds
Situational Judgement	26 minutes	69	22 seconds

The table above is the timing for each section. I also included a breakdown of the time per question for those who may want. For example, if you wanted to work on your speed in the AR subtest you could set a mini-test, say of 20-questions, and would aim to complete it in 5 minutes. See calculation below:

$$Time \ (mins) = \frac{No \ of \ Questions \times Time \ per \ Question}{60}$$

i.e.

$$Time \ (mins) = \frac{20 \times 15}{60} = 5 \ mins$$

What to do if speed is not improving: I recommend tracking how long it takes you to complete the subtest of concern at normal pace whilst maintaining 80% accuracy, then gradually cutting down your time with every practice. For example, say at your normal pace you complete a full QR subtest in 50 minutes, shave off a minute or two with every practice until you get down to the 24 minutes time limit of the exam. Ensure you maintain 80% accuracy, if at any point your accuracy drops severely, pause and practice at that time limit until accuracy goes back up. For instance, say you manage to get timing down from 50 minutes to 38 minutes whilst maintaining an 80% average, but then went down to 34 mins and accuracy drops to 40%. Continue to practice at 34 minutes until you've fixed underlying uses and brought your accuracy back up.

Advice from Mike: When working on speed, it's not enough to be able to complete the subtest in time but completing it in time with a low error rate.

Strategy: Using a UCAT Question Log

UCAT question logs are hugely underrated when preparing for the exam. They can be an absolute asset if used properly. A question log is basically an excel spreadsheet where you track your UCAT study by recording questions you answer incorrectly (or correctly). By doing this, you can spot patterns and begin to apply elaborative interrogation. Thus, allowing you to assess your performance effectively – you can challenge your assumptions, ask new questions, make sense of results and process what you've learned into deeper memory. There isn't one universal approach to using a UCAT question log. It really depends on your objective during mock review. To help explain, I have broken this down into 3 key goals, they are as follows:

1. Identifying natural capabilities under testing conditions

This is where you aim to identify which types of questions are your strongest and most difficult. It also involves recognising the default strategies and tactics you employ when attempting these questions. It is good to identify this early as possible to help dictate how you prepare for the UCAT.

Using a UCAT question log: Record every UCAT question you attempted during timed practice and tag them as either answered 'right' or 'wrong'. Also include information on your reasoning (i.e. why you selected your answer) and include a brief summary of the evidence for the correct solution.

Advice from Mike: I recommend at the beginning of prep to record at least the first 100 UCAT questions attempted for each subtest to help identify where your natural capabilities lie. Analyse patterns in the questions that you get right and wrong. Use data to identify your strengths and weaknesses.

2. Identifying underlying weaknesses

This is where you aim to recognise any shortcomings in skill or approach that results in answering a specific type of question incorrectly. It involves deep-diving into the questions you answered wrong and making sense of the result and approach adopted.

Using a UCAT question log: Record ONLY questions that you answer wrong, include information on your reasoning and include a summary of the evidence that supports the right answer.

Advice from Mike: I recommend doing this for the remainder of your preparation, after you have identified where your natural capabilities lie. When analysing questions answered incorrectly try finding particular skews and biases in your reasoning. Make sure to challenge your approach.

3. Improving Accuracy / Reducing Error Rate

This is where you aim to improve your accuracy in answering a specific type of question. Once you have identified the underlying issue resulting to incorrect responses and have done the necessary steps to combat this. Do more practice and record performance.

Using a UCAT question log: Adopt ONLY one tip (tactic, technique or strategy) at a time and test it as you attempt questions. Record results and tag questions as either answered 'right' or 'wrong', include information on your reasoning and tactic (i.e. why you selected your answer and the technique(s) used) as well as a brief summary of the evidence for the correct solution.

Advice from Mike: Remember that no tip or tactic works 100% of the time. The key thing is that it improves your error rate no matter how significant. I recommend analysing performance with the 'Pareto lens', that is trying to spot the 20% of tactics that resulted to 80% of the desired outcome. In other words, which 2 out of 10 strategies resulted to the most improvement?

How to deal with inconsistent Mock Scores

UCAT preparation is all about progress, so it can be frustrating to see your mock performance go up and down. When facing inconsistent mock scores, embrace the reality that it is indeed part of the process and a key part of your learning. Instead of feeling anxious or uncertain about "where you stand," look for ways to turn score inconsistencies into valuable learning:

Look for what was significant about low vs high scoring days

Was there a particular issue on a day of a low score such as fatigue or ability to focus? Did you feel particularly good on days when you got higher scores? Look for clues as to what daily habits (sleep, stress, caffeine intake) affect your performance. You'll want to optimize these for test day.

Address low vs high scoring content

Was there a substantial difference in what was tested from one test to another? Perhaps you were more/less familiar with the topics covered in a subtest on a single test in a way that impacted the outcome. Variation in test content can happen, so take notes of what topics you should be focusing more on.

Doubling down on inconsistencies

You can immediately and significantly improve the impact of your mocks by merely doubling down and reviewing each mock after you take it. Be attentive to the underlying reason for choosing an option, whether it's right or not. You can catch poor habits that occasionally lead to losing easy marks. Ensure that you keep track of such issues and if necessary, spend additional time fixing them.

What does this mean for test day?

Mock scores can go up and down. What matters is how you perform on test day. Use your mocks to your advantage by taking lessons from each experience — be it test-taking skills or identifying strengths and weakness. Use what you learn to adjust your prep both in terms of content review and daily habits. Look to each mock test, regardless of its score, as an opportunity to reflect on your progress and make adjustments. Understanding how you got to a low (or high!) mock score may help ease the uncertainty of inconsistent performance. Then you can apply that understanding and get back to work!

Choosing and Discarding Exam Strategies

Choosing exam strategies for the UCAT is like building a house. First, you need to lay a good foundation before putting up the walls and windows. In the same vein, you need to understand why you're making mistakes in order to choose a set of tips and strategies to use on test day. From recognising this, you can test different strategies until you find one that fixes or greatly improves the issue. **How you test and choose exam strategies will greatly depend on whether the goal is to fix one of the issues mentioned on pages 81-82:**

Step 1 –Review Mock results: Review incorrect answers until you understand absolutely why the correct answer is better than the one you picked. Also, be sure to review and understand each and every question in the mock, you might have got some questions right by luck.

 Step 2 - Identify the underlying issue: Dig deeper and look carefully at what tripped you up and the underlying cause for your mistake. Try to categorise the mistake into one of the 4 categories.

Strep 3 – Pick an exam strategy and goal: Focus on one issue at a time and decide whether the strategy you will adopt will **improve your accuracy, speed or both**. The book contains hundreds of exam strategies and tips, so I expect you to discard plenty - don't get bogged down on trying everything shared in this guide. Pick ONE at a time and practice it.

Step 4 – Practice exam strategy: Do as many questions as possible until you become comfortable using exam strategy. If you intend to adopt the strategy to improve accuracy, then practice the questions untimed. If the goal is to improve speed, practice the questions timed. If it's to improve both, start with untimed practice then work your way to timed practice.

Step 5 – Test exam strategy: Set a mini-test (full or partial) and apply strategy wherever possible (for how to set mini-tests check out step 5: Practice).

Step 6- Review performance: Again, review answers and make sure understand each and every question, especially the ones you got wrong. Remember to assess carefully how much strategy improved performance and address the underlying issue. Did it work? If not, why? Use elaborative interrogation to get to the bottom of this. If you are not satisfied with the strategy, test it again before completely discarding it. Most of the time, students add or take out elements that do not work for them and possibly create an entirely unique approach and strategy.

Step 7 – Record in Game Plan: Record the strategies that work. Make sure to have an attack plan for each question-type and how you intend to finish each subtest on time.

I strongly recommend writing an outline of the tips and strategies you intend to use for each question-type in the exam. It primes the brain before test day. Here is my UCAT game plan for the VR subtest when I took the test:

Subtest	Question-Type	Game Plan
Verbal Reasoning	True/False or Can't Tell	*Keyword Strategy*
	Incomplete Statements	*Keyword Diary & Mapping*
	According To The Passage	*Keyword Diary & Mapping*
	Except Question	*Elimination & Keyword Strategy*
	Most Likely	*Elimination Technique*

It takes a lot of practice to find the right set of strategies to use in the exam. Since everyone is different what might work for me may not work for you, so be sure to test as many strategies as possible until you find the right one.

30-DAY UCAT STUDY SCHEDULE

DAILY STUDY SCHEDULE TO PREPARE
FOR THE UCAT TEST

Day 1

Task: Attempt the Verbal Reasoning Question Banks

Estimated Time: 2 hours

Reason: They are the only official verbal practice questions available; they reflect the same difficulty you can expect in the exam.

Study tip: Do not time yourself when attempting questions. Just focus on accuracy. Record your answer on a sheet of paper and check them against the explanations once finished.

Advice from Mike:
- Attempt VR questions with no prior preparation to determine where your natural capabilities lie.
- Review answers and identify difficult question types.
- Identify which skills you struggle with the most (e.g. comprehension, critical reading, speed etc.).
- Take note of your Strengths, Weakness, Opportunities and Threats. Suggest how to improve.
- After completing each question bank reflect and think about how you can improve your accuracy in the next bank of questions

Tips from other top scorers:
- At the very least glance at the question first. It makes you read passage with a purpose rather than wondering what you need to know.
- Though the average is 30 seconds per question throughout VR, the reality is some can be done quicker, and some take longer. Take note of the question-types that regularly take you longer and work on speeding them up
- Have an approach to picking and scanning keywords during VR. Practice. Also, have a plan for when you cannot find keywords
- When reading a passage try to summarise the topic of each paragraph in 1-2 words in your head. It helps with recall and retention.

Day 2

Task: Attempt the Decision Making Question Banks

Estimated Time: 2 hours

Reason: They are the only official decision making questions available, they reflect the same scope and difficulty you can expect in the exam.

Study tip: Do not time yourself when attempting questions. Just focus on accuracy. Record answer on a sheet of paper and check them against the explanations once finish.

Advice from Mike:
- Attempt DM questions with no prior preparation to determine where your natural capabilities lie.
- Review answers and identify difficult question types.
- Identify which skills you struggle with the most (e.g. deductive reasoning, evaluating arguments, statistical reasoning, etc).
- Take note of Strengths, Weakness, Opportunities, Threats and suggest how to improve.
- After completing each question bank reflect and think about how you can improve your accuracy in the other question banks.

Tips from other top scorers:
- Draw diagrams when possible. You can almost always visualise logical puzzles better than reading it out.
- There is no overall solution that works for every question-type in the decision making subtest, so having a strategy for each type is really important. Think of ways to improve accuracy for now (then later speed).
- Probability is an important concept – Independent and dependent events, conditional probability and mutually exclusive events, as well as multiplication and addition rules.

Day 3

Task: Attempt the Quantitative Reasoning Question Banks

Estimated Time: 2 hours

Reason: They are the only official quantitative reasoning questions available.

Study tip: Do questions untimed, only focus on accuracy for now.

Advice from Mike:
- Do not time yourself when attempting questions.
- Practice using the on-screen calculator provided.
- Practice using mental arithmetic tricks to save more time.
- Don't over complicate questions (questions are GCSE standard and require use of fairly basic mathematical operations).
- Take note of Strengths, Weakness, Opportunities and Threats; and suggest how to improve.
- After completing each question bank reflect and think about how you can improve your accuracy in the other question banks.

Tips from other top scorers:
- Beware of examiner tricks where they provided details in a scenario using one unit but the answers in another unit. The correct answer is usually dressed up in different unit to confuse students.
- Practise using the on-screen calculator but beware of typos when using it. Leave yourself time to double-check when doing complex calculations
  Don't overcomplicate questions. Questions typically require use of fairly basic Maths. If you are overcomplicating things, then it's very likely you are heading down the wrong track.
- Think of mental maths calculations that you struggle to do quickly in specific scenarios. For example, squaring a two-digit number when doing compound interest problems.

Day 4

Task: Attempt the Abstract Reasoning Question Banks

Estimated Time: 2 hours

Reason: They mimic the scope and question-types you can expect in the exam.

Study tip: Do questions untimed, only focus on accuracy for now. Don't be intimidated by a set you cannot solve instantly. Record answer on a sheet of paper and check them against the explanations once you finish.

Advice from Mike:

- Attempt questions with no prior preparation to determine where your natural capabilities lie.
- Review answers and Identify difficult question types.
- Identify which skills you struggle with the most
- Reflect on your pattern finding approach (e.g. mnemonic etc.).
- Take note of Strengths, Weakness, Difficult question types and come up with suggestions on how to improve.
- After completing Question Bank 1 reflect and think about how you can improve your accuracy in the next bank of questions.

Tips from other top scorers:

- The more abstract reasoning questions you practise, the easier you'll find the subtest. Once you start to get better at spotting patterns you'll naturally pick up the pace over time.
- When working out patterns try starting with the simplest box because it will most likely contain the fewest distractors.
- Most students instinctively start at Set A when trying to work out patterns, it might be easier to start at Set B instead. Start with the set that looks easier (i.e. less patterns per box)

Day 5

Task: Attempt the Situational Judgement Question Banks

Estimated Time: 2 hours

Reason: They mimic the scope and question-types you can expect in the exam.

Study tip: Do questions untimed, only focus on accuracy for now. Do not worry if you have little or no knowledge of the key principles of medical professionalism. Record answer on a sheet of paper and check them against the explanations once you finish.

Advice from Mike:
- Attempt questions with no prior preparation to help gauge your level of understanding on key medical/dental principles.
- Always read the scenario first.
- Double check you know whose point of view you are answering from.
- When reviewing answers try to categorise incorrect responses in terms of the medical principle. For example, a question on patient safety.
- After completing Question Bank 1 reflect and think about how you can improve your accuracy in the next bank of questions.

Tips from other top scorers:
- A scenario will sometimes feature more than one 'character'. Check you know whose point of view you are answering from.
- It's important to that medical (or dental) students are NOT doctors yet and shouldn't behave as if they are.
- Always remember that patient safety is of utmost importance
- Always answer according to what you **should** do not what you would do.
- It can be difficult at times but judge each possible answer independently and not as if it is the only thing you do.

Day 6

Task: Analyse performance for all Question Banks

Estimated Time: 1 hour

Reason: To find out the underlying causes for wrong answers during untimed practice.

Study tip: Please note that learning the solutions is not what we are doing today. The goal here is to go one step further and understand *why* you answered questions incorrectly. Use strategies recommended in step 4 of the Preparation Guide to help.

Advice from Mike:

- Try to identify which question-type you regularly get wrong and figure out why. Use strategies such as 5 why technique or Grid Method to help with this.
- Think about what mental processes or skill you struggled with? For example, slow at mental arithmetic? If so, which one? (percentages, addition of three-digit numbers? When it comes to identifying skills in each subtest, use the information covered in step 2.
- From your analysis create a list of topics, concepts or areas within each subtest that are top priority that you intend to work on.
- Think of ways on your own on how you can improve this. Do not use any of the exam strategies recommended in the guide yet – try to work it out on your own. This is a great way to challenge your understanding and develop approach.

Tips from other top scorers:

- For every question you miss, identify what type of question it is. When you notice patterns to the questions you miss, you must then devote extra practice to those sub-skills.

- If you don't understand **exactly** why you missed a question, you'll make the same mistake over and over again.
- Make sure to adopt a no-mistake-left-behind policy when analysing performance. Letting one go can mean you make the same mistake on test day.
- Get help with difficult areas by asking questions in the UCAT study group, forums or leaving comments on a related article on the MEDIC BLOG.

> **Heads up:** Over the next 3 days we will attempt the official practice tests under exam conditions. Please allow 2 hours of uninterrupted practice time for each day.

Day 7

Task: Attempt Practice test A under exam conditions and Review Answers

Estimated Time: 3 hours

Reason: To identify weaknesses under timed conditions

Study tip: Pick up the pace and try to complete each subtest within the time limit. Answer questions as quickly and accurate as possible

Advice from Mike:

- Review your performance in questions banks and suggest ways to save time and compensate for shortcomings before attempting practice test A.
- Treat practice test A as the real test, do not take any break during the duration of the test.
- Pace yourself so you can attempt all the items in each section.
- Once test is completed review all questions not just the ones you answered incorrectly.
- Record your score in each subtest (you will need the UCAT conversion table).
- What did you find most difficult in each subtest? Write this down as we will go over this soon.

Tips from other top scorers:

- Be ruthless in eliminating distractors from study time. Some helpful tips include: turning off your phone, avoiding social media, locking your door and asking people not to disturb.
- Familiarising yourself with the pace required in each subtest is an essential component of revising for the exam. During timed full practice test try to practice keeping an eye on the clock and assessing how far along you are.
- Try using the flagging and keyboard shortcuts during mocks

Day 8

Task: Attempt Practice test B under exam conditions and Review Answers

Estimated Time: 3 hours

Reason: Continue with identifying weaknesses under timed conditions

Study tip: Continue to pick up the pace and try to complete each subtest within the time limit. Answer questions as quickly and accurate as possible

Advice from Mike:
- Review your performance in Practice test A and suggest ways to improve for Practice test B.
- Treat practice test B as the real test, do not take any break during the duration of the test.
- Pace yourself so you can attempt all the items in each section.
- Once test is completed review all questions not just the ones you answered incorrectly.
- Record your score in each subtest (you will need the UCAT conversion table).
- What did you find most difficult in each subtest? Was it the same as what you struggled with in Practice Test A? If so, try to understand why you still struggle with this, write this down as we will go over this soon.

Tips from other top scorers:
- The 1-minute instructions never change; so do not waste your time reading them. Instead think about your game plan for the subtest.
- Get used to keeping an eye on the clock, but you need to figure out what works best for you, but generally avoid checking the time more than once every few questions – otherwise, you'll end up wasting time obsessing over the clock.
- During UCAT practice establish a feedback loop by testing strategies, reviewing your mistakes, and testing again.

Day 9

Task: Attempt Practice test C under exam conditions and Review Answers

Estimated Time: 3 hours

Reason: Further identify weaknesses under timed conditions

Study tip: Continue to pick up the pace and try to complete each subtest within the time limit. Answer questions as quickly and accurate as possible

Advice from Mike:

- Review your performance in Practice test B and suggest ways to improve for Practice test C.
- Treat practice test C as the real test, do not take any break during the duration of the test.
- Pace yourself so you can attempt all the items in each section.
- Once test is completed review all questions not just the ones you answered incorrectly.
- Record your score in each subtest (you will need the UCAT conversion table).
- What did you find most difficult in each subtest? Was it the same as what you struggled with in Practice Test A and B? If so, try to understand why you still struggle with this.

Tips from other top scorers:

- You will be provided with a marker and note board. It can be helpful to jot notations down but be careful not to get into the habit of writing too many things.
- Learn how to play the exam, beyond knowing what the exam looks likes – recognise common tricks used by examiners to waste your time and catch you out.
- Triage hard questions: Get comfortable skipping hard questions and coming back to them later.

Day 10
You're on a Roll!

Well done on completing the official question banks and practice tests. Today, take a break, only review performance - complete exercise 3 in Step 2 (Identify) to identify your **true weakness**.

Do not get demotivated if your scores are low, it is expected as you have not learned many techniques. Remember, the point of this exercise is to identify your natural abilities so that you can work on your weakest areas.

Advice from Mike:
- Convert practice test results and Calculate your score in each subtest out of 900 using the conversion table on the blog.
- Compare your score to previous year candidate results.
- Identify your strongest and weakest subtests.
- Within each subtest recognise your weakest areas
- Identify any trends or patterns that occurs.
- Create a priority table (optional)

Tips from other top scorers:
- Your average score on the official practice tests will most likely be below your target score at this point. Do not be put off by this, it is expected at the beginning of revision.
- Create a To-do-list (TDL) for each subtest. It must include the areas you intend to work on to improve accuracy and speed.
- Once sufficient time has passed, re-attempt the official UCAT questions and compare results to first attempt.

Heads up: Over the next 4 days you will focus on learning tips, techniques and strategies to improve your TWO weakest subtests. Then on Day 15 you will attempt a full mock test under timed conditions (please ensure you have at least 2 hours of uninterrupted revision time).

Day 11

Task: Improve Accuracy in Weakest subtest.

Estimated Time: 3 hours

Study tip: Learn strategies to improve accuracy and tweak them accordingly. In some cases, you may need to learn new concepts to improve.

Advice from Mike:

When I was preparing for the UCAT in 2015, I discovered the Verbal reasoning subtest was my weakest section. I spent the majority of my time learning techniques and strategies to improve my accuracy in answering questions.

I looked at the error rate for each question-type and looked into the underlying reasons to why I got questions wrong. In addition, I worked on my reading strategy, I also took time to recognise some of the common methods and tricks used by UCAT examiners and figured out how to avoid them. Once I had gathered a few strategies I practised implementing them by attempting questions untimed and tweaked them accordingly until I reached an accuracy level I was happy with.

The aim for today is to improve your accuracy in your weakest section, test strategies by doing practice questions untimed. If there is a specific question-type that is an issue work mostly on it until your accuracy improves. Refer to the strategies chapter of the guide to learn new tips and techniques.

Action Points:

- Rank your areas of weakness from most frequently observed to least.
- Start fixing things in order of which mistakes will respond the fastest to corrective prep measures.
- Set a mini test (untimed) to see whether you've improved (for advice on setting mini-tests see step 5 of the preparation guide).

- Repeat the process of taking mini-tests and assessing your mistakes until you reach a score level that makes you happy.

Tips from other top scorers:

- You're not going to be able to raise your UCAT score until you get to the bottom of what's holding you back.
- Get familiar with the type of tricks and methods examiners use in the UCAT. This will provide a psychological advantage of comfort and visual familiarity.
- Get into habit of recognising simple and complex questions before you begin to solve it. You can triage questions more effectively if you are able to recognising how long it will take to answer.

Day 12

Task: Improve Speed in Weakest subtest.

Estimated Time: 3 hours

Study tip: Learn strategies to improve speed and tweak them accordingly.

Advice from Mike:

In order to make the most out of practice, you'll have to use test-taking strategies that work to your advantage. Many improvements are dependent on adjusting your strategy, especially when it comes to issues with running out of time. The most effective strategies may differ depending on overall performance in each subtest.

The aim for today is to improve your speed in answering questions in your weakest subtest, implement strategies by doing practice questions timed. If there is a specific skill or mental process that takes you longer than necessary, learn shortcuts to save time. In addition, develop a triage strategy -i.e. your approach to streamline through questions. For my weakest subtest, my triage strategy included skipping specific question-types and coming back to them later.

The best way to look at improving your speed is to consider it at two levels:

Micro level: Timing issues due to specific shortcomings in skill e.g. slow at converting Km/hr to m/s, slow at converting decimals accurately, reading regression, etc.

Macro level: Timing issues due to poor exam-taking techniques e.g. not adopting questions triage, wasting time on difficult questions, no flagging strategy etc.

Action Points:
- Rank micro and macro level timing issues frequently observed to least.
- Learn techniques and strategies to fix each issue methodically
- Take a timed mini-test to see whether you've improved

- Repeat the process of taking timed tests and assessing your timing issues until you reach a level that makes you happy.

Tips from other top scorers:

- If you run out of time to answer all the question in a subtest. Continue answering questions, record how long it takes you normally and begin to cut it down gradually until you reach the time limit of the exam.
- Try to adopt speed strategies that also help with improving accuracy. This way you are killing two birds with one stone.
- Keep a record of all the strategies that work and don't work. Be open to combining techniques and trying different things until find a set of techniques that improve your speed and accuracy to a level that you are pleased with.

Day 13

Task: Improve Accuracy in 2nd Weakest subtest.

Estimated Time: 3 hours

Study tip: Learn strategies to improve accuracy and tweak them accordingly. In some cases, you may need to learn new concepts to improve.

Advice from Mike:

The Quantitative Reasoning subtest was my second weakest section. In terms of accuracy, I wasn't too bad. I needed to brush up on statistics and dealing with complex money calculations such as compound interest. I evaluated my error rate for each question-type and looked into the underlying reasons to why I got questions wrong. In most cases, I was pressed for time and made careless mistakes.

The aim for today is to improve your accuracy in your 2nd weakest subtest, test strategies by doing practice questions untimed. If there is a specific question-type that is an issue work mostly on it until your accuracy improves. Refer to the strategies chapter of the guide to learn new tips and techniques.

Action Points:

- Rank your areas of weakness from most frequently to least observed.
- Start fixing things in order of which mistakes will respond the fastest to corrective prep measures.
- Take a mini test (untimed) to see whether you've improved
- Repeat the process of taking mini-tests and assessing your mistakes until you reach a score level that you are happy with (i.e. target score reached).

Tips from other top scorers:

- It comes with practice but learn to use the clues in both the question and the answer choices to help find the right answer when guessing strategically. Often (though not always), a little strategy will allow you to eliminate at least one or two answer choices and make an educated guess.
- For numerical problems in the Quantitative Reasoning and Decision Making subtests, be comfortable picking an answer without completing the entire calculation. Sometimes you can narrow down the correct answer by eyeballing and using a bit of common sense.
- When analysing graphs and tables it's always good idea to eyeball the information and answer options. Sometime you may be able to pick the correct answer without doing any calculations.

Heads up: On day 15 you will attempt a full mock test under timed conditions (please arrange at least 2 hours of uninterrupted practice). Aim to implement all the newly learned strategies.

Day 14

Task: Improve Speed in 2nd Weakest subtest.

Estimated Time: 3 hours

Study tip: Learn strategies to improve speed and tweak them accordingly.

Advice from Mike:

The aim for today is to improve your speed in answering questions in your 2nd weakest subtest, implement strategies by doing practice questions timed. If there is a specific skill or mental process that takes you longer than necessary, learn shortcuts to improve. In addition, develop a triage strategy -i.e. your approach to streamlining through questions. For my 2nd weakest subtest, my triage strategy included often strategically guessing questions (though not always) that presented information in a straightforward graph or tabular format. Also, I would skip questions that required complex calculations and come back to them if I had time.

When improving your speed consider timing issues at both the micro and macro levels (for explanation on both levels refer to Day 12).

Action Points:
- Rank micro and macro level timing issues from frequently observed to least.
- Learn techniques and strategies to fix each issue methodically
- Take a timed mini-test to see whether you've improved
- Repeat the process of taking timed tests and assessing your timing issues until you reach a level that you are happy with.

Tips from other top scorers:
- Double down on exam tricks and doing independent practice of the question-types under timed conditions.
- If you're struggling with a question and notice yourself allocating a lot of time to it, make an educated guess and move on. Make sure to take

note of the question-type so you can allocate some time improving this later.

- Have a triage strategy for each subtest based on the question-types you have identified as strengths and weaknesses.
- Have a rough idea on the time you are meant to spend on each question in a subtest. Use it to set time markers on the test day (strategy #36).

Heads up: Tomorrow you will attempt a full mock test under timed conditions (please arrange at least 2 hours of uninterrupted practice). Aim to implement all of the newly learned test strategies.

Day 15

Well Done!

Task: Attempt and Review a Practice test under exam conditions (Practice Test 1)

Estimated Time: 3 hours

Study tip: Implement exam and triage strategies to improve accuracy and pace. Use an online course for this exercise to mimic testing conditions.

Advice from Mike:

Well done! You are halfway through the study schedule. Today, we will attempt another full practice test under exam conditions. Please ensure to mimic the testing conditions and ensure you are not disturbed for the entire 2 hours.

The goal today is to implement the newly learned exam and triage strategies to boost both your accuracy and speed in your two weakest sections. Do the other 3 subtests as normal. During review, take note of any issues or threats that arise, and we will address them soon.

Action Points:
- Go over your 'game plan' for each subtest (particularly the two weakest sections).
- Attempt a practice test under exam conditions
- Mark and revise the practice test
- Audit strategies adopted (what works and what doesn't work)
- Identify threats (these are areas that didn't improve despite practice)
- Compare test results to previous mock results on Day 7- 9
- Propose plan to improve

Tips from other top scorers:

- Double down on exam strategies that improve your performance in the exam and discard the ones that do not work. What might work for one student might not work well for you. So be sure to test and validate strategies with practice.

- Regularly perform an audit of the tips, techniques and strategies you decide to adopt for exam day under exam conditions.

- When reviewing the answers of the questions you got wrong in a practice test, try to attempt them again before looking at the answers. This will help you figure out if the issue is a timing or accuracy problem. If you got a question wrong the first time but answered it right the second time then its most likely a timing issue. However, if you answer it wrong both times then it's clearly an accuracy issue.

Day 16

Task: Address 'Threats' in Practice Test 1

Estimated Time: 4 hours

Study tip: Make sure to get to the bottom of all 'threats' before moving onto Day 17.

Advice from Mike:

The aim for today is to work on the areas that you have identified as 'Threats'. These are areas that you have practised and done as much as you can to improve but efforts seem futile. The key to improving these areas is to assess your current process in solving them and figuring out which element you need to work on to reduce the likelihood of making the same mistake again.

Must Read: Due to the depth of this process I have provided an exclusive feature on the blog at www.themedicblog.co.uk/evaluate-ucat-process.

In the article I also provide tips on how to improve some of the most common areas that have been identified as 'threats' by past candidates.

Action Points:
- Review all incorrect responses in practice test 1
- Assess process for all questions answered incorrect and spot 'Threats'
- Learn tips and strategies to combat 'Threats'
- Practice techniques to fix 'Threats'. Recommend practising questions on the UCAT user interface.
- Repeat the process of taking timed tests and assessing your timing issues until you reach a level that you are pleased with.

Tips from other top scorers:
- Review practice tests to the point where it switches from merely practice

to actually teaching yourself.
- When reviewing your UCAT practice results, make sure to review all the questions - including the ones you answered correctly, double check you followed the same process as the solutions.
- Do not focus on what you did well and ignore what you did wrong. This is a common mistake by many students.

Day 17

Task: Improve Accuracy in 2nd strongest subtest.

Estimated Time: 3 hours

Study tip: Learn strategies to improve your accuracy and tweak them accordingly.

Advice from Mike:

When I was preparing for the UCAT in 2015, I discovered that the Decision Analysis section was my second strongest section. I spent time learning techniques and strategies to reduce my error rate.

The aim for today is to improve your accuracy in your 2nd strongest subtest, test strategies by doing practice questions untimed. If there is a specific question-type that is an issue, work mostly on it until your accuracy improves. Refer to relevant strategies from guide to learn new tips and techniques.

Action Points:
- Rank your areas of weakness from most frequently observed to least.
- Start fixing things in order of which mistakes will respond the fastest to corrective prep measures.
- Take a mini test (untimed) to see whether you've improved
- Tweak strategies accordingly until you see improvement
- Repeat the process of taking mini-tests and assessing your mistakes until your accuracy improves.

Tips from other top scorers:
- Controlling your mental status is important during the UCAT. Just like a pro athlete or performer, you need to be confident about your skills. You already put in a ton of work, and you've learned a lot so the last thing you want to do is ruin your performance. Instead of dwelling on a single question, do your best, clear your head and move on.

- The process of preparing for the UCAT can teach you a lot about yourself and your limits. Use that to your advantage- always think of ways you can capitalise on strengths and compensate weaknesses.
- Eliminate distractors during UCAT revision, if you're studying and you glance at your phone every 3 minutes, you are NOT STUDYING.

Day 18

Task: Improve Pace in 2nd strongest subtest.

Estimated Time: 3 hours

Study tip: Learn strategies to improve speed and tweak them accordingly.

Advice from Mike:

The aim for today is to improve your speed in answering questions in your 2nd strongest subtest, implement strategies by doing practice questions timed. If there is a specific skill or mental process that takes you longer than necessary, learn shortcuts to improve. In addition, develop a triage strategy -i.e. your approach to streamlining through questions. Make sure to identify and fix all timing issues at both the micro and macro levels (for explanation on both levels refer to Day 12).

Action Points:

- Rank micro and macro level timing issues from frequently observed to least.
- Learn techniques and strategies to fix each issue methodically
- Take a timed mini-test to see whether you've improved
- Repeat the process of taking timed tests and assessing your timing issues until you reach a level that you are pleased with.

Tips from other top scorers:

- Don't be tricked into spending too much time on a particularly difficult question. Examiners include them on purpose to weed out those that cannot triage questions.
- You feel less time pressure in the UCAT if you know the method you need to solve each question.
- You won't be able to memorise or comprehend all materials at once. Balance is key - ensure that you reward learning with break times to recharge and relax.

Day 19

Task: Improve Accuracy in strongest subtest.

Estimated Time: 3 hours

Study tip: Learn strategies to improve accuracy and tweak them accordingly. In some cases, you may need to learn new concepts to improve.

Advice from Mike:

I discovered the abstract reasoning subtest was my strongest section. I spent the majority of my prep learning techniques and strategies to improve my speed but I also worked on accuracy as well.

I looked at the error rate for each question-type and looked into the underlying reasons to why I got questions wrong. In addition, I worked on my pattern finding strategy. I also took time to recognise some of the common relationships used by UCAT examiners and figured out how to avoid red herrings. Once I had gathered a few strategies I practised implementing them by attempting questions untimed and tweaked them accordingly until I reached an accuracy level I was happy with.

The aim for today is to improve your accuracy in your strongest section, test strategies by doing practice questions untimed. If there is a specific question-type that is an issue work mostly on it until your accuracy improves. Refer to the strategies chapter of the guide to learn new tips and techniques.

Action Points:
- Rank your areas of weakness from most frequently observed to least.
- Start fixing things in order of which mistakes will respond the fastest to corrective prep measures.
- Take a mini test (untimed) to see whether you've improved
- Repeat the process of taking mini-tests and assessing your mistakes until you reach your target score level.

Tips from other top scorers:

- For the QR and DM subtests you need to thoroughly understand all of the common topics that are tested and supplement with other resources to improve.
- Compile and learn formulas for concepts that come up regularly in the QR and DM subtests. Some common ones include percentage change, income tax, median, etc.
- Avoid strategy errors – this is when you understand the content/topic that's being tested, but make mistakes in your approach to solving it.

Day 20

Task: Improve Speed in strongest subtest.

Estimated Time: 3 hours

Study tip: Learn strategies to improve speed and tweak them accordingly.

Advice from Mike:

The aim for today is to improve your speed in answering questions in your strongest subtest, implement strategies by doing practice questions timed. If there is a specific skill or mental process that takes you longer than necessary, learn shortcuts to improve. In addition, develop a triage strategy -i.e. your approach to streamlining through questions.

Make sure to identify and fix all timing issues at both the micro and macro levels (for explanation on both levels refer to Day 12).

Action Points:
- Rank micro and macro level timing issues from frequently observed to least.
- Learn techniques and strategies to fix each issue methodically
- Take a timed mini-test to see whether you've improved
- Repeat the process of taking timed tests and assessing your timing issues until you reach a level that you are pleased with.

Tips from other top scorers:
- There's no negative marking in the UCAT so it's in your best interest to answer every single question in a subtest, even if you plan to come back to it later.
- Have a timing contingency plan for each subtest in case you ever in a position where you are running out of time.
- The UCAT has a particular style of asking questions that you'll want to become closely familiar with. Thus, each section has its own distinct set of question types and formats that you will face on test day. How

to prepare for QR subtest will be different than how to prepare for the VR subtest, which will be different than how to prepare for STJ subtest.

Heads up: Tomorrow you will attempt a full mock test under timed conditions (please arrange at least 2 hours of uninterrupted practice). Aim to implement all newly learned strategies.

Day 21

Keep it Up!

Task: Attempt and Review a Practice test under exam conditions (Practice Test 2)

Estimated Time: 3 hours

Study tip: Implement exam and triage strategies to improve accuracy and pace.

Advice from Mike:

Today, we will attempt another full practice test under exam conditions. Please ensure to mimic the testing conditions and ensure you are not disturbed for the entire 2 hours.

The goal today is to implement the newly learned strategies and review any issues or threats that arise. We will address them tomorrow.

Action Points:

- Go over your 'game plan' for each subtest (at this point, it should be all subtests except the STJ section)
- Attempt a timed practice test
- Mark and Review practice test
- Audit strategies adopted (what works and what doesn't work)
- Identify threats (these are areas that didn't improve despite practice)
- Compare test results to previous mock results on Day 15
- Propose plan to improve.
- Update game plan accordingly.

Tips from other top scorers:

- The reality is that analysing your performance on each practice test is the key to improving. Tally up all the reasons for your mistakes on a practice test and look into at least at the top three reoccurring errors.
- Do not take any mistake for granted, your score will not magically improve without consistently working on underlying issues during practice.
- When you have finished a practice test, reattempt questions you missed before looking at the answer explanations.

Day 22

Task: Address 'Threats' in Practice Test 2

Estimated Time: 4 hours

Study tip: Adopt a no-mistake-left-behind policy. Letting one slip through can mean you make the same mistake in the real UCAT.

Advice from Mike:

The aim for today is to work on the areas that you have identified as 'Threats'. These are areas that you have practised and done as much as you can to improve but efforts seem futile. The key to improving these areas is to assess your current process in solving them and figuring out which element you need to work on to reduce the likelihood of making the same mistake again.

Action Points:
- Review all incorrect responses in practice test 2
- Assess process for all questions answered incorrect and spot 'Threats'
- Learn tips and strategies to combat 'Threats'
- Practice techniques to fix 'Threats'. Recommend practising questions on the UCAT user interface.
- Repeat the process of taking timed tests and assessing your issues until you reach a level that you are pleased with.

Tips from other top scorers:
- During QR practice, if a topic can use multiple solving methods for its problems, try all the different ways in order to find the one most comfortable for you.
- Once you've brushed up on the topic, take practice problems in multiples at a time, as if you were truly working on the test. As you solve your practice questions, don't solve questions one at a time and stop to look up the answer after each one. Though you may be tempted to

know exactly how well you've done after solving each problem, this kind of pacing does NOT give you an accurate picture of how you'll do on test day and can hamper your progress.

- For every question that you miss, you need to identify the type of question it is. When you notice patterns to the questions you miss, you then need to find extra practice for this sub skill.

Day 23

Task: Improve Accuracy in Situational Judgement

Estimated Time: 4 hours

Study tip: Learn the key principles of medical professionalism using official practice questions and GMC documents.

Advice from Mike:

The aim for today is to work on the Situational Judgment subtest. It is the 5th and final section of the UCAT. It is designed to test your judgment of medically relevant situations and is marked in bands, where band 1 is the highest and band 4 is the lowest.

Go over all the situational judgment questions you have attempted to date (including the official questions banks and practice tests), reattempt questions you missed before looking at the answer explanations. Categorise all the questions you answered incorrectly or guessed into one of the following:

- Integrity
- Team work
- Patient care
- Dealing with Colleagues/Professional behaviour
- Drug Misuse
- Medical ethics - Beneficence, Autonomy, Consent, Confidentiality, etc
- Coping with pressure
- Other

Rank categories in terms of weakness from most frequently observed to least. Try to spot any patterns in misunderstanding or strategies used by examiners to catch you out. Starting with the most occurring threat, use the *good Medical practice* and *tomorrows doctor* guides to learn key principles.

Tips from other top scorers:

- Don't read the GMC guide or Tomorrows guide cover-to-cover, this can be tedious and a waste of time. instead focus on areas where you have weak understanding.

- When reading a scenario always try to understand the conflicting issue before looking at the question. There is always the temptation to quickly scan the text. Avoid this!

Day 24

Task: Improve Speed in Situational Judgement

Estimated Time: 4 hours

Study tip: Use an online course that mimics the official UCAT exam interface.

Advice from Mike:

The aim for today is to improve your speed in attempting STJ questions. If there is a specific question-type that is an issue work mostly on it until your accuracy improves. Refer to the strategies chapter of the guide to learn new tips and techniques to improve pace.

Make sure to identify and fix all timing issues at both the micro and macro levels (for explanation on both levels refer to Day 12).

Action Points:
- Rank micro and macro level timing issues from frequently observed to least.
- Learn techniques and strategies to fix each issue methodically
- Take a timed mini-test to see whether you've improved
- Repeat the process of taking timed tests and assessing your timing issues until you reach a level that you are pleased with.

Tips from other top scorers:
- The first thing you need to identify in every scenario is the character or profession involved. This is particularly important when looking at the duties of a medical student compared to a fully trained medical doctor – as they are not the same.
- All decisions that affect patient care should be made to benefit the patient. Of secondary importance are your work colleagues. Finally, of lowest importance is yourself. Remember the key principles of professional conduct and you will do well. Of utmost importance is

patient safety.

- No one knows exactly how the Situational judgement is scored; however you still get partial marks even if you select the wrong answer. For example, if you the correct answer for a response is Very Appropriate and you select "Appropriate, but not ideal" you will still get some marks if you are on the right side of the conflicting issue- so if you are ever torn between two answer options on the same side go with your gut. Chances are you'll still awarded some points.

Day 25
5 Days left!

Task: Attempt and Review a Practice test under exam conditions (Practice Test 3)

Estimated Time: 3 hours

Study tip: Implement exam and triage strategies to improve accuracy and pace.

Advice from Mike:

Today, we will attempt another full practice test under exam conditions. Please implement learned strategies and take note of any issues.

Action Points:

- Go over your 'game plan' for each subtest (at this point, it should be all subtests including the STJ section).
- Attempt practice test under exam onditions
- Mark and Review practice test
- Audit strategies adopted (what works and what doesn't work)
- Identify threats (these are areas that didn't improve despite practice)
- Compare test results to previous mock results on Day 21
- Propose ways to improve and update 'game plan' accordingly.

Tips from other top scorers:

- Inconsistencies in test performance can be expected, and in such instances do not panic, try to figure out what elements need improvement and look for ways to turn score inconsistencies into valuable learning. In most cases, it either a strategy or pacing issue that can be fixed once you recognise the underlying problem.

Day 26

Task: Address 'Threats' in Practice Test 3

Estimated Time: 4 hours

Study tip: Stay focus on improving on your accuracy and reducing the chances of spending too long on any one question.

Advice from Mike:

Aim to work on the areas that you have identified as 'Threats' in yesterday's mock. Assess your current process in solving them and figure out which element you need to work on to reduce the likelihood of making the same mistake again.

Action Points:

- Review all incorrect responses in practice test 3.
- Assess process for all questions answered incorrect and spot 'Threats'
- Hone tips and strategies to combat 'Threats'
- Practice techniques to fix 'Threats' on the UCAT user interface.
- Repeat the process of taking timed tests and assessing your issues until you reach a level that you are pleased with.

Tips from other top scorers:

- Practise using the on-screen calculator before test day. Also be aware of typos when you use the on-screen calculator. On test day, try to develop a method to double-check complicated calculations.
- Never overcomplicate questions. Always use shortcuts, educated guesses and common sense whenever possible.
- Keep moving methodically through each subtest. There will be ambiguous questions that will make you doubt your answers.

Day 27

3 Days Left!

Task: Attempt and Review a Practice test under exam conditions (Practice Test 4)

Estimated Time: 3 hours

Study tip: Implement exam and triage strategies to improve accuracy and pace.

Advice from Mike:

Today, we will attempt another full practice test under exam conditions. Please ensure to mimic the testing conditions and ensure you are not disturbed for the entire 2 hours. The goal today is to implement the newly learned exam and triage strategies to boost both your accuracy and pace in all the sections that you have worked on. During the review, take note of any issues or threats that arise, and we will address them tomorrow.

Action Points:

- Go over your 'game plan' for each subtest
- Attempt practice test under exam conditions
- Mark and Review practice test
- Audit strategies adopted (what works and what doesn't work)
- Identify threats (these are areas that didn't improve despite practice)
- Compare test results to previous mock results on Day 25
- Propose a plan to improve in each subtest.

Tips from other top scorers:

- Remember if you don't know the answer, make an educated guess! You can't actively lose marks.
- Practice enough questions to the point where at a glance you can identify whether a question is likely to be easy or take some time.

- When you go back to a flagged question, try to remind yourself the context of the question and pick up where you left off. It is easier said than done, but having that mindset helps.

Day 28

Task: Address 'Threats' in Practice Test 4

Estimated Time: 4 hours

Study tip: Start fixing things in order of which mistakes will respond the fastest to corrective prep measures.

Advice from Mike:

Work through the threats from yesterday's practice test and assess your mental process in solving them.

Action Points:

- Review all incorrect responses in practice test 4
- Assess process for all questions answered incorrect and spot 'Threats'
- Learn tips and strategies to combat 'Threats'
- Practice techniques to fix 'Threats' on the UCAT user interface.
- Repeat the process of taking timed tests and assessing your issues until you reach a level that you are pleased with.

Tips from other top scorers:

- In the QR subtest, examiners can include questions that have large amount of data that would take a few minutes just to read it all and understand it. In such cases, scan through to quickly understand the 'type' of information then read the question. This allows you to quickly determine what you need when you go over the data again.
- In the VR subtest, keep an eye out for key words such as 'may', 'can', 'should' etc that are usually overlooked but can change the validity of a statement.

Day 29

1 Day Left!

Task: Attempt and Review a Practice test under exam conditions (Practice Test 5)

Estimated Time: 3 hours

Study tip: Implement exam and triage strategies to improve accuracy and pace.

Advice from Mike:

Today, we will attempt another full practice test under exam conditions. Please ensure to mimic the testing conditions and ensure you are not disturbed for the entire 2 hours. Implement the newly learned exam and triage strategies to boost both your accuracy and pace in all the sections that you have worked on. During the review, take note of any issues or threats that arise, and we will address them tomorrow.

Action Points:
- Go over your 'game plan' for each subtest
- Attempt practice test under exam conditions
- Mark and Review practice test
- Audit strategies adopted (what works and what doesn't work)
- Identify threats (these are areas that didn't improve despite practice)
- Compare test results to previous mock results on Day 27
- Propose plan to improve

Tips from other top scorers:
- Repeat the process of taking timed mini-tests and assessing your mistakes until you reach your desired score level

- When you have finished a practice test or mini-test, reattempt questions you missed before looking at the answer explanations.
- if you're not thinking about the problems, concepts, and strategies that you're weak in, you're missing out on valuable opportunities to improve your score.

Day 30

Task: Address 'Threats' in Practice Test 5 and Tie up loose Ends.

Estimated Time: 5 hours

Study tip: Remember to adopt a no-mistake-left-behind policy.

Advice from Mike:

The aim for today is to work on the areas that you have identified as 'Threats'. These are areas that you have practised and done as much as you can to improve but efforts seem futile. The key to improving these areas is to assess your current process in solving them and figuring out which element you need to work on to reduce the likelihood of making the same mistake again.

Today, also go over game plan for each subtest and do some practice on areas that you are a little concerned about. When working on game plan have strategies (both exam and triage techniques) for how you are going to attempt each question-type.

Action Points:
- Review all incorrect responses in practice test 5
- Assess process for all questions answered incorrect and spot 'Threats'
- Learn tips and strategies to combat 'Threats'
- Practice techniques to fix 'Threats'. Recommend practising questions on the UCAT user interface.
- Repeat the process of taking timed tests and assessing your issues until you reach a level that you are pleased with.
- Go over performance in all practice tests and mini-tests attempted to date.
- Work on Game plan.

Tips from other top scorers:
- During QR practice, if a topic can use multiple solving methods for its

problems, try all the different ways in order to find the one most comfortable for you.

- Once you've brushed up on the topic, take practice problems in multiples at a time, as if you were truly working on the test. As you solve your practice questions, don't solve questions one at a time and stop to look up the answer after each one. Though you may be tempted to know exactly how well you've done.

UCAT EXAM STRATEGIES

TIPS, TACTICS AND STRATEGIES TO BOOST YOUR PERFORMANCE IN EACH SUBTEST

UCAT Exam Strategies

Introduction

Getting a UCAT score in the top percentile isn't easy. But with hard work and honing the right strategies you'll be able to do it. I've provided over 200 exam strategies in this chapter and links to articles on the blog that provide additional tips which you can access at www.themedicblog.co.uk/my-ucat-study. Unfortunately, it was impossible to include all the exam tips in the book, so I shortlisted the most essential ones for each subtest that would be enough to help you achieve your desired UCAT score. These are the strategies and tactics recommended by myself and other past candidates that scored highly in the exam. I strongly recommend you perfect the ones that help improve your speed and accuracy in answering questions in the exam. It is important to note that each strategy is different, and to help ensure you navigate through them properly I've broken them down into 4 main types, they are as follows:

Type 1: Preparation tactics

These are strategies you can adopt during preparation to improve a skill deemed important for the exam. They are not necessarily tactics you can use in the live test but will provide a solid foundation for honing final techniques used in the exam. For example, I provide advice on experimenting with different reading techniques for the verbal reasoning subtest (strategy #1). This is classified under Type 1, because you will have to work on it during preparation, but it is also a Type 2 (live exam strategy) because once you have found the right technique you can adopt it in the exam. However, there are some strategies that are solely type 1, like my advice on how to set exercises with newspapers to improve speed reading (strategy #32) or how to improve your reading comprehension (Strategy #6).

Type 2: Live Exam Strategies

These are strategies you can adopt in the live test. They may require a bit of practice to master and are great for saving time, improving accuracy or both. For example, the keyword strategy when attempting questions in the verbal reasoning subtest (Strategy #12) or using 'Guesstimation' when rounding or approximating values in the quantitative reasoning subtest (Strategy #142). These Type 2 strategies can also be Type1 where they can also be adopted during preparation, such as how to skim text passages (Strategy #9), which is classified as both Type 1 and Type 2, because you will have to work on it during prep and also adopt it in the exam.

Type 3: Timing Strategies

These are exam strategies to improve your pace or speed in a subtest. For example, my advice on how to scan text (Strategy #10) or using the process of elimination (Strategy #21). There are many time saving strategies recommended in this guide which can be beneficial if you are struggling to complete a subtest within the time allocated

Type 4: Accuracy Strategies

This is another class of exam strategies, primarily focused to improve your accuracy in answering questions in a subtest. For example, my advice on categorising your reaction in the situational judgement subtest (Strategy #202) or using the SCAN method to spot patterns in the abstract reasoning subtest (Strategy #166). There are many accuracy strategies recommended in this guide that can be beneficial if you are struggling to improve error rate.

Complete Breakdown by Type

I strongly advice not to read the exam strategies in order or cover to cover, skip liberally and pick relevant strategies to address issues you've spotted in your performance. To help with this, I have provided a complete breakdown of all the strategies in this guide according to their type.

KEY

Find below a meaning of Icons to give you an idea of what the text is about, this should be used to help find relevant information to help address areas you intend to work on during your UCAT preparation.

For example, if you were looking to improve your pace in the situational judgement subtest you would look for content that included both the timing and situational Judgement icons, for example:

	Icon	Meaning
Verbal Reasoning		Tip, tactic or strategy to improve VR performance.
Quantitative Reasoning		Tip, tactic or strategy to improve QR performance.
Abstract Reasoning		Tip, tactic or strategy to improve AR performance.
Decision Making		Tip, tactic or strategy to improve DM performance.
Situational Judgement		Tip, tactic or strategy to improve STJ performance.
Preparation Strategy		Adopt during preparation
Live Exam Strategy		Adopt in live test

| Timing strategy | ⏱ | Improves pace or speed |
| Accuracy Strategy | 🎯 | Improves accuracy |

	🛠	🖥	🎯	⏱
📖	1, 4, 5, 6 , 7, 9, 10, 11, 12, 13, 14, 15, 16, 17, 18, 19, 20, 21, 22, 23, 24, 25, 26, 27, 28, 29, 30, 31,32, 33, 34, 34, 35, 37, 38, 39, 40, 41, 42, 44, 45, 47, 48, 49	1, 2, 3, 8, 9, 10, 11, 12, 13, 14, 15, 16, 17, 18, 21, 23, 25, 26, 27, 29, 36, 37, 38, 39, 41, 42, 43, 45, 46	4, 5, 6, 7, 11, 13, 14, 15, 17, 18, 19, 20, 21, 26, 27, 36, 43, 45, 49	1, 2, 3, 8, 9, 10, 12, 29, 37, 38, 39, 40, 41, 42, 47, 48
🧩	50, 57, 58, 59, 60, 61, 62,63, 64, 65, 66, 67, 68, 69, 70, 71, 72, 73, 74, 75, 76, 77, 78, 79, 80, 89, 90, 91, 92, 96, 98	51, 53, 54, 55, 56, 57, 58, 59, 61, 63, 66, 69, 71, 72, 73, 74, 75, 76, 77, 81, 82, 83, 84, 85, 86, 87, 88, 91, 93, 94, 95, 97, 99	51, 53, 54, 55, 56, 57, 58, 59, 61, 63, 66, 71, 75, 76, 77, 79	52, 61, 62, 41, 42, 47, 48

⊞ (calculator)	101, 102, 103, 110, 113, 114, 115, 116, 117, 118, 119, 126, 127, 141, 143, 144, 146, 147, 148, 149, 150, 151, 152, 154, 155, 156, 157, 158, 159, 160, 161, 162, 163	100, 104, 105, 106, 107, 108, 109, 110, 116, 117, 118, 119, 120, 121, 122, 123, 124, 125, 128, 129, 130, 131, 132, 133, 134, 135, 136, 137, 138, 139, 140, 142, 145, 153, 154, 160, 161, 162, 163, 164	102, 108, 109, 142, 143, 161	111, 112, 117, 118, 119, 120, 121, 122, 123, 124, 125, 128, 129, 130, 131, 132, 133, 134, 135, 136, 137, 138, 139, 140, 141, 145, 153, 154, 155, 163, 164, 41, 42, 47, 48
🔍 (magnifier)	166, 167, 168, 169, 170, 190	166, 167, 168, 169, 170, 171. 172, 173, 174, 175, 176, 177, 178, 179, 180, 181, 182, 183, 184, 185, 186, 187, 188, 191, 192, 193, 194, 195, 197	166, 167, 168, 169, 170	183, 189, 196, 41, 42, 47, 48
🩺 (stethoscope)	201, 204 206, 207, 208	198, 199, 200, 202, 203, 205, 209, 210	198, 199, 200, 202, 203, 205, 209, 210	41, 42, 46, 47, 48

VERBAL REASONING

TIPS, TACTICS AND STRATEGIES TO IMPROVE YOUR UCAT VERBAL REASONING SCORE

#1. Experiment with Different Reading Strategies and Pick One

There are different strategies for how to read a passage and answer questions in the verbal reasoning subtest. Some candidates read the questions before reading the passage. Others read the passage first. The one you pick should line up with your strengths and weaknesses perfectly, or else you'll make mistakes or run out of time. To do this, **you need cold, hard data from practice.** Try each reading strategy when practising VR questions. If one of them is a clear winner for you, then hone that method further.

Method 1: Skim the Passage, then read the questions

Skim the passage on the first read through. **Don't try to understand every single line**, or write notes predicting what the questions will be. Just get a general understanding of the passage. You want to try to finish skimming the passage in 1 minute, if possible. The goal with this method is that you are trying to map key ideas to where they appear on the text so that you save time later on when scanning the passage to answer questions.

Next, go to the questions. If the question refers to content in a specific paragraph, then go back to where it is located in the paragraph and understand the reading around it. The key to mastering this method is by improving your ability to skim effectively. Skimming (strategy #9) works because questions in the exam will ask about far fewer lines than the passage actually contains. **Therefore, if you spend time trying to deeply understand an entire passage, you'll be wasting time.** By only drawing out information from parts of the passage that are being tested, you guarantee reading efficiency.

You must be able to skim effectively. This means being able to quickly digest a text without having to slowly read every word. If you're not quite good at this yet, practice on newspaper articles and VR practice questions.

There is no universal method to skimming, find what works for you, be creative if you have to, as long as it works. For example, check out the unconventional skimming method recommended by a past candidate that scored 740 in the VR subtest (total score: 3150):

I must reiterate that there is no one-size-fits all, do not shy from tweaking or adding to the proposed methods included in this strategy.

Method 2: Read the question first, then scan the passage

Read the question first and understand what is being asked of you before finding the relevant information in the passage. With this method, you save time by scanning parts of the passage that aren't asked about, only reading the sentences that include the information needed to answer the question. Many past students recommend this method because it saves time to know what you are looking for in the passage.

Make sure when using this technique, you read the question carefully and have a clear understanding of what is being asked – for instance; What kind of information will you need to gather when you read? Will you be looking for facts? Or will you be reading between the lines to come up with your own conclusion?

In addition to skimming effectively, the key to mastering this method is by improving your ability to spot and scan for keywords (strategy #11). This can be a word or phrase – nouns (such as names, countries, places), dates and figures are common examples. It is important to scan for all the appearance of the keyword. If a keyword appears more than once you may have to combine information to determine the correct answer.

strategy works best for you in answering each question-type. In the actual test, I always took a quick glance at the question, if it is was a T/F/C question then I knew the remaining 3 questions associated with the passage will also be T/F/C question-types as the test is set up that way – so I would switch to method 2. If the questions were any other question-type, then I would switch to method 1.

Method 3: Read the passage in detail, then answer questions

Since most people have a reading speed of about 250 words per minute, this method is pretty much impossible to adopt in the real test, as you won't have enough time to read an entire passage in detail. Additionally, you waste time reading parts of the passage that isn't being tested so it is not an efficient reading method. However, this is a good method to adopt during practice to help identify gaps in critical thinking and comprehension when working on accuracy.

Reading a passage in detail should only be reserved for practising questions at your own pace when assessing accuracy. As you prepare for the exam you ideally want to increase your speed and thus shift from Method 3 to either Method 1 or 2 over time

#2. Take note of the length of the Passage

You will be presented with eleven passages in the VR subtest, each associated with 4 questions. Some passages are longer than others, always take a mental note of the length of the passage. This should prompt you to adopt an appropriate reading strategy and skimming method when you are under exam conditions. Test different methods and find what works best for the respective scenarios:

- **Scenario 1:** Short passage with True, False or Can't Tell questions
- **Scenario 2:** Short passage with Multiple-choice questions
- **Scenario 3:** Long passage with True, False or Can't Tell questions
- **Scenario 4:** Long passage with Multiple-choice questions

Short passages are pieces of text with less than 300 words and have 1 paragraph. Long passages are pieces of text with more than 400 words with three or more paragraphs. Also note that the type of question may also influence how you approach reading and skimming the passage.

#3. Take note of the first question of the passage

The VR subtest follows a peculiar structure that can give you a strategic advantage. If the first of four questions is a **True, False or Can't tell question then the remaining 3 questions accompanying the passage are also T/F/C questions**. By spotting this, you are prompted to adopt an appropriate strategy for reading the passage and dealing with T/F/C questions. In cases where the first question is a multiple-choice question, then the accompanying questions can be any of the other question-types, thus prompting you to read the passage more carefully.

#4. Understand the meaning of True, False and Can't Tell (and recognise Examiner Traps)

For some of the questions in the verbal reasoning section you'll be given a statement and asked to decide whether it's TRUE, FALSE or CAN'T TELL. To help tackle these types of questions let's consider what each option means:

TRUE means that the statement is correct based on the passage. There are two main ways a statement can be true, firstly it can be directly stated in the passage. This is simple and easy to find in the passage. Let's consider the excerpt below:

KPMG has grown significantly since its launch in 1987. To date, a huge number of firms in the UK are using KPMG to run their auditing operations.

Statement: KPMG was founded in 1987

The statement is TRUE as it is a direct match since it clearly states in the passage KPMG launched in 1987.

The second way a statement can be true is through inference from the passage. Based on the information the passage you can infer something is true, this is where the line can get blurred between True and Can't Tell. This is more difficult to answer, look at the statement below:

Statement: KPMG are a popular auditing firm in the United Kingdom

Even though the passage above doesn't directly say that KPMG are a popular auditing firm, you can infer from the passage that this is the case since *"a huge number of firms are using KPMG to run their auditing operations"*. Thus, this statement must be true.

FALSE means that the statement contradicts the passage. Again, it may not be explicitly shown to be wrong, but instead you can detect it using inference. There are two main ways a statement can be false. Firstly, through a contradiction, this is a direct mismatch where a statement goes against the passage factually or in terms of general opinion. The other way is when a statement goes beyond the 'premise' of the passage. Let's consider the statement below:

Statement: KPMG is solely an investment management firm

The passage states that KPMG is an auditing firm, so the statement directly contradicts the passage. Therefore, it is False. However, if the statement had been 'KPMG is an investment management firm' - remember that just because a statement is saying something different than the passage, this doesn't necessarily make it a false one. If it doesn't explicitly contradict the passage, it may still be a "Can't Tell" answer.

Statement: KPMG has slowed in growth recently.

The passage states that KPMG has grown significantly since its launch in 1987. The text alone does not give any indication how the firm is doing recently. However, the next sentence, starts with "To date..." which gives some indication on recent developments, so you can infer that KPMG is still growing. So, the statement is false.

CAN'T TELL means you cannot be certain based on the information provided in the passage. The statement you are asked about is simply not given in the passage, or there's no premise for correctly inferring the truth or falsity of the statement. Consider the statement below:

Statement: KPMG is the best auditing firm in United Kingdom.

Even though the paragraph states that a huge number of firms in the UK are using KPMG, it will be too much of a leap to infer that KPMG is the best auditing firm in the UK. So, we Can't Tell as we do not have sufficient information. To determine that the answer is can't tell, you must ensure that the information needed to give a True or False answer is simply not available within the text.

Common Examiner Tricks

The above examples are very simple problems to help explain each concept, and most, if not all, candidates should be able to answer these easily with a bit of practice. In other cases, statements can be more difficult and may require **making inference or drawing on multiple sources of text**. These questions tend to take longer to answer, and usually contain traps. There are two main approaches used by examiners to trick candidates when answering T/F/C questions, they are as follows:

- **Broadening Scope:** This is where they take a statement or keyword from the text and then make it broader in scope than the passage. This is usually to confuse you to pick 'True' or 'False' instead of Can't Tell. For example, the statement KPMG is an investment management firm.
- **Shift in Context**: This is where examiners might use qualifiers to make a subtle change of the context, sometimes by wrongly paraphrasing, to give a different twist or meaning to a statement. For example, the statement: KPMG is the most popular auditing firm in the UK.

By understanding the tricks used by examiners, you can reduce the likelihood of falling victim to them. When reviewing practice try to recognise traps you fell for and think of ways you can avoid falling victim to them in the future.

Common Mistakes to Avoid

Avoiding just a few of the most common mistakes students often make can really help improve your error rate when answering T/F/C questions. Let's go through them one at a time:

Misunderstanding the meaning of each option: One of the main reasons as to why many candidates struggle with this question-type is that they are not fully clear on the meaning of each option. Attempt a lot of T/F/C questions untimed to get your head around the meaning of each answer

option before doing timed practice.

Waste time searching for information that is not provided: Another common mistake is that candidates tend to search for information that is not in the passage. This is usually the case when we can't tell what is the correct answer. Remember, a statement may be slightly off topic and the passage does not provide enough information. Thus, don't spend too long searching for facts that you can't find. The rule of thumb is that if you cannot find the information right away, cut your losses - pick "Can't tell" and move on.

Using External Knowledge: Another common mistake is that candidates tend to use external knowledge to answer questions. Remember, you are only allowed to work with the information in the passage.

Not paying close attention to the text: At times some questions in the verbal reasoning subtest are written in somewhat of a tricky way to catch out candidates that do not pay close attention to detail. For example, statement may involve a very subtle change in wording that will shift the correct answer from true or false to can't tell. Make sure to review how passage adjustments (strategy #18) and, extreme language (strategy #17). can make a difference between right and wrong answers.

#5. Have a strategy for answering each type of Multiple-Choice Question

Unlike True/False/Can't Tell questions, other questions in the VR subtest include four answer options, where students are required to pick one correct answer. These question-types are split into 4 main types, they include: *Incomplete Statements, According to the passage, Except questions and Most likely questions.* During practice, I strongly recommend having an approach to dealing with each one. Here are a few things to consider when working through each type of multiple-choice question:

- Reading strategy

- Skimming
- Scanning for textual evidence / proving (or disproving) answer options
- Elimination strategy (how you eliminate wrong options)
- Guessing strategies (for time-consuming or difficult questions)

#6. Improve Reading Comprehension

Comprehension is the understanding of what a particular text means and the ideas the author is attempting to convey, both textual and subtextual. In order to read any text, your brain must process not only the literal words of the piece, but also their relationship with one another. You must also consider the context behind the words, how subtle language and vocabulary usage can impact emotion and meaning behind the text as well as how the text comes together as a larger, coherent whole. For instance, let's look at the first line from Jane Austen's novel, Pride and Prejudice:

"It is a truth universally acknowledged, that a man in possession of a good fortune, must be in want of a wife."

Now, a completely literal interpretation of the text, just based on word-meaning, would have us believe that 'all rich men want wives.' But the context, word choice, and phrasing of the text actually fails to justify that interpretation. By using the phrases "universally acknowledged" and "must be in want of", the text is conveying a subtle sarcasm to the words. Instead of it being an actual truth that 'rich men want wives,' this one sentence instantly tells us that we're reading about a society preoccupied with marriage, while also implying that the opening statement is something people in that society may believe, but that isn't necessarily true. In just a few short words, Austen conveys several ideas to the reader about one of the main themes of the story, the setting, and what the culture and people are like. And she does so all the while seeming to contradict the literal words of the piece.

Without practice, nuances like these can become lost. As you can see, reading comprehension involves many processes happening in your brain at once, and thus it can be easy for some aspects of a text to get lost in the muddle. But the good news for anyone who struggles is that reading comprehension is a skill just like any other. It can be learned through practice, focus, and diligence.

How to Improve Comprehension: Three Steps

Because reading comprehension is a skill that improves like any other, you can improve your understanding with practice and a game plan. I recommend dedicating yourself to engaging in a combination of both "guided" and "relaxed" reading practice for at least two to three hours a week. Guided practice will involve structure and focused attention, like learning new vocabulary words and testing yourself on them, while relaxed practice will involve merely letting yourself read and enjoy reading without pressure for at least one to two hours a week. Ensure that if you already read for pleasure, add at least one more hour of pleasure-reading per week. By combining reading-for-studying and reading-for-pleasure, you'll be able to improve your reading skill without relegating reading time to the realm of the "UCAT" alone. Reading is a huge part of our daily lives and improving your comprehension should never come at the cost of depriving yourself of the pleasure of the activity. So, what are some of the first steps for improving your reading comprehension level in time for the exam?

Step 1: Understand and re-evaluate how you currently read

Before you can improve your reading comprehension, you must first understand how you're currently reading and what your limitations are. Start by selecting excerpts from different texts with which you are unfamiliar - text books, essays, novels, news reports, or any *kind* of text you feel you particularly struggle to understand - and read them as you would normally. As you read, see if you can notice when your attention, energy, or comprehension of the material begins to flag. If your comprehension or concentration tends to lag after a period of time, start to slowly build up your stamina. For instance, if you continually lose focus at the 20-minute mark every time you read, acknowledge this and push yourself to *slowly* increase that time, rather than trying to sit and concentrate on reading for an hour or two at a stretch. Begin by reading for your maximum amount of focused time (in this case, twenty minutes), then give yourself a break. Next time try for 22 minutes. Once you've mastered that, try for 25 and see if you can still maintain focus. If you can, then try for thirty.

Improvement comes with time, and it'll only cause frustration if you try to rush it all at once. Alternatively, you may find that your issues with reading comprehension have less to do with the time spent reading, than with the

175

source material itself. Perhaps you struggle to comprehend the essential elements of a text, the context of a piece, or textbooks with densely packed information. If this is the case, then be sure to follow the tips in the next page to improve these areas of weakness. Remember, improving your reading comprehension level takes time and practice but understanding where your strengths and weaknesses stand now is the first step towards progress.

Step 2: Improve Your Vocabulary

Reading and comprehension rely on a combination of vocabulary, context, and the interaction of words. So, you must be able to understand each moving piece before you can understand the text as a whole. If you struggle to understand specific vocabulary, it's sometimes possible to pick up meaning through context clues (how the words are used in the sentence or in the passage), but it's always a good idea to look up the definitions of words with which you aren't familiar. As you read, make sure to keep a running list of words you don't readily recognize and make yourself a set of flash cards with the words and their definitions. Dedicate fifteen minutes two or three times a week to quizzing yourself on your vocab flash cards. In order to retain your vocabulary knowledge, you must practice a combination of practiced memorization (like studying your flashcards) and make a point of *using* these new words in your verbal and written communication. Guided vocabulary practice like this will give you access to new words and their meanings as well as allow you to properly retain them.

Step 3: Read for Pleasure

The best way to improve your reading comprehension level is through practice. And the best way to practice is to have fun with it! Make reading a fun activity, at least on occasion, rather than a constant chore. This will motivate you to engage with the text and embrace the activity as part of your daily life (rather than just your study/work life). As you practice and truly engage with your reading material, improvement will come naturally. Consider reading materials that are slightly below your age and grade level (especially if reading is frustrating or difficult for you). This will take pressure off and allow you to relax and enjoy the story. Once you feel more comfortable reading and practicing your comprehension strategies (tips in the next page), go ahead and allow yourself to read at whatever reading or age level you feel like.

Reading Comprehension Tips

Improving your vocabulary and increasing the amount of time you spend reading overall will help you to improve your reading comprehension over time, but what should you do to help comprehend a particular piece of text?

Stop when you get confused and try to summarize what you just read: as you read, let yourself stop whenever you lose focus or feel confused. Just stop. Now, without re-reading, summarize aloud or in your head what you've comprehended so far (before the place where you became confused). Skim back through the text and compare how you've summarized it with what's written on the page. Do you feel you've captured the salient points? Do you feel a little more focused on what's going on now that you've put the material into your own words? Keep reading with your summation in mind and let yourself stop and repeat the process whenever the piece becomes confusing to you. The more you're able to re-contextualize the work in your own words, the better you'll be able to understand it and lock the information in your mind as you keep reading.

If You're struggling, try reading aloud: sometimes, we can form a sort of "mental block" that can halt our reading progress for whatever reason (maybe the sentence looks complex or awkward, maybe you're tired, maybe you feel intimidated by the word choice, or are simply bored). Reading these problematic passages aloud can often help circumvent that block and help you to form a visual of what the text is trying to convey.

Re-read (or Skim) previous sections of the text: for the most part, reading is a personal activity that happens entirely in your head. So, don't feel you have to read just like anyone else if "typical" methods don't work for you. Sometimes it can make the most sense to read (or re-read) a text out of order. It is often helpful to glance backwards through a piece of text (or even re-read large sections) to remind yourself of any information you need and have forgotten - what happened previously, what a particular word means, who a person was...the list is endless. Previous sentences, sections, or even whole chapters can provide helpful context clues. Re-reading these passages will help to refresh your memory so that you can better understand and interpret later sections of the text.

Discuss the text with a Friend (or Imaginary friend): Sometimes discussing what you read can help clear up any confusion. If you have a friend who hasn't read the text in question, then explain it to them in your own words, and discuss where you feel your comprehension is lacking. You'll find that you've probably understood more than you think once you've been forced to explain it to someone who's completely unfamiliar with the piece. Even if no one else is in the room, trying to teach or discuss what a passage says or means with "someone else" can be extremely beneficial.

#7. Work on ability to read and think critically (Aim, tone & summary)

Critical thinking requires approaching texts with a critical eye: evaluating what you read for not just what it says, but how and why it says it. This is central to dealing with inference question and questions centered on an author's opinion and tone. For example, questions in the exam like *which of the following will the author most likely agree with, which of the following can be inferred from the passage* or *which of the following can be deduced from the passage*. Being a critical reader means exercising your judgement about what you are reading – that is, **not taking what you read at face value.**

Critical thinking means being able to reflect on what a text says, what it describes and what it means by scrutinising the style and structure of the writing, language used as well as the content. When reading a passage to answer inference or author-based questions your ability to read and think critically comes into play.

How to Improve Critical Thinking: Four Steps

Step1: Evaluate your thinking process and work on it - It is vital that you evaluate how you read as well as how you take in what you read – and make judgements about how to improve, and when it comes to reading develop a mindset where you don't just accept everything as if it were absolute truth. Your judgements should include whether the claims are reasonable, whether the evidence is strong, whether the conclusions are sound, whether the ideas can be applied in the real-world, and so on.

Step 2: Engage with text or reading material - Read with a pen or pencil, highlighting key statements, parts, or points – even those you find confusing. Also, make note of words or terms you don't understand so you can look them up later. Write down your reactions to the text while you read. It is important to record not just what the author said, but also what you think about it. As you read, ask yourself questions about the text, such as what is the main thesis? What is the supporting evidence? What are the counterpoints? What's the authors opinion?

Step 3: Practice explaining both 'What the text says" and "what it does" - in other words, practise summarising and recognising the aim of each paragraph in a passage, seek to also understand the purpose of each sentence within a paragraph. Over time this will help build on your ability to solve complex author-based questions in the exam.

Step 4: Practice Reading between the lines - reading a text critically requires that you ask questions about the writer's authority and agenda. You may need to put yourself in the author's shoes and recognize that those shoes fit a certain way of thinking. Practice determining and understanding an author's context, purpose, and intended audience when reading.

#8. Develop an eye for spotting time-consuming questions

Some questions in the VR subtest are longer to answer than others, by recognising these time-consuming questions early (before you even try to solve them) you can adopt appropriate strategies to increase your chances of finishing the subtest on time. For example, questions that use phrases like *"which of the following can be inferred"*, *"which of the following can be deduced"* or *"which of the following will the author most likely agree/disagree with"* tend to take longer to answer, this should prompt you to deploy triage. For example, you may want to flag and skip these questions an come back to them later. Here are a few things to consider when deploying triage:

- Type of question
- Strengths and weaknesses identified in the VR subtest
- Number of questions left in subtest
- Amount of time left

- Level of understanding of text in passage

#9. Experiment Skimming Methods and Pick the most appropriate

Skimming should not to be confused with scanning (strategy #10). It involves discovering the main ideas of a text, whilst scanning on the other hand is searching for important words, facts or phrases to find specific information. In my opinion, skimming is one of the most important skills to develop when preparing for the UCAT. It goes hand-in-hand with developing your reading strategy (strategy #1) for the exam. Every person processes information differently, so you have to figure this out on your own through testing. If your current approach isn't working, you might want to consider switching it up. The most suitable skimming method is one that decreases **regression** (the number of times that you go over what you have read in the passage) and increases **retention** (ability to recall and remember the main points of each paragraph).

Common Misconceptions with Skimming

There is some confusion as to what skimming is and when to use it. Before we dive into how to skim, I would like to address some of the common misconceptions with skimming.

Misconception #1: Skimming is reading every word fast

A lot of students think skimming means reading every text in a passage quickly. This is a serious misunderstanding, when you read every word of a passage you take up too much time and memory space focused on unimportant parts of the passage. This is extremely dangerous when one assigns too much attention to trivial details and forgets about the key points. At worse, we glance over details and forget what we just read – we obviously want to avoid this. When skimming our goal is to read fewer words but get more meaning.

Misconception #2: Skimming to search for keywords

Skimming should never be carried out to find words in a paragraph. Instead, **draw out the main idea within the text.** There are one of four things you want to accomplish when skimming, they include:

Purpose: what is the point of the passage? Is it meant to argue a point? Explain a concept? Compare two conflicting viewpoints? Or analyse a course of action. In other words, you want to understand what the passage does.

Main Idea: what is the passage about? What is each paragraph about? We want to capture the main focus of each paragraph and overall passage.

Structure: how is the passage structured? Does it lay out an argument to start then present a counterpoint before rebutting that counterpoint. Or does it start with background information on a trend, then dig into it by providing historical examples before finally projecting trend into the future. Basically, find the purpose of each paragraph within a passage.

Tone: how does the author feel about the main idea? Does the author feel anything? Sometimes the answer is no. If it's yes, how do they feel? Is it positive or negative? Are they excited or cautiously optimistic? Are they not in favour or hesitant? This can apply to people in the passage as well.

How to Skim: Two Key Rules

Getting the essence from a passage without reading all the words boils down to practice and adopting a couple key rules:

Rule #1: Read ONLY Important Sentences

There are certain sentences in the passage that we know will be relevant to the purpose, main idea, organisation and tone of a passage. These major sentences include the **first sentence of a paragraph, the last sentence of a paragraph** and **sentences with extreme transition words**. When you skim, it is good idea to read the first sentence in each paragraph properly as it usually describes what follows. Every passage is different, so it may be appropriate to also read the last sentence of a paragraph. The final sentence usually concludes or summarises what was covered and may prove to give more context to the main idea of the passage. If you see transition words such as 'However', 'Therefore', 'In contrast', 'As a result', 'But',' Should', 'Must', 'Since' etc, it is worth giving the whole sentence a read as well. On the other hand, sentences with 'For instance", 'For example' or 'such as' should be skipped. These important sentences should provide a solid framework to build your skimming strategy for the UCAT verbal reasoning

181

subtest.

Rule #2: Interpret as you go

Take a second at the end of each paragraph to summarise what you've read in a few words. What did it say? What role does it serve in the passage? If you have long paragraphs, it might be a good idea to take a pause at each transition word. What is the part before the transition word compared to after the transition word? Incorporate that shift into your summary. This is a great time to think about purpose, main idea and tone of the passage. Interpreting as you go will help you stay engaged and help with retention.

If while skimming, you feel you are grasping the main ideas, then you are skimming correctly. If you are unable to recognise the main idea, tone or structure of the passage then you are not skimming effectively. Always have a goal each time you attempt to skim the passage and assess afterwards if you have achieved it.

Methods of Skimming

I strongly recommend trying each skimming method below and picking the one that works the best for you under timed conditions. You may find yourself using one method to answer a specific question-type and another method for another. Do not shy from combining methods and creating your own unique approach. Try to find which approach works best for the respective scenarios:

- **Scenario 1:** Short passage with True, False or Can't Tell questions
- **Scenario 2:** Short passage with Multiple-choice questions
- **Scenario 3:** Long passage with True, False or Can't Tell questions
- **Scenario 4:** Long passage with Multiple-choice questions

Method #1: Read First Sentences ONLY

The introductory sentence of each paragraph usually describes what follows in the paragraph. When skimming, read only the first sentence in each paragraph and take a second to interpret it as you go. Think about the main idea and purpose of each paragraph as well as the structure of the overall passage. See the image below highlighting the only parts of the passage a candidate would read using this method:

Most educated people of the eighteenth century, such as the Founding Fathers, subscribed to Natural Rights Theory, the idea that every human being has a considerable number of innate rights, simply by virtue of being a human person. When the US Constitution was sent to the states for ratification, many at that time felt that the federal government outlined by the Constitution would be too strong, and that rights of individual citizens against the government had to be clarified. This led to the Bill of Rights, the first ten amendments, which were ratified at the same time as the Constitution. The first eight of these amendments list specific rights of citizens. Some leaders feared that listing some rights could be interpreted to mean that citizens didn't have other, unlisted rights. Toward this end, James Madison and others produced the Ninth Amendment, which states: the fact that certain rights are listed in the Constitution shall not be construed to imply that other rights of the people are denied.

Constitutional traditionalists interpret the Ninth Amendment as a rule for reading the rest of the constitution. They would argue that "Ninth Amendment rights" are a misconceived notion: the amendment does not, by itself, create federally enforceable rights. In particular, this strict reasoning would be opposed to the creation of any new rights based on the amendment. Rather, according to this view, the amendment merely protects those rights that citizens already have, whether they are explicitly listed in the Constitution or simply implicit in people's lives and in American tradition.

More liberal interpreters of the US Constitution have a much more expansive view of the Ninth Amendment. In their view, the Ninth Amendment guarantees to American citizens a vast universe of potential rights, some of which we have enjoyed for two centuries, and others that the Founding Fathers could not possibly have conceived. These scholars point out that some rights, such as voting rights of women or minorities, were not necessarily viewed as rights by the majority of citizens in late eighteenth century America but are taken as fundamental and unquestionable in modern America. While those rights cited are protected specifically by other amendments and laws, the argument asserts that other unlisted right also could evolve from unthinkable to perfectly acceptable, and the Ninth Amendment would protect these as-yet-undefined rights.

***Skimming Method 1:** Read first sentences ONLY*

Method #2: Read First and Last Paragraphs ONLY

Most educated people of the eighteenth century, such as the Founding Fathers, subscribed to Natural Rights Theory, the idea that every human being has a considerable number of innate rights, simply by virtue of being a human person. When the US Constitution was sent to the states for ratification, many at that time felt that the federal government outlined by the Constitution would be too strong, and that rights of individual citizens against the government had to be clarified. This led to the Bill of Rights, the first ten amendments, which were ratified at the same time as the Constitution. The first eight of these amendments list specific rights of citizens. Some leaders feared that listing some rights could be interpreted to mean that citizens didn't have other, unlisted rights. Toward this end, James Madison and others produced the Ninth Amendment, which states: the fact that certain rights are listed in the Constitution shall not be construed to imply that other rights of the people are denied.

Constitutional traditionalists interpret the Ninth Amendment as a rule for reading the rest of the constitution. They would argue that "Ninth Amendment rights" are a misconceived notion: the amendment does not, by itself, create federally enforceable rights. In particular, this strict reasoning would be opposed to the creation of any new rights based on the amendment. Rather, according to this view, the amendment merely protects those rights that citizens already have, whether they are explicitly listed in the Constitution or simply implicit in people's lives and in American tradition.

More liberal interpreters of the US Constitution have a much more expansive view of the Ninth Amendment. In their view, the Ninth Amendment guarantees to American citizens a vast universe of potential rights, some of which we have enjoyed for two centuries, and others that the Founding Fathers could not possibly have conceived. These scholars point out that some rights, such as voting rights of women or minorities, were not necessarily viewed as rights by the majority of citizens in late eighteenth century America but are taken as fundamental and unquestionable in modern America. While those rights cited are protected specifically by other amendments and laws, the argument asserts that other unlisted right also could evolve from unthinkable to perfectly acceptable, and the Ninth Amendment would protect these as-yet-undefined rights.

***Skimming Method 2:** Read First and Last Paragraph ONLY*

All passages in the UCAT are organised with an introduction, main body and

183

a conclusion. The introductory paragraph gives context and introduces the main idea of the passage whilst the conclusive paragraph generally summarises what has been said about the main idea. You can therefore get a good idea of the overall content of a passage by reading the first and last paragraphs. For some questions that will be enough to answer them, but if it isn't, you will now have a good idea of the content and will find it easier to read in detail.

Feedback from top scorer: Method 2 worked really well for small passages (3 paragraphs or less) with multiple-choice questions (i.e. Most likely questions, Except questions, According to the passage and Incomplete statements). If I didn't know the answer to a question, I assumed the information required to answer it was in the main body (2nd paragraph).

Method #3: Advanced Pseudo-Skimming

Most educated people of the eighteenth century, such as the Founding Fathers, subscribed to Natural Rights Theory, the idea that every human being has a considerable number of innate rights, simply by virtue of being a human person. When the US Constitution was sent to the states for ratification, many at that time felt that the federal government outlined by the Constitution would be too strong, and that rights of individual citizens against the government had to be clarified. This led to the Bill of Rights, the first ten amendments, which were ratified at the same time as the Constitution. The first eight of these amendments list specific rights of citizens. Some leaders feared that listing some rights could be interpreted to mean that citizens didn't have other, unlisted rights. Toward this end, James Madison and others produced the Ninth Amendment, which states: the fact that certain rights are listed in the Constitution shall not be construed to imply that other rights of the people are denied.

Constitutional traditionalists interpret the Ninth Amendment as a rule for reading the rest of the constitution. They would argue that "Ninth Amendment rights" are a misconceived notion: the amendment does not, by itself, create federally enforceable rights. In particular, this strict reasoning would be opposed to the creation of any new rights based on the amendment. Rather, according to this view, the amendment merely protects those rights that citizens already have, whether they are explicitly listed in the Constitution or simply implicit in people's lives and in American tradition.

More liberal interpreters of the US Constitution have a much more expansive view of the Ninth Amendment. In their view, the Ninth Amendment guarantees to American citizens a vast universe of potential rights, some of which we have enjoyed for two centuries, and others that the Founding Fathers could not possibly have conceived. These scholars point out that some rights, such as voting rights of women or minorities, were not necessarily viewed as rights by the majority of citizens in late eighteenth century America but are taken as fundamental and unquestionable in modern America. While those rights cited are protected specifically by other amendments and laws, the argument asserts that other unlisted right also could evolve from unthinkable to perfectly acceptable, and the Ninth Amendment would protect these as-yet-undefined rights.

Skimming Method 3: *Advanced Pseudo-Skimming*

Advanced Pseudo-skimming is where you read only the first and last paragraphs, as well as the first sentence of all the paragraphs in the main body. The idea is that you put a little time upfront reading the passage but will save time overall answering the set of four questions related to the passage, because you will be able to quickly refer to relevant sections for each question. This method is essentially combining skimming method 1 and 2. Pseudo-skimming works really well if you can increase your reading speed. You can build on this method by also reading the last sentences of each paragraph in the main body, this should give more context in most cases.

Advice from top scorer: Method 3 worked really well for long passages (4 paragraphs and more) with multiple-choice questions. I realised that spending a little bit of time reading the passage meant I could answer the corresponding questions quicker

Method #4: Transition Skimming

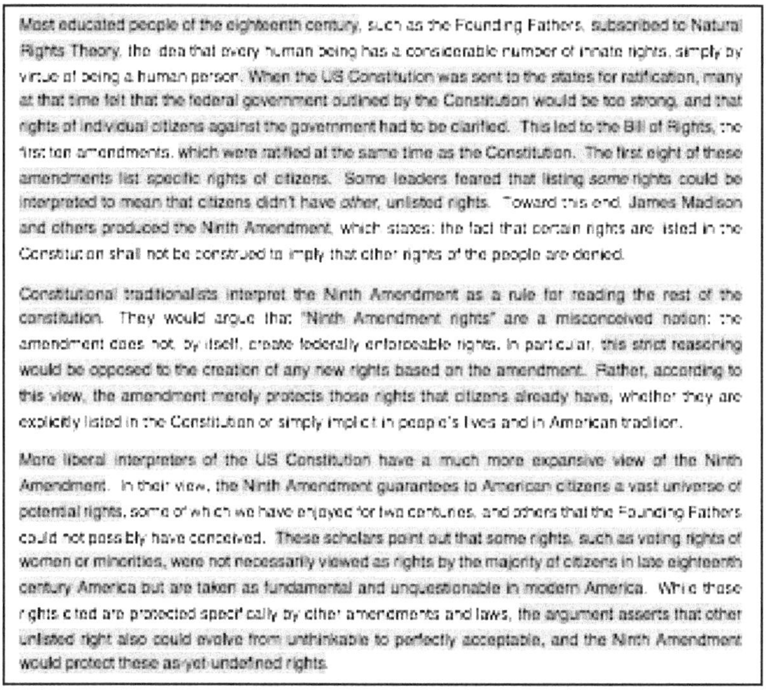

Most educated people of the eighteenth century, such as the Founding Fathers, subscribed to Natural Rights Theory, the idea that every human being has a considerable number of innate rights, simply by virtue of being a human person. When the US Constitution was sent to the states for ratification, many at that time felt that the federal government outlined by the Constitution would be too strong, and that rights of individual citizens against the government had to be clarified. This led to the Bill of Rights, the first ten amendments, which were ratified at the same time as the Constitution. The first eight of these amendments list specific rights of citizens. Some leaders feared that listing some rights could be interpreted to mean that citizens didn't have other, unlisted rights. Toward this end, James Madison and others produced the Ninth Amendment, which states: the fact that certain rights are listed in the Constitution shall not be construed to imply that other rights of the people are denied.

Constitutional traditionalists interpret the Ninth Amendment as a rule for reading the rest of the constitution. They would argue that "Ninth Amendment rights" are a misconceived notion: the amendment does not, by itself, create federally enforceable rights. In particular, this strict reasoning would be opposed to the creation of any new rights based on the amendment. Rather, according to this view, the amendment merely protects those rights that citizens already have, whether they are explicitly listed in the Constitution or simply implicit in people's lives and in American tradition.

More liberal interpreters of the US Constitution have a much more expansive view of the Ninth Amendment. In their view, the Ninth Amendment guarantees to American citizens a vast universe of potential rights, some of which we have enjoyed for two centuries, and others that the Founding Fathers could not possibly have conceived. These scholars point out that some rights, such as voting rights of women or minorities, were not necessarily viewed as rights by the majority of citizens in late eighteenth century America but are taken as fundamental and unquestionable in modern America. While those rights cited are protected specifically by other amendments and laws, the argument asserts that other unlisted right also could evolve from unthinkable to perfectly acceptable, and the Ninth Amendment would protect these as-yet-undefined rights.

Skimming Method 4: *Transition Skimming*

This skimming method takes a lot of practice, it is where you read only major sentences by recognising transition words and using a bit of common sense. The goal is to **skip sentences that elaborate on the preceding sentence**. A good starting point is to skip sentences that start with transition words like

'For instance", 'For example' or 'Such as'. You only want to pull out the main idea not the finer points within it. Make sure to take a second at the end of each paragraph to summarise what you've read. This technique is really good if you have good retention, i.e. are able to remember what you've read later on, as you'll be taking in more information from the passage than any other skimming method.

If you are new to skimming, I would recommend starting with method 1 then building yourself up to method 4. For worked through examples of each method of skimming visit www.themedicblog.co.uk/ucat-skimming-method. Try each one during practice and pick the one that works best under timed conditions. You may find yourself using a method to answer a specific question-type.

#10. Experiment Scanning Methods and Pick the most appropriate

Scanning goes hand-in-hand with skimming and reading in detail. Don't be afraid to go ahead and peek at the question before reading a passage. The question might indicate relevant keywords, ideas, or phrases that you will encounter. First, skim the passage to get a bird's-eye-view of the main idea in each paragraph. Read the question properly then go back and scan the passage to identify the information or keywords. When scanning, **don't read every word, you are only looking for the location of the text within the passage**. Pay attention to important information in the form of dates, places, names, and technical terms. Once you find the keyword read the referenced line or paragraph, whichever is appropriate. Finally, return to the question and pick your answer based on the details gathered from the piece of text.

Unlike skimming, when scanning, you are looking only for a specific piece of information without really digesting the text - **your level of comprehension should be kept as minimal as possible to save time**. For scanning to be effective, you need to combine it with your reading and skimming strategy. Thus, effectively mapping out the passage in terms of how it is laid out and overall structure. If the referenced sentence confuses you, reread it and the adjacent sentences to fully absorb the information to the fullest extent.

How to Scan: Five Key Rules

Rule #1 establish a goal

This would be a keyword, idea or phrase you are searching for within the passage. Sometimes when eliminating options or picking the final answer, you may want to refer back to the passage and scan for phrases or words that prove or disprove an option.

Rule #2 look don't read

Scanning is not Skimming, don't read the words or sentences – just look. Only read when you find the relevant information to help answer a question. Keep your level of comprehension as minimal as possible when looking through words and sentences.

Rule #3. keep your eyes moving quickly

Keep thinking about the words or phrases you are looking for and keep your eyes moving quickly. If you don't do it quickly then you are not really scanning, and probably stopping to read the other words. Avoid this at all cost!

Rule #4: if you don't find the Keyword don't Panic

If you don't find it first time, try again. There is always a chance examiners are trying to trick you by using a different alternative to the phrase used in the passage (e.g. residential properties instead of home, vehicle instead of car, etc), or maybe introduce a topic not covered in the text. This is common, these questions will require to think more about context or potentially choose the "Can't Tell' option as they are not in the passage.

Rule #5: reduce Subvocalization and Fixation

The smaller the number of words being subvocalized (i.e. saying words in your head or out loud while reading), the faster scanning will become. Also, reduce to number of fixations on irrelevant texts, i.e. stopping and focusing on text without the keyword.

Common mistakes to avoid when scanning text

Mistake #1: skimming and scanning at the same time -This is where you are reading the text as you try to find a keyword or phrase, this is detrimental as it can waste time, students tend to not comprehend what their reading well enough if they do not find the keyword. Focus on one task at a time –

when you are skimming do not scan, and when you are scanning do not read the text until you find the relevant keywords or phrase.

Mistake #2: not checking other mentions of the keyword

It is common for students once they find a keyword not to double check it's not mentioned in other parts of the passage. Always double check the remainder of the passage as you may need to combine information from separate parts to make a decision.

Mistake #3: not reading surrounding sentences for more context

Once you find the keyword or phrase you are looking for, don't only read the referenced line. As a minimum, read the line preceding it as well as the line after to get more context. If that is not enough to make a decision, it may be appropriate to read or skim the entire paragraph.

Scanning Methods:

Method #1: eye movement

This is the standard method for scanning the text. When we scan text, our eyes move in quick jerky movements called saccades. This rapid eye movement allows us to move quickly though the text. It might not seem like it, but scanning requires concentration and can be surprisingly tiring. You may have to practice at not allowing your attention to wander or fixate on irrelevant text. If you find yourself in a position where this is difficult then consider one of the other methods of scanning

Method #2: reverse eye movement

This is the same as method 1, but instead of moving through the text from left-to-right as you do when you read a text. You scan the text backwards from right-to-left. This forces you not to read the passage. It is a great method to reduce subvocalization and fixation.

Method #3: finger or pointer method

Learning to use your finger or the mouse pointer in the exam as a visual aid to scan the passages can be helpful when dealing with challenging material. This reduces the likelihood of reading and fixations as well - therefore, increasing overall scanning speed. Keep your eye fixated above the tip of your finger or pointer. It serves as a pacer to help maintain consistent speed. If you prefer using your finger go for it, the UCAT is computer-based so holding your finger against the screen might seem a bit weird at first but could prove beneficial.

#11. Scan for Textual Evidence more Effectively

Always back up your decision with evidence direct from the passage. When eliminating options or picking the right answer, refer back to words or phrases in the passage that justify your decision. This way, you know you're basing your answer on the information provided in the passage, rather than on your own assumptions. If that is not enough to make a decision, it may be appropriate to read/skim the entire paragraph. In cases where you cannot identify exactly where in the passage you found evidence for your decision; it is likely you are making an assumption.

#12. Master the Keyword Method

The Keyword method builds on the scanning method (strategy #10), where instead of starting at the passage, you first read the question and choose a keyword to scan for in the text.

Step 1: read the question and pick a Keyword

Pick a keyword from the statement or question. This keyword will help you find the information you are looking for in the passage.

Step 2: scan passage for the Keyword and carefully read the relevant sentence(s)

Scan for the keyword in the passage. When you find it, read/skim the surrounding sentences, i.e. the sentences before and after the keyword sentence. This small section of text should contain the answer. If necessary, read more sentences in the paragraph until you solve the problem.

Step 3: pick an option

Eliminate the wrong answers and select the correct one. There may be cases where you cannot find the keyword in the passage, in that case I would recommend quickly looking again in case you've missed it, also consider synonyms (e.g. 'holiday' may be found as 'trip' or 'vacation').

Choosing a Good Keyword: Five Key Rules

Rule 1: keyword should be seldom - When picking a keyword make sure it doesn't appear too many times in the passage, because it will make it difficult to narrow down the information you need to answer the question.

Rule 2: easy to find by Visual Inspection - Make sure to pick keywords that are easy to find by visual inspection – Dates, numbers, names and places make very good keywords.

Rule 3: consider alternative keywords – Keywords do not necessarily have to be a 'word'. It can instead be a 'phrase', or 'made up' from the idea or concept presented in the question. You can choose a different keyword if the first one isn't working.

Rule 4: consider Keywords in Answer Options - For some questions in the VR subtest it may be more appropriate to search for keywords from the answer options to help eliminate wrong answers and pick the correct one.

Rule 5: Gauge the topic of the passage before carrying out the keyword method – This could help when choosing a relevant keyword. For example, imagine you had a passage about the rise of hip-hop music as the most popular genre of music. Each paragraph discussed the different eras, such as 80's, 90's and most popular songs in the last decade. Your Question: *"Conscious rap in hip-hop is becoming more popular in recent years" True, False or Can't Tell?* In this scenario, a good keyword is 'conscious rap', and a weak keyword is 'Hip-hop' as it will be mentioned multiple times in the passage. This shows you the value of gauging the main topic of the passage before carrying out the keyword method.

The quickest way to gauge the passage is by reading the first two lines of the passage. Feel free to adapt your reading strategy (strategy #1) or skimming method (strategy #9) accordingly to improve the keyword method.

Keywords Appearing Multiple times

When you find the keyword, carefully read the sentences around it. If you find a reference to the question information, then you can be generally satisfied that you have found the right section of text. However, be aware that the keyword may appear again later on in the passage, so do a quick scan to see if there is another reference of the information you are looking for. This is a common mistake many candidates make in the exam, they do not check for this. Always check for multiple appearances of a keyword or information that relates to the keyword.

Keywords that do not appear in the text

Sometimes the keyword will not appear in the passage. In this situation do not panic, as it is common in the exam. You have to assess the text in the passage and decide on your approach appropriately. If you feel that the answer is hidden somewhere, try a different approach to find it: check again if you have rushed your search, it is sometimes worth scanning the passage again for the keyword. Also consider synonyms or rephrasing of the keyword. Alternatively, consider choosing a different keyword from the question. Be aware that the examiners might include questions that are beyond the scope of the text, if you believe this is the case the answer is 'Can't Tell', choose this and move on.

Pros and Cons with the Keyword Method

The Keyword method is great for True/False/Can't Tell questions. However, it can be a waste of time when dealing with *hypothetical questions* (strategy #16) or a poor technique on its own when dealing with multiple-choice question-types (e.g. *According to the passage, Except questions, Incomplete statements and Most Likely questions*) as it may become too time consuming as you may find yourself going back and forth proving or disproving each option. It is more efficient to use it in combination with other techniques (strategy #5).

#13. Perform Mental Recaps when Reading Passages

Due to the time pressure in the exam it is not uncommon for students to instantly forget what they've read in a passage. This problem creates the need to improve one's ability to recall information. One popular method is mental recaps. After reading a paragraph, stop and take a second or so to summarize to yourself what you just read. If you can't remember the main points, you can go back and skim the material again to refresh your memory. Practice this when reading generally and when you get more comfortable, use it when skimming passages under timed conditions.

#14. Predict Answer before Looking at the Answer Options

It's also helpful after reading the passage to answer questions in your own words first before looking at the answer options. That way you'll already have a rough idea of what the answer should be and are less likely to be tricked into choosing an answer that is slightly off. Many students get tripped up by answer choices that are plausible interpretations of information in the text but aren't supported by direct evidence. Don't let that be you! Remember questions in the VR subtest require you to use only information provided in the passage, not any external knowledge you already have. This strategy **works particularly well for incomplete statements**. To answer questions correctly, it's crucial that you turn off your personal biases or opinions and base your understanding completely on the text at hand. Luckily, the *According to the passage* questions are a good reminder to base responses only on the information provided in the passage.

#15. Paraphrase – Simplify Answers in your own words

This strategy is extremely helpful when dealing with multiple-choice questions with long-text options. It involves **simplifying the answer options in your own words to avoid confusion or loss in train of thought.** Long text answers tend to include slight adjustments and potential traps, so stay sharp! Paraphrasing each option consolidates understanding and reduces the likelihood of falling for traps.

#16. Develop an eye for spotting Hypothetical Questions

Examiners might include questions where you have to apply information in the text to solve a hypothetical scenario. These questions usually present a scenario not presented in the passage, thus, strategies such as scanning or the keyword method may prove futile. Rather **you need to understand the premise and apply it.** Although these questions are phrased differently, they can be in any form (i.e. T/F/C or multiple-choice). A common example includes - *If the information in the passage is presumed to be true, which of the following must be true?* This should prompt you to either deploy triage or adopt an appropriate strategy. Remember, strategies such as the keyword method may be a waste of time as information provided in the question may not be present in the text itself. **Although other types of questions may start with the word "if", Hypothetical questions typically start with this word**. During practice develop an eye for spotting them and dealing with them strategically. Things to consider:

- Level of understanding of the premise
- Number of questions left in subtest (when deploying triage)
- Amount of time left in the subtest (when deploying triage)

#17. Evaluate Extreme Language

You must be able to spot and distinguish between extreme and soft claims when reading text in the UCAT verbal reasoning subtest. Your ability to evaluate extreme language is an important skill to develop before test day.

Evaluating extreme language in the UCAT verbal reasoning subtest is all about spotting subtle differences in sentences or phrases. It consists of assessing a wide range of qualifiers that are extreme (i.e. never, always, all, only) or soft words (i.e. closely, nearly, less, fewer) which are often incorporated into text passages, statements or answer options to evaluate candidate's attention to detail to spot subtle differences in meanings or arguments. These qualifiers can be easily overlooked when reading quickly in the exam. Let's first look at how qualifiers are used in the exam before diving into some of the most common examples.

193

How are Qualifiers used in the UCAT?

Qualifiers are words or phrases used to limit or enhance another word's meaning, as well as affect the certainty and specificity of a statement. There are a number of key ways they are used in the UCAT, they are as follows:

Time: This is when words or phrases are used to specify time. For example, 'occasionally', 'sometimes', 'now and again', 'usually', 'always', 'never'.

Necessity: This is when words or phrases are used to specify the state of an event or object being required. For example, 'must', 'should', 'ought', 'required', 'have to'.

Quality: This is when words or phrases are used to specify relative quality. For example, 'best', 'worst', 'finest', 'sharpest', 'heaviest'.

Quantity: This is when qualifiers are used to specify relative quantity or proportion. For example, 'some', 'most', 'all', 'none'.

Possibility: This is when words or phrases are used to specify the possibility of an event. For example, 'could', 'may', 'likely', 'possible', 'probable'.

Common Words used in the UCAT

The table below shows some of the commonly used extreme words in the verbal reasoning subtest and their softer alternatives. For example, the words "May", "Might" and "Could" mean that is possible for an event to take place without any reference to frequency or probability. Consider the statement "Smoking may lead to lung cancer", it suggests that is possible for smoking to cause lung cancer, however it is not definite as opposed to "Smoking will lead to lung cancer". The second statement uses an extreme tone and assumes that the evidence is conclusive. It's very important for the verbal reasoning subtest to be able to spot and distinguish between **extreme claims** (in which the text is asserting that something is unconditionally true) and **softer claims** (where the text is asserting something but recognizing that the claim has limits). These claims can be found in the **passage, question or answer options,** and are easily missed when reading quickly.

Extreme Words	Softer Words
Will	May, Might, Could
All, Every	Many, Most, Some, Majority
None	Few, Minority
Always	Often, Frequently, Commonly, Usually, Sometimes, Repeatedly
Never	Rarely, Infrequently, Seldom
Certainly	Probably, Possibly
Impossible	Unlikely, Improbable, Doubtful

Common Mistakes to Avoid

To help explain some of the most common mistakes to avoid, let's solve some verbal reasoning questions related to the passage below:

Childhood obesity has become an urgent and expensive health problem in Lisbon and the schools have a significant role to play in its mitigation along with partners in the community. Many public and private schools organise sport related events to promote health and well-being of their students. For example, at a Lisbon public school the physical fitness program was established for all students to maintain a level of fitness to reduce the probability of obesity and other related illnesses. Students regularly meet at campus once a week and get involved in a wide range of competitive and leisure activities, organised by the student union. Moreover, at these events, students have the opportunity to socialise, get to know each other or share their experiences.

Mistake #1: Misinterpreting Quantifiers, Qualifiers and Modifiers

This is the most common mistake candidates make when evaluating extreme language. Attempt the problem below:

Most public and private schools in Lisbon organise sport events.

o   True

o   False

o   Can't Tell

If you picked *True*, then you are misinterpreting quantifiers. Quantifiers are qualifiers used to indicate the amount of something. The passage says "Many public and private schools organise sport related events to promote health and well-being of their students" – the use of "Many" suggests a large number but necessarily the majority. Whereas, the statement in the question uses the qualifier "Most" which means the majority. Since no other sentence in the passage gives any indication that an overwhelming majority of schools organise sport events the correct answer is **CAN'T TELL**. There can also be similar confusion with other quantifiers like "few", "fewer", "some", as well as modifiers such as "can", "could" or "might" used in the exam that might shift statement from 'True' or 'False' to 'Can't Tell'.

Mistake #2: Only Searching for Qualifiers in a Statement

Qualifiers are usually incorporated in the statement but can be found in the passage and answer options as well. Be sure to keep an eye out for them at all times as they can shift the meaning of a sentence. Consider the problem below:

According to the passage, which of the following is True?

(A) Childhood obesity has become the most expensive health problem in Lisbon.

(B) Most private schools in Lisbon organise sports related events

(C) Schools have a huge influence over the health and well-being of their students.

(D) Sport events are usually organised once a week at the campus auditorium.

Using the process of elimination, we can deduce the following:

Option A – Childhood obesity has become the most expensive health problem in Lisbon. The passage says, "Childhood obesity has become an urgent and expensive health problem in Lisbon". The answer option uses the extreme word "most", which cannot be concluded from the passage. Therefore, option A is Incorrect.

Option B – Most private schools in Lisbon organise sport related events. The passage says, "Many public and private schools organise sport related events to promote health and well-being of their students". However, it doesn't indicate what proportion of private school organise sport events. Therefore, Option B is incorrect.

Option C – Schools have a huge influence over the health and well-being of their students. The passage says "schools have a significant role to play in its mitigation along with partners in the community" which suggests that schools may have influence over their student's well-being. Therefore, option C is Correct.

Option D – Sport events are usually organised once a week at the campus auditorium. The passage says, "Students regularly meet at campus once a week and get involved in a wide range of competitive and leisure activities, organised by the student union". However, there is no information provided where at the campus events held. Therefore, Option D is Incorrect.

Please note: Options A, B and D are incorrect because we 'Can't Tell' based on the information provided in the passage, not because they are 'False' i.e. contradicts the information in the passage.

Mistake #3: Not Keeping an eye out for subtle claims in the passage

There will be cases where an extreme or soft claim may be used in the passage without it being obvious. In cases like this it is important to **establish the conditions or rules set in the passage before picking an answer.** This can help with solving questions that require you to make inference. Consider the problem below:

Local communities in Lisbon might have some influence on helping childhood obesity

o True

o False

o Can't Tell

If you picked Can't Tell, then you missed a subtle claim in the passage. In the first sentence the text says, "Childhood obesity has become an urgent and expensive health problem in Lisbon and the schools have a significant role to play in its mitigation along with partners in the community". This is subtle, but you can infer that local communities might have a role to play.

The Statement in the question uses soft qualifiers so it not beyond the scope of the passage. Therefore, the statement is **True**.

Golden Rule for Extreme Language

The golden rule when evaluating extreme language is as follows; **soft statements tend to be True whilst extreme statements tend to be False or Can't Tell.** This should be used with caution and students must always find textual evidence to back-up decisions. Unless the passage makes it absolutely clear, a statement with an extreme qualifier is more likely False or Can't Tell.

Soft Phrases	Extreme Phrases
Tend to be True	Tend to be False or Can't Tell
Many, Most, Some, Majority, etc.	Always, Never, None, the best, etc.
"The ozone layer may be depleted in the next century"	"The ozone layer will definitely be depleted in the next century"

#18. Beware of Passage Adjustment

Beware of subtle changes in text that might change the overall meaning of a statement. During practice develop an eye for spotting changes in text. Passage adjustment is a common trap laid by examiners; it involves slightly adjusting the statement to trick readers into picking the wrong answer. This is very common in True/False/Can't tell questions. Consider the passage excerpt and attempt the question below:

> In 2010, FIFA officially announced that the 2018 world cup will be held in Russia. It will be the first world cup held in Eastern Europe, and the 11th time that it has been held in Europe.

Question: FIFA announced the 2018 world cup will be held in Moscow. True, False or Can't Tell?

You might have been tricked and thought it was True. You can see that there is a slight adjustment here where the statement says <u>Moscow</u>. Even though, Moscow is the capital of Russia we cannot say definitely that the world cup will be held there. Therefore, the correct response is Can't Tell. Obviously, it is easy to spot in the above small passage but in the exam, you might miss small details due to the longer text and time pressure.

Examiners might also use broader context where the passage might refer to a specific situation, but the statement may refer to the broader context or vice versa. Consider the excerpt below and the corresponding question:

> The housing bubble affected over half of the U.S states. Housing peaked in early 2006, and started to decline mid 2006 and 2007, and reached new lows in 2012. 2008 saw the biggest housing market crash with over 35% of residential properties reclaimed by the banks.

Question: Over a third of properties were reclaimed by banks. True, False or Can't Tell?

The passage says, "over 35% of residential properties were reclaimed by banks". However, the statement is broad and does not specify which type of property, so it is not definite to assume that all properties were reclaimed by the banks. If the statement said 'over one third of homes were reclaimed by the banks' then we could infer the answer would be True.

Tips for Dealing with Passage Adjustment

Tip #1: Always read both the passage and statement carefully - Once you have scanned the passage and found the keyword. Read the text carefully and compare wording with the statement. If you see the same wording with a slight word change be on the alert and assess problem accordingly.

Tip #2: Avoid using external knowledge - This is a mistake you may be making without realising it. Avoid using pre-existing knowledge not included in the passage. For example, if you picked True for the above problem about the FIFA 2018 world cup in Moscow. Then this might be something you may need to work on.

#19. Recognise the Most Common type of Wrong Answers in the exam

By developing an eye for spotting wrong answers, you reduce the likelihood of falling for them. Let's go over the main types used in the UCAT verbal reasoning subtest and strategies to help spot them!

Type #1: Too Extreme, Extra Information or Slightly Off

Answer options that provide extra details that aren't backed up by the passage. Even one unsupported descriptive word can make an answer incorrect. Sometimes, an answer might contain an extreme language (such as 'none', 'always', 'every time', 'must', 'definitely' etc.) that may shift the context of the statement and make it incorrect. Make sure you look at wording carefully and cross it out if you think it's extreme (unless its explicitly stated in the passage).

Type #2: Opposite or Contradicts

These are answer options that are opposite to what is stated in the passage. Even if you don't know the exact answer to a question, you should be able to tell by assessing context cues and tell if relationships in the passage is reversed. These answer choices can be tricky because if you're reading quickly, you might miss it. That's why it's so important to double check your answers! Always scan for textual evidence in the passage.

Type #3: Vague, Irrelevant or Concept Confusion

Vague and irrelevant answers can be tricky because they prey on one's tendency to overthink the question and twist any choice into a plausible answer. If something seems unrelated to what you've read, it's wrong. Don't doubt yourself! Again, if you're going too fast these can be a problem for you. Never choose an answer just because it contains key words.

Type #4: Plausible Interpretation but illogical

These ones can be tough to eliminate, especially if you're used to viewing literature in the context of standard English GCSE level, where many interpretations are valid. Again, you should only rely on direct evidence to answer questions.

#20. Improve Reading Retention

Retention is the ability to use short term memory to recall information you have just read to answer questions in the exam. There are many ways to improve retention during practice. A great starting point during untimed UCAT practice is to make short bullet point summaries when reading passages before attempting questions. It may seem odd because it's not applicable in the exam. However, this forces your brain to think about the material a lot more. Thus, training the parts of the brain used for short term memory recall. Additionally, you want to gradually cut down what you write whilst still being able to recall finer points in the passage. If you find yourself going back to the passage to answer a question, its fine. Practice until you get better and the number of times you regress reduces. Keep practising until you are able to recall without taking notes. Other strategies to help with retention include mental recap (strategy #13) and reciting (strategy #35).

#21. Master the Process of Elimination

There is no negative marking for incorrect answers in the UCAT, this means you should guess on any question you can't answer, because **you won't be penalised**. However, that doesn't mean that guessing completely randomly is a good idea. You should always use the process of elimination as much as you can to increase your chances of getting the right answer. If you guess randomly on a verbal reasoning question with four choices, your chances of guessing the correct answer is 25%. If you can eliminate one wrong answer, those chances jump to 33%. If you can eliminate two, those chances jump even higher to 50%. This means that even if you can't definitively identify the correct answer, eliminating wrong answers will be a huge help. However, in order to eliminate correctly, you have to first be able to identify which answers are incorrect. You will find yourself more than often in situations where you have skimmed the passage and found the relevant information but still are stuck choosing the answer. No matter how difficult a statement, you can always eliminate one answer choice by thinking about it differently. For example, with True/False/Can't Tell questions: If the statement does not contradict the passage - eliminate false. Then it comes down to either 'True' or 'Can't tell'. Your chance of guessing the right answer is now at 50%. For multiple choice questions: think about what you fully grasp from the passage then try mentally paraphrasing each option in your own words into a simple sentence. At this point, make a quick judgement call and eliminate options that do not fit the same premise or may seem 'extreme' in context. Most of the time, you'll find yourself eliminating options that are subjective and vague. Strategies to help with elimination include evaluating extreme language (strategy #17), True, False or Can't Tell test (strategy #36) and recognising common wrong answers (strategy #19).

#22. Get good at spotting Inference Questions

This builds on spotting hypothetical questions (strategy #16). Some questions in the verbal reasoning subtest tend to include questions that test your ability to logically infer information from the text. These questions closely mimic a specific idea in the text - it is your task to read in between the lines to decide an appropriate conclusion. Unlike direct VR questions, the answer options will not be directly stated in the text, which is why inference questions use wordings like "*inferred from*" or "*deduced from*". I strongly recommend you look out for phrases like this, it will prompt you to realise two things – firstly, the question is **time-consuming** so you might want to deploy triage, and secondly, **direct textual evidence does not exist so going back to the passage for direct evidence is a waste of time.** Thus, ensuring you act appropriately before attempting the question. Depending on the strategy you choose to adopt, you may want to flag and skip these questions and come back to them later (triage) or may be make an educated guess based on what you already know from the passage. Better yet, you may understand the text enough to eliminate answer appropriately. Whatever your tactic, spotting inference questions and adjusting your approach before attempting them can help save valuable time.

#23. Have a strategy for dealing with Threats and Weaknesses

Finding an appropriate strategy to deal with difficult questions takes practice, make sure to drill into the underlying reasons to what's holding you back from answering them correctly and spend additional time improving. It may be due to shortcomings in a specific skill, question format or type. If you find yourself in a position where you are not improving despite putting in loads of effort to improve, then consider guessing strategies (strategy #49) and elimination strategies (strategy #21) to increase probability of selecting the right answer.

#24. Do Additional Practice focussed ONLY on Inference Problems

We earlier touched upon improving your ability to spot inference questions before attempting them (strategy #22) as they tend to be time consuming. When attempting these types of questions, you will be required to make logical deductions from sentences, where you cannot infer too far and make a big assumption. However, this is easier said than done. I strongly recommend spending extra time doing inference reading questions of any type to build on your deductive skills. During practice, try to find gaps in your cognitive process and how you think when drawing inference (strategy #28) – monitor comprehension and repair misunderstanding. Start by doing questions at your own pace and as you start to improve accuracy pick up the pace! Helpful strategies to aid with answering inference questions includes rephrasing to reach a logical conclusion (strategy #26), constructing a mental syllogism (strategy #27) and elimination techniques (strategy #12)

#25. Have a Strategy for Dealing with Writer Questions

Writer questions are verbal questions centred on the author's opinion or the opinion of others in the passage. They can cover anything from basic comprehension such as "According to the author..." to more unclear questions such as "What is tone of the author?" which requires a good understanding of the entire text. Inferences are required to answer broader type of writer questions such as "Which of the following is the author more likely to agree with?" or "The author most likely would not agree with: …". I strongly recommend during practice to review the different type of writer questions in the exam and develop a strategy for answering the different forms. They require you to recognise the writer's opinion(s) quickly and worry only about their view. *Find below a sample game plan from a contributor who took the UCAT 2018:*

Writer Question-Type	Strategy
According to the author…	Keyword Method
Which of the following will author agree/disagree with…?	Textual Evidence, Keyword method & Elimination
What is the tone of the author…	Textual Evidence & Elimination
What is the author's most strongly stated option…	Flag, Guess and come back to it later.

#26. Deduction – Rephrase to Reach a logical Conclusion

This technique is great for answering inference or writer questions based on an overarching opinion. It involves **rephrasing the literal text in the passage from a slightly different angle**, and making a **logical extension**. To help explain this let's look at an easy problem:

> Amazon has become one of the most popular book retailers in the world, having a best-seller on the platform is becoming a dream for many established authors

Question: Amazon is the best book retailer in the world. True, False or Can't Tell?

Thought process: From the excerpt, Amazon is one of the most popular book retailers in the world. The key phrase from this is "one of the most popular". In other words (rephrasing), "Amazon is one of many other book retailers that are popular". Therefore (logical extension), it's <u>possible</u> Amazon could be the best. However, there could be other book retailers that are as popular if not more. Therefore (conclusion), it is too much of a leap to infer it is the best book retailer in the world based on the information in the passage. Answer is Can't Tell.

Rephrase → Logical extension → Conclusion

#27. Deduction – Construct a Mental Syllogism

This is another technique for dealing with inference problems and it is based on **constructing a mental syllogism, from two known premises in the text, but with a third missing. You solve the syllogism by supplying the missing premise, which is the inference**. Thus, this method draws a valid conclusion from multiple premises. For example, imagine a passage in the exam about pets, and you were given the question *"According to the author, it can be inferred that dogs make good pets. True, False or Can't Tell?"*. This is not directly stated in the passage. However, from reading the passage you have deduced two things:

Premise 1: Cats make good pets (directly stated in the text)
Premise 2: Dogs and cats are equally as good as pets (also directly stated in the text)

From these two premises you can construct a mental syllogism, where the goal is to create a conclusion from premises 1 and 2. If *cats make good pets*, AND *dogs and cats are equally good as pets*. Then it follows that *dogs make good pets (inference)*. Answer is True.

#28. Find gaps in Cognitive Process when Drawing Inference

In strategy #24 I recommend spending additional time attempting inference comprehension questions to help improve familiarity and skill. However, it's important that you are pinpointing your strengths and weaknesses when drawing inference. One the best ways to help with this, is by understanding the types of inferences used in the exam. By understanding this, you can effectively pinpoint gaps and improve your cognitive process. There are four main categories of inference used in reading comprehension, they include:

Type	Example	Explanation
Text-connecting	*Jake begged his mother to let him go to the party.*	Realise that the pronouns (such as 'his' and 'him') refer to a noun (Jake) to fully understand a sentence.
Gap-filling	*Rachel dropped the vase. She ran for the dustpan and brush to sweep up the pieces.*	Draw upon life experience and general knowledge, you would have to realise that the vase broke to supply the connection between these sentences.
Syllogistic	*Chickens are mammals. Chickens lay eggs.*	Draws upon 2 premises in the passage to draw a final conclusion, mammals lay eggs.
Over-arching	*Inferences about the theme, main point or tone of a passage or author.*	Create a coherent representation of the whole text, the reader would infer over- arching ideas by drawing on local pieces of information.

#29. Reduce Re-reading as much as Possible

When reading a passage commit to reading sentences or pieces of text only once. Imagine you will not get another chance to read it again. This shift in mindset will force you to concentrate more when skimming and closely reading text. Strategies to help with reducing regression (another name for re-reading) includes passage mapping (strategy #30), improving retention (strategy #20) and keyword diary (strategy #31).

#30. Passage Mapping

Reading comprehension is a multifaceted process that depends on multiple skills, including your ability to make inference. That's probably why, when you Google "How to improve reading comprehension," you're bombarded with a list of articles filled with esoteric verbiage about mental frameworks, remediation and reading attitudes. It's difficult to find concrete tips you can immediately apply for the UCAT. Luckily, there's one technique that's both simple and effective: passage mapping.

It is a visual representation of a passage that shows the main idea surrounded by connected branches of associated topics split according to paragraphs or ideas. In a classic passage map, you'll always find the main idea of the passage, prominently placed in the centre of the map canvas, with all other ideas and keywords arranged around the centre in a radiant structure. See template below:

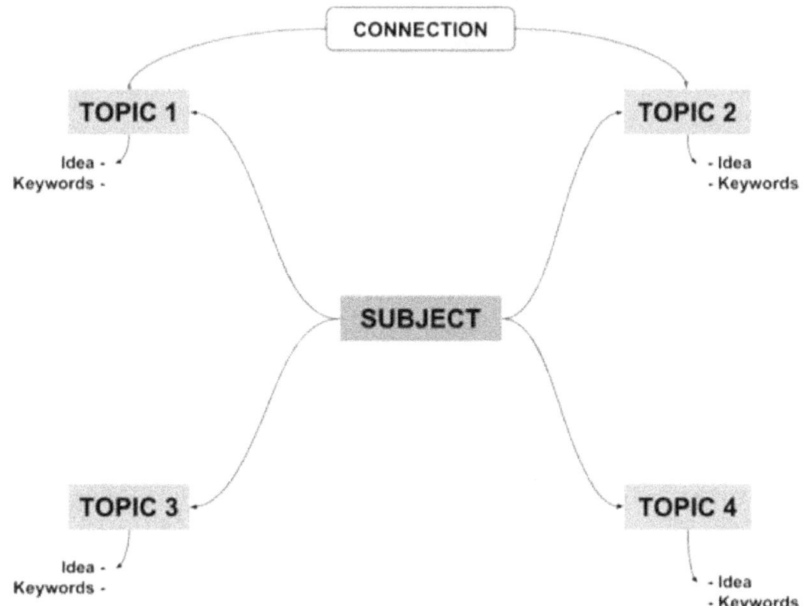

From the above template, we can see the main idea or subject of the passage is placed in the centre, linked to 4 individual topics, with each topic having its own list of keywords and idea. There is also the use of arrows to indicate connections between the topics.

How does Passage Mapping improve Comprehension?

Identifying the main idea of each paragraph is a great skill to develop for the verbal reasoning subtest. Passage maps aid with this and offers a number of benefits that can aid your ability in comprehending and retaining the information read. They are as follows:

- Passage maps help with structuring your thoughts. No matter how complex an idea or text, a passage map helps by forcing you to organise the information.
- Passage mapping provides a clear overview of a topic. It enables you see the bigger picture, find connections and detect hierarchies between individual pieces of information.
- Passage mapping enhances memory by utilising mental recaps. Because they encourage the use of single keywords instead of whole sentences, you are able to review core concepts and ideas at a glance.

How to create a Passage Map

No matter how complex the passage, the steps for creating a passage map are simple:

Step 1: Skim text or passage

Step 2: Write subject or main idea in the centre of canvas

Step 3: Draw branches that point away from the centre. Each branch symbolises one thought or idea related to the subject. Use connectors wherever applicable.

Step 4: From each branch, more ideas can branch off. List meaningful keywords for each branch.

Now that you know how to create a basic passage map, check out a worked through example on the blog, visit www.themedicblog.co.uk/passage-mapping.

#31. Keyword Diary

Regression is when you go back to the passage to re-read a piece of text you have already read. In the UCAT it can't be avoided, however, it **must be kept minimal and used as a last resort**. The main issue with regression is that it is a waste of time, think about it, you're essentially reading text that you've read over again. It's a common reading habit for many students and researchers propose it's a mechanism of laziness, where students rely on the fact that they can go back and re-read at any time, so the brain relaxes and does not concentrate properly. Another cause of regression is doubt in one's skills, where students do not trust that they fully comprehend what they read. Whatever your reason, practice reducing regression, this will not only improve reading concentration, but it will also drastically improve your pace in the exam. A simple and effective technique to help control regression is the Keyword diary method. **Instead of only looking for a specific keyword every time you refer to the passage, simultaneously keep an eye out for other keywords in the passage and write them down**, these are other names, dates, places or key phrases mentioned in the passage - list them according to the paragraphs where they are found in the passage.

Benefits and How to create a Keyword Diary:

You reduce regression by referring straight to this 'diary' instead of re-skimming through the passage to find the target keyword. Depending on your reading strategy (strategy #1) you could create the keyword diary before you attempt questions or whilst you attempt them.

Students that skim or read passage before looking at questions:

Step 1: Count the number of paragraphs and write them down (e.g. paragraph 1 is P1, Paragraph 2 is P2 and so on).

Step 2: Skim the passage and simultaneously write potential keywords you come across in the passage, placing them to the paragraph where they are found. Make sure to only include keywords where you understand the information - commit to reading sentences only once.

Step 3: Read question as normal and pick a keyword. If the keyword is listed in the diary mentally recall what you read and answer the question straight away. Only refer to the passage as a last resort.

Step 4: If target keyword is not included in the diary then its either you missed it, or it's not covered in the passage. Scan the passage again to double check. Save time by using the keyword dairy wherever possible to find *relatable keywords*. For example, let's assume you read a passage about the rise of the internet and you had a question with the keyword 'Spotify', which was not included in the diary. However, you included the keyword 'iTunes' in paragraph 3 of your diary. It is more likely if information about Spotify exists in the passage, it will be in the third passage, since they are both relatable (music streaming services). Rather than scanning the entire passage from the beginning, start scanning from paragraph 3.

Students that read question before skimming passage:

Step 1: Count the number of paragraphs and write them down (e.g. paragraph 1 is P1, Paragraph 2 is P2 and so on).

Step 2: Read question as normal and pick a keyword.

Step 3: Scan the passage for the target keyword and simultaneously write potential keywords you come across in the diary. Don't bother with understanding the information of non-targeted keywords as you don't have time to dive into them.

Step 4: When you find target keyword, read/skim the surrounding sentences, i.e. the sentences before and after the keyword sentence. This small section of text should contain the answer. If necessary, read more sentences in the paragraph until you solve the problem. Commit to reading sentences only once and adding more keywords to diary from the surrounding text.

Step 5: If a keyword in the diary is included in a later question check diary to find where it is located in the passage and scan the located paragraph to answer the question. This is more efficient that scanning the entire passage again.

If you struggle with picking a keyword or remembering what's in the passage, take a moment after each paragraph to do a mental recap of what

For a worked through example using the keyword diary technique visit the blog at www.themedicblog.co.uk/keyword-diary-method.

#32. Read Newspaper – Speed Reading Exercise

A common piece of advice you may have come across when preparing for the UCAT verbal reasoning subtest is to read broadsheet newspapers. I remember reading news articles from various sources like the Economist, BBC news app to the Guardian for several months leading to the exam when I took the test. However, I soon realised that reading widely without a goal in mind was a waste of time. In my opinion, it is far more effective to treat news reading as an exercise to improve skills that you will need in the exam. One of the main challenges in the verbal reasoning subtest is timing. When reading news article consider setting exercises to improve your ability to become proficient at reading large chunks of text quickly. There are many ways to improve this, but here are a few exercises that helped significantly improve my skills:

Exercise – Reduce Subvocalization

When we say the words in our minds, it's called "subvocalization". However, subvocalization doesn't allow us to read faster because we can only go as fast as we speak. The average speaking rate is about 150 words per minute (wpm), while the average reading speed is about 200-300 words per minute. So, to read faster, we need to silence that voice inside. How? Listening to music while reading helps. At first, it will affect your comprehension. But soon you'll notice your concentration increase.

Exercise - Read groups of words

As children we learn to read by joining syllables. Later, we join words to understand sentences, but we often stop there. However, there is another level—absorbing groups of words at once. Here's how to get started: Grab a pencil and divide text into 3 columns, so each of them has 2 to 4 words in a row. Try to read them together jumping from one column to another. It is easier than you think. Once you get the hang of it, you won't need the columns. We are applying the same rule from comprehending words. We don't read every letter, but we recognise the whole word. Now, instead of reading separate words read groups at once.

Exercise - Calculate wpm and track progress
Try to consistently read sections of the same word-count and time your results. Slowly push yourself to get faster. Start with a baseline of how many pages/words you are reading per-minute and set yourself a goal of
 how many words-per-minute (wpm) you would like to reach. For the UCAT a 300 - 400 wpm range is a good level to aim for.

#33. Read Newspaper – Skimming and Scanning Exercise

Set exercises to improve your ability at pulling out the key details of each article, thus this trains your eyes and brain to become more efficient when reading passages or searching for keywords. This can be done by improving your skimming and scanning skills. It is important to note that scanning and skimming are not the same thing (see strategy #9). As you read an article, skim through the text, set questions you want to find answers to. Then scan for the answers to your questions. Focus on what you want to take away from the reading and skip irrelevant information. It is impossible to remember everything you read, so learn to pull out what is relevant to your needs.

#34. Read Newspaper- Critical Reading & Comprehension Exercise

Critical reading involves breaking an article down into its parts, striving to understand how it relates to one another, and examining the role of each sentence or paragraph. For example, you might begin by identifying the conflict and resolution of a story, and then assess what role each paragraph plays. A practical starting point therefore, is to consider anything you read not as fact, but as a plot (or argument) of the writer. A great starting point is the opinion columns of broadsheet newspapers, as they present logical arguments rather than neutral facts. At the end of a few paragraphs in an article, pause and recall what you just read. Write a few key words in the margin. This will help you with comprehension. When doing this also think critically not just descriptively; I used to be a descriptive thinker, I would read an article and pay only attention to 'what' and 'who'. For example, I might read an article on Donald Trump about his rise to presidency and only take away things like 'Hillary Clinton' (who he ran against), 'Republican Party' (what party he ran for), 'Melania' (who is his wife) and '20th January 2017' (his inauguration date). A critical thinker would pay more attention to the author's tone, how they convey information and why they use certain words or sentences. By paying attention to these additional variables, one could potentially deduce whether the author is a Republican or Democrat supporter, which might not be directly stated or described from the text.

#35 Recite without looking

After reading a passage, look away and try to recite the main points of the passage. If you can't recall the information from the passage, look at the text and try again. Take note how many times you viewed the passage and work on actively cutting this number down. This is a good strategy to improve retention

#36. Mental True, False & Can't Tell Test (Elimination Strategy)

A student that scored 3200 in the exam recommended this method of identifying wrong answers. It's a proven method to help eliminate answer options when dealing with multiple choice questions such as According to the passage, Except questions, Incomplete statements and Most Likely questions. The idea is that **as you read each answer option, you ask yourself whether the statement is True, False or Can't Tell.**

True: You are certain answer is correct based on what you remember from the passage.

False: Answer is incorrect and contradicts what you remember from the passage.

Can't Tell: Beyond the scope of the passage OR not sure and may need to review passage again.

In a scenario where you must pick the correct answer option you select the choice that is true, whereas questions that you must pick the INCORRECT answer option (negative questions) you select the choice that is either false or can't tell.

Task	Examples	Aim
Pick CORRECT answer option	<ul><li>According to the passage which of the following is true…</li><li>Which of the following is the author most likely to agree with…..</li></ul>	Select **TRUE** option

Pick INCORRECT Answer option	• According to the passage which of the following is incorrect…., • The following are opinions expressed by the author <u>except</u>… • Which of the following the author is most likely to disagree with… • Which of the following cannot be inferred…	Select **FALSE** or **CAN'T TELL** option

#37. Practice Monitoring Your Time

The first step to improving your ability to finish the verbal reasoning subtest is to keep track of your time. The best ways to do this is by recording **how long you're taking to answer each question-type** and being aware of the **average time you take to complete an entire test** i.e. 44 questions.

Know how long you're taking for each question-type

During practice if you find you're taking too much time on a particular question, mark it and come back to it in review. But what is "too much time?" Well, it depends how you look at it, the VR subtest is made up of 44 questions expected to be completed in 21 minutes, so that would mean you have about 30 seconds per question or about 2 minutes per passage, since the test is made up of 11 passages with 4 accompanying questions. When reviewing a practice test, mark questions or passages you end up spending a long time on. Really break down what stumped you about the question. Was it the wording? The question-type (e.g. most likely, except or inference) ? Were you just tired and misread the passage, so you didn't know the answer? There is always a pattern, find it and fix it.

Know your Average time to complete VR test

The best way to find this out is by doing a full VR test untimed and tracking how long it takes you to complete it at your own pace. You'll need a timer, but my advice is to avoid checking the time until you complete the subtest. It is essential that you treat it like the real UCAT, make sure you are not distracted, do not pause the timer or take any breaks until you complete the subtest. Once you know your average time, begin cutting it down by doing timed VR practice. For example, if it takes you 60 minutes to complete a VR subtest at your own pace, try to shave a little bit of time off the subtest each time you practice. Continue cutting a minute or two until you get down to 21 minutes. If at any point your accuracy drops severely again, pause and practice at that time constraint for a while until the accuracy comes back. Say you manage to get your timing in VR down from 60 minutes to 45 minutes whilst maintaining an 80% accuracy average, but then went down to a 50% average at 40 minutes. Continue to practice at 40 minutes until you've fixed the issues and your accuracy goes back up.

#38. Reduce Subvocalization when Reading

Subvocalization is a very common habit amongst readers. It involves saying words in your head or out loud while reading and it's one of the main reasons why people read slowly and have trouble improving their reading speed. Numerous studies have shown that eliminating this habit completely is not possible. However, minimizing subvocalization will help you boost your reading speed, and it will also help you increase your skimming and close reading speed. Reading isn't even about words, but rather about extracting ideas, absorbing information, and getting details. Words by themselves don't mean much unless they're surrounded by other words. When you read the words "New York City", do you even think of it as three words? Probably not. Many of the words we see are simply there for grammatical purposes (e.g. 'the',' a', 'an' etc). They don't provide you with the same kind of meaning as words like "university". You have to minimize subvocalization in-order to boost our reading speed because it limits how fast we can really read. Think about it this way: if you are saying each word in your head, doesn't that mean that you can only read as fast as you can talk? If you're saying every single word in your head, your limit is going to be your talking speed. The average reading speed is about 150-250 words per minute (wpm) and the average talking speed is exactly the same because most people say words in their head while reading (subvocalization), they tend to read at around the same rate as they talk. You can test this out for yourself if you like. Try reading for one minute normally, and then try reading out loud for one minute. If you're like most people, your reading speed and talking speed will be similar (within 50 words higher or lower). If your reading speed exceeds your talking speed, that's a good thing to notice. For the UCAT, we don't want to be limited to our talking speed.

Changing the habit of subvocalization is easier said than done you can't just turn this voice in your head off. Instead of eliminating this habit, you want to minimize it. For example, let's say you're reading some text that said, "The boy jumped over the fence". To minimize subvocalization, you might just say in your head, "Boy jumped fence," three words rather than six words in that sentence. **Some people think this means skipping words, but you aren't actually skipping them. Your eyes still see all the words. You are simply just saying a few of the words. This is how you minimize subvocalization**. Keep in mind that there are a lot of words in sentences and paragraphs that are not essential to the meaning of that paragraph. We are reading for ideas, not words. Saying words in your head can sometimes be helpful. For example, when you are reading material that has technical terminology or vocabulary that you are not familiar. In situations like this, saying words in your head, or even out loud, can be a useful way to digest complex information.

#39. Reduce Fixation when Reading

Reading is possible through eye movement but there are four different types of eye movement. For instance, there's something call smooth pursuit, which our eyes do when we are tracking a moving subject. There is also vergence when your eyes move closer together to focus on a subject in the middle of your field of vision. There's also vestibular eye movement which is what happens when your eyes are fixed upon a fixed subject, but your head moves, and your eyes compensate for the head movement. But when we read our eyes move in quick jerky movements called saccades.

When we are reading silently to ourselves the average saccades length is about two visual degrees which equates to about eight letters on a page. This takes about 30 milliseconds to do. When your eyes stop and focuses on a text that's called fixation. To understand fixation, you need to understand the three ranges of vision your eyes have. The Foveal which spans about two visual degrees right in the centre of the retina. The Parafoveal which goes about five degrees on either side of any given fixation. Finally, your Peripheral vision which is pretty blurry and can make out shapes and movement, but it can't pick up a whole lot of detail. The foveal, by contrast, picks up detail very well and this is absolutely critical for reading. Most of what you can understand in any given fixation needs to be in that Foveal range. Maybe one or two letters can be in the Parafoveal range but that's it. The average fixation when you're reading silently takes about 225 milliseconds, though it's an average. The range is typically anything from 100 milliseconds to 500 milliseconds.

Furthermore, your reading speed isn't just determined by fixation and saccades. There is also the actual cognitive processing time that you have to go through in order to understand what you just read. When reading passages in the UCAT save time by reducing fixations, a great method is the finger method. It involves using your finger or mouse pointer as a visual aid to read the passages during the exam. This reduces the likelihood of regression, back-skipping and the durations of fixations - therefore, increasing overall reading speed. Keep your eye fixated above the tip of your finger (or pointer). It will serve as a tracker and pacer to help maintain consistent speed and decrease fixation duration.

#40. Speed Reading – Rapid Serial Visual Presentation (RSVP)

I began exploring speed reading during my preparation for the UCAT back in 2015, I am a natural slow reader, so it is no surprise that I found the UCAT verbal reasoning section the most difficult. I dedicated a lot of time working on my speed at reading passages and statements. However, I noticed that it came at the expense of my comprehension and retention of the information I read. Even though I was able to "increase" the speed at which I was reading the passage I noticed when answering questions, I found myself regressing a lot, i.e. re-reading the passage. This obviously wasn't a feasible approach for the exam as I was wasting more time. It was this problem that lead me down the path of speed reading. The RSVP technique is scientifically proven to increase speed reading, it stands for Rapid Serial Visual Presentation (RSVP). In rapid serial visual presentation, words are shown one-by-one in quick succession, rather than being all on the page in a block of text. It's easy to be skeptical that something so simple would have such a big effect on reading speed, but studies have shown that using Rapid Serial Visual Presentation helps increase reader's reading speed because it trains the brain to stop reading out loud inside their head (subvocalization), and suppresses the tendency for eyes to backtrack the line while reading and searching for the end of the sentence.

Technique: During preparation for the UCAT, read articles on an RSVP reader such as Spreeder (www.spreeder.com). Start with small articles (less than 300 words) at 200 words per minute (wpm) or the speed you feel most comfortable and comprehension is roughly 100%. I challenge you to read for pleasure through this tool for a whole week and gradually increase the wpm. Pay attention to your inner voice, work on suppressing it, avoid saying each word after one another. Once you've finished reading a text summarise the text in your own words. Rapid serial visual presentation does have its downsides though. For one, paying attention to text displayed this way can be tiring. Then, there's a thing called "attentional blink," where if the words are presented too quickly together the brain will skip a beat, missing some of the text. However, with enough practice you will be fine. At the time of writing this book I improved my reading speed from 200 words-per-minute (wpm) to 325 wpm. Start at 200 wpm (or the speed you feel comfortable and comprehension is roughly 100%) then work on increasing it, ideally you want to reach at least 300 – 400 wpm for the UCAT.

#41. Have a Flagging Strategy

In the UCAT you can mark questions and come back to them later using the flagging function. It is extremely beneficial because you do not waste time dwelling on questions you find difficult. However, flagging must be done effectively – here are 5 key tips to follow when using the function:

Tip #1: have a preferred method of flagging

There are two ways to flag a question in the UCAT, you can either click on the 'Flag for Review' button on the top right corner of the screen or use the keyboard shortcut 'ALT + F'. When attempting questions on the UCAT platform be sure to pick a preferred flagging method and practice using it so that it comes more natural to you on test day. This will ensure you maintain a steady pace throughout the exam.

Tip #2: know the reason for flagging a question

Be selective on what you flag in the exam. Ideally, you want to only flag questions that you can remember why you marked them in the first place. Some students only flag questions that are completely guesses, others flag questions they feel with a bit more time they could answer correctly. Whatever your approach, try to be consistent so that when you come back to it, you know why it's been flagged in the first place. This allows you pick up from where you left off and dive into the problem quicker.

Tip #3: save time with the 'ALT + V' keyboard shortcut

After completing a subtest, you will be taken to the review screen, if you want to go back and look through only questions you have flagged, you can use the keyboard shortcut 'ALT + V'. This will take you back into the test only showing you questions you've flagged. This function will save you a ton of time in the test, I strongly recommend becoming familiar with it during practice.

Tip #4: Consider using the whiteboard provided

It's a popular approach for students to write down difficult questions on the whiteboard provided in the exam to distinguish between questions you completely guessed and the ones you may need more time on. For instance, questions you have no clue what to answer you could flag and also write on the whiteboard, so that when you review all the questions later you know which ones you completely guessed on and can probably start dealing with them first.

Tip #5: Always put in an Answer

Never flag a question without putting in an answer, even if it is a guess. If you do not get time to come back, at least you will have an answer prepared.

#42. Take Advantage of the Keyboard Shortcuts

Keyboard shortcuts can be used to navigate the verbal reasoning test if you find it preferable. Nevertheless, with limited time, awareness and implementation, keyboard shortcuts can be essential and help save a bit of time. The shortcuts can be used at any time depending on the current screen being viewed. However, they cannot be used to pick your answer, this can only be done with a mouse to select an option. I strongly recommend to **practice adopting shortcuts when attempting questions on the UCAT platform.** You don't have to use all of them, just test each shortcut and pick a few that feel natural and are most helpful in improving overall speed:

Shortcuts on Questions Screen:

ALT + P = Previous Question

ALT + N = Next Question

ALT + F = Flag Question*

ALT + C = Calculator

Shortcuts on Review Page

ALT + V = Review only Flagged Questions

ALT + I = Review Incomplete Questions

ALT + A = Review all questions

ALT + S = Return to Review Screen

ALT + E = End Review

#43. Never use External Knowledge, but Prior Knowledge is fine

As a general rule, **always separate your external knowledge from the information provided in the passage,** and only use the latter to answer questions in the verbal reasoning subtest. However, it is important to realise that prior knowledge, i.e. knowledge obtained solving an earlier question from the same passage, is different from external knowledge. This strategy can be used to make educated guesses on time consuming questions – the idea is that you use prior knowledge gathered from attempting an easier question to guess difficult and time-consuming question-types (such as writer questions, except questions, inference questions, etc.) and move on. With a bit of common sense you can narrow down answer options based on what you already know from the passage. Be careful not to make any assumptions!

#44. Monitor Your Logical Reasoning and fix Misunderstanding

The verbal reasoning subtest measures how well you can extract and work with meaning, information and implications from text. It's all about **logic expressed verbally.** Logic let's you analyse an argument or statement and work out whether it is likely to be correct or not. In the verbal reasoning section, examiners create questions that build on two approaches of logic: deductive reasoning and inductive reasoning.

Deductive reasoning works from the more general to the more specific. Sometimes this is informally called a "top-down" approach. We might understand the main idea or concept in a passage. We then have to narrow that down into more specific hypotheses to solve problems in the exam.

Inductive reasoning works the other way, moving from specific observations to broader generalizations and theories. Informally, we sometimes call this a " bottom-up" approach. In inductive reasoning, we begin with our understanding of specific observations read in the passage, then have to develop a broader conclusion to solve a problem.

During practice try to **recognise which of the two approaches of logical reasoning you struggle with in the exam**. It can help set the foundation to how you go about dealing in logical certainties and answering certain questions in the exam.

#45. Differentiate between Correlation and Causation

It's important to recognise and distinguish between causation and correlation when reading text. <u>Causation is when A causes B</u>, for example: "Since the early 80s, the rise in sugar consumption has led to an increase in the number of reported cases of childhood diabetes", whilst <u>correlation is when A and B have both changed in a certain way, but they could be unrelated</u>. For example: "Since the early 80s, there has been a rise in sugar consumption and rise in reported cases of childhood diabetes". The first example presents the information showing there is a direct link. However, the second statement is more ambiguous, it shows there may be a relationship, but you should be careful not to over-extrapolate. Such reasoning forms the basis of numerous questions in the exam.

#46. Trust your Instincts (Avoid Systematic Approach)

The multiple-choice verbal questions usually take longer to answer because you have to choose between four different statements, thus the need to check whether each statement is true or not. This could take up valuable time. I strongly recommend not to go systematically through all answers if you can avoid it. Read all four options as quick as possible and **select the option that you instinctively think may be the correct answer. Test it against the text. Then proceed to your next best guess.** In other words, never try to validate or prove each statement in order. Start with your gut choice then test it against the text before moving onto the next one.

#47. Build Confidence in Deploying Question Triage

You are going to have to fight the urge of doing verbal reasoning questions in order. Examiners intentionally include a few *time wasters*; these are questions that take far longer than the average time per question to answer properly. Rather than following the usual time limit, spend no more than 15 seconds on them. Make a strategic guess (strategy #49), flag for review and move on. I recommend to **triage question-types that you have recognised take you too long to answer during practice**. Certain question-types can be considered as 'threats', i.e. despite your efforts you don't seem to improve. I would recommend triaging them in the real test. When I took the UCAT I would triage writer inference questions as I was really bad at them. You need to practise for triage and build up your confidence in deploying triage as a test-taking strategy in the exam. During review identify which of the 4 question-types that you found most difficult. Create a triage strategy based on this, here are some example of triage strategies you can adopt, test them and see which one works best for you:

- **Strategy #1:** Skip and come back to passages with long text
- **Strategy #2:** Skip and come back to question-types identified during preparation as threats and weakness
- **Strategy #3:** Skip and come back to questions you cannot answer within 15 seconds.

Please note: *Never skip a question without putting in an answer, even if it is a guess. At the end go back to skipped and guessed questions and refine your answer as necessary*

#48. Have a Timing Contingency Plan

With the tips, techniques and strategies in this guide you should improve both your accuracy and pace in the verbal reasoning subtest. However, have a plan in place to ensure you finish the subtest on time in non-ideal cases. In a scenario where you are behind on questions and have 5 minutes or maybe 15-20 questions left what would you do? Have a plan in place to give you the best possible chance of answering questions correctly. For instance, if you had 5 minutes left to answer 15 questions you could guess the remaining questions by only evaluating extreme language and using the keyword method together, where you are looking for keywords and using extreme language to eliminate answer options if the passage doesn't give obvious hints.

#49. Hone Your Guessing Strategy

When some people hear the word "guess", they think of surrendering. They imagine a frustrated student who simply throws in the towel and picks an answer at random. However, the savvy candidate realises that guessing involves strategy too. Even when you cannot definitively select a correct answer, you can often eliminate several options that are obviously wrong. This approach is guessing done right. While you cannot earn a strong score on the verbal reasoning subtest by selecting answers at random, working the odds by removing wrong responses will boost your score more than you might think. Never resort to blind guessing too quickly when you get frustrated with a question; you'll end up selling yourself short. Here are some helpful guessing strategies for the verbal reasoning test.

Strategy #1: Spotting Extreme language

Spotting extreme language can be used when narrowing down answer options. The golden rule when evaluating extreme language is as follows; **soft statements tend to be True whilst extreme statements tend to be False (or Can't Tell).** For example, consider these two answer options, one states, "Technology <u>may</u> be responsible for the decline in GCSE grades" and another option states "The Internet is <u>solely</u> responsible for the decline in GCSE grades". The first statement uses a softer tone with the use of the qualifier "may", so it is more likely to be the correct answer than the second statement which uses an extreme qualifier "solely" (for more on evaluating extreme language see strategy #17). This approach can also be used when guessing on negative questions where you have to pick the option that is NOT TRUE, in this case you want to pick the option with an extreme qualifier.

Strategy #2: Pick 'Can't Tell' Strategically

The verbal reasoning section is sprinkled with True/False/Can't Tell questions. In situations where you have skimmed the passage and have good understanding of the main idea but cannot decide which of the options to pick, then go with the 'Can't Tell' option. The reason you cannot decide on an answer is probably due to the information not being provided in the passage. If you feel that this is not the case, then consider quickly re-skimming the passage. It is likely you may need to combine multiple pieces of information or make inference from the text. Nonetheless, use context clues (hints or words that the author uses to help define an idea) and a bit of common sense to pick between True or False. Remember, for a statement to be 'True' it must be directly stated or inferred from the passage. For it to be 'False' it must contradict text either directly or indirectly.

Strategy #3: Use Common Sense and 'Prior' Knowledge

Prior knowledge from answering easier questions can be used to make logical deductions when answering more difficult problems. With a bit of common sense you can eliminate answer options based on what you already know from the passage.

Strategy #4: Do an O.L.F.S Evaluation

This is where you evaluate each answer and shortlist the ones that are *objective, logical, factual and/or specific.* More often than not (except when dealing with questions based on an opinion), the correct answer meets at least two of these requirements. When guessing, ask yourself whether the answer is objective? Logical? Factual? and Specific? If it doesn't, check at least two then it is most likely wrong. This can be used as an elimination strategy when guessing.

Strategy #5: Go with your gut (Pick Option that you AGREE with)

In situations where you have a decent understanding of the text, go with your gut! If you find that there's one out of the four options that makes you want to to go back and do close reading, chances are it is the right answer (if it passes the O.L.F.S check).

Strategy #6: Avoid picking vague and/or subjective options

Vague and subjective answer options tend to be incorrect so avoid picking them when guessing.

Strategy #7: Chose longer answer options that pass the O.L.F.S check

This can be applied to multiple-choice questions, where there is a significant difference in the length of the answer options. Longer answer options tend to be correct. So, go with the long answer that seems objective, logical, factual and/or specific.

DECISION MAKING

#50. Logical Puzzles – Develop an eye for Spotting Question-type

The main type of Logical puzzle in the UCAT are "logic grid" puzzles. With this question-type, you are presented with information and are required to work through a set of rules to solve it. They typically include a series of categories, and an equal number of variables. Your goal is to figure out which variables are linked together based on a series of given clues. Information may be given in the form of text, tables or graphs. These questions are usually easy to spot due their **distinct layout that include a list of clues that are listed separately from the main stem**. Another way to recognise logical puzzles in the exam is by the question itself: if *there is a series of variables: like names, places,* etc it is most likely a logical puzzle you are dealing with. I strongly recommend you look out for this, it will prompt you to realise the question might require a complex logic grid so you might want to deploy triage. Thus, ensuring you act appropriately before attempting the question. Depending on the strategy you choose to adopt, you may want to flag and skip these questions and come back to them later (triage), or adopt the appropriate strategy to solve problem. Whatever your tactic, spotting logical puzzles before attempting them can help prompt you to manage time better.

#51. Logical Puzzles - Write or Draw Out the Information

It is very easy to make mistakes when solving a logical puzzle, the best way to reduce this is by writing or drawing out the information. This helps you keep track of matches you have deduced and ensure you are placing things in the right order, thus reducing the likelihood of mistakes. You will be provided a whiteboard and marker on test day make sure to use it to help visualise things. Let us look at an example: *Mrs Suzano has five children: Anthony, Brian, Charlie, Daniel and Erica who are 18, 17,16,15 and 14 (not in this order). Each of the five kids has a distinct favourite colour (blue, green, yellow, orange and red), not necessarily in the same order.*

- *Erica is younger than Anthony, with one of them liking yellow*
- *The 17-year old likes blue and has elder brother, Charlie*

- *The orange lover and Brian are two years apart*
- *Daniel is a year older than the red lover who is in turn a year older than the green lover.*

Question: What is Anthony's favourite colour?

Clue 2 tells us that the child who likes blue is the second oldest. Since there is only one sibling older than the 17-year-old's older brother, Charlie must be none other than the first child. We have:

18	17	16	15	14
Charlie	???	???	???	???
???	Blue	???	???	???

Considering clue 4, there are two possible arrangements:

18	17	16	15	14
Charlie	Daniel	???	???	???
???	Blue	Red	Green	???

Or

18	17	16	15	14
Charlie	???	Daniel	???	???
???	Blue	???	Red	Green

If we take the second possibility, then we realise that the only two possible people who like yellow are Charlie and Daniel, but clue 1 tells us that either Erica or Anthony likes yellow, resulting in a contradiction. Hence only the first arrangement is possible. This means that the child who likes yellow must be the youngest. It cannot be the first child as the first child is Charlie. This means Charlie likes orange as that is the only colour left. We have:

18	17	16	15	14
charlie	Daniel	???	???	???
orange	Blue	Red	Green	Yellow

Clue 3 tells us Brian is the middle child. Since Erica is younger than Anthony, we deduce that Erica is the youngest while Anthony the second youngest. We have:

18	17	16	15	14
charlie	Daniel	Brian	Anthony	Erica
orange	Blue	Red	Green	Yellow

Therefore, Anthony's favourite colour is **Green.**

This was an example of a logical puzzle where you had to complete the grid in order to arrive at the correct answer. In the UCAT, expect problems where you do not have to complete the grid to pick the correct answer. For example, if the question asked us to find Daniel's favourite colour we would have finished the above problem earlier. Also note that the above problem was textual, questions in the UCAT can also be in tabular or graphical format.

#52. Logical Puzzles – Minimise Text Regression as much as you can

For beginners, It is almost impossible to solve a logical puzzle in the exam without regressing (i.e. re-reading the text over and over again) when starting out. However, as you practice more puzzles and become more comfortable with the question-type, commit to going back to the text no more than 5 times. Imagine you will not get another chance to read it again. A helpful technique is to quickly recognise the variables (or categories) on the first skim then draw out information from the second read. When solving the problem only refer to your drawing to solve the puzzle, this shift in mindset will force you to concentrate more when reading text.

#53. Logical Puzzles - Always start drawings with the Sequential Variable

You would have noticed from our example in Strategy #51 that we used the age of the children as the starting point in our deduction. This is because it follows a sequence i.e. 18, 17, 16, 15 and 14. Before drawing out a logical puzzle try to spot the sequential variable and list that out first in order before placing the other variables. Examples of sequential variables include age, months of the year, days of the week and position in a race. During practice, try to identify the sequential variable in a problem before drawing the information. This will help with reaching conclusions quicker and reduce the likelihood of confusion.

#54. Logical Puzzles – Begin with Direct and Straightforward Facts

There will be 1 or 2 of the clues that you can place straight way. Always start from here. I would recommend having this inputted in drawing before looking at the answer options. Sometimes, you may be able to eliminate 1 or 2 options based on this.

#55. Logical Puzzles – Use Known Clues as Reference Points

Always use the clues provided in the question as reference points to deduce and infer other positions in your drawing. With each position you work out refer back to the clues to double check reasoning is valid. Then check answer options to see if there is anything you can eliminate. Typically, with each position, you will find you should be able to eliminate one answer option. Therefore, you only have to fill about 75% of the grid to be able to pick the correct answer. Sometimes 50% is enough to eliminate three options. So do not waste time and only deduce what you need.

#56. Logical Puzzles – Look out for 'Must 'or 'Might 'in the Question

In most cases, you'll be asked *which of the following options MUST be true?* In this instance, you will be given a logical puzzle that you can complete and select the appropriate answer. Please note that you don't need to finish the puzzle in order to eliminate wrong options and pick the correct answer. In other cases, you may be asked *which of the following MIGHT be true?* Where you'll be given a logical puzzle where you are not been given enough clues to complete. In this scenario you must eliminate and pick the appropriate option based on what you can deduce.

> *Which of the following options MUST be true? – Look for Certainty*
> *Which of the following options MIGHT be true? – Look for Possibly*

This is good to spot as it indicates the amount of evidence you need to work out to prove the answer. In cases where you're looking for possibility you do not have to do as much deduction and can pick options quicker than when proving for certainty. Always double check there are no qualifiers in answer options as this might influence meaning. Options with soft qualifiers are more likely to be correct (for more on evaluating extreme language see strategy #17).

#57. Logical Puzzles – Drawing Tables for Sequential Variable Problem

Logical puzzles come in many forms in the Decision-Making subtest, they can be in the form of text, graphs or illustrations where you'll be asked to infer the information provided to solve the puzzle. The table method is a signature technique that can be applied to answering most puzzles in the exam. Let's go through the process of creating one to solve a problem in the exam.

Four Rugby players (Matt, John, Jake and Paul) won 'Player of the month'

at the Hackney Rugby Club in February, March, April and June. Each got a customised colour ball upon winning (from Red, Black, Orange and Green). John won his award two months before Matt (who got an Orange ball)

The Red ball was given first, the green one was given last

Which of the following statements must be True?

> *A.   Jake won the black ball*
>
> *B.   Paul won his award In June*
>
> *C.   The Black ball was won before the Orange one*
>
> *D.   John won his award one month before Jake*

Step 1: Identify and write out the sequential variable in order

The sequential variable is the information that follows a sequence or logical order, in the example that would be the months that the players won (Feb, March, April and June). (For examples of sequential variables see strategy #53).

Feb	**Mar**	**Apr**	**June**

Step 2: Include other variables and Direct facts

Before looking at the answer options input the other variables and facts. Most tables follow the layout below, where you have variable 1 in the first row, variable 2 in the second and variable 3 in the final row. From the question we can deduce the other two variables are the *players names* (Matt, John, Jake and Paul) and the *colour of the balls* (Red, Black, Orange and Green).

235

Feb	Mar	Apr	June	
???	???	???	???	← *Sequential*
???	???	???	???	← *Variable 2*
???	???	???	???	← *Variable 3*

From the direct facts provided in the question the red ball was given first and the green one was given last. We have:

Feb	Mar	Apr	June	
???	???	???	???	← *Months*
???	???	???	???	← *Player*
Red	???	???	Green	← *Colour*

Considering the next clue that John won his award 2 months before Matt (who got the orange ball), there are two possible arrangements:

Feb	Mar	Apr	June
???	John	???	Matt
Red	???	???	Orange

Or

Feb	Mar	Apr	June
John	???	Matt	???

Red	???	Orange	Green

If we take the first possibility, it results in a contradiction to the fact that the green ball was given last. Hence only the second arrangement is possible. This means that John won first (Feb) and Matt won in April.

Step 3: Look through answer options to see if you can eliminate any of the choices before continuing with drawing.

Option A: Jake chose the black ball
Looking at the table this is possible, but it may not be true either. It is also possible that Paul chose the black ball.

Option B: Paul won his award In June
This is possible but it may not be true either. It is also possible that Jake chose the black ball.

Option C: The Black ball was won before the Orange one
This MUST be True, since the only colour left in our table is Black, which is in March, before Orange (April) - so it is the right answer

Option D: John won his award one month before Jake
Again, looking at the table – this may be true, but it also may not be.

Option C is the correct Answer.

#58. Logical Puzzles – Drawing Tables for Non-Sequential Variable Problems

The strategy in #57 can solve most logical puzzles in the exam. Unlike the worked through example in strategy #57, you may get a logical puzzle that doesn't have a sequential variable.

Pre-schoolers Chris, Sophie, Daniel, Rachel and Mike have one bike each. Their bikes are either red, blue or green in colour.

Three of the bikes are tricylces and the rest are bicycles
All bicycles are green
Tricycles are either blue or red

Michael and Chris do not have Tricycles

Amongst Sophie, Daniel, and Rachel, only Daniel has a blue bike.

Which of the following is True?

A. *Rachel has a red bicycle*

B. *There are three red bikes*

C. *There are two blue bikes*

D. *Sophie has a red tricycle*

Step 1: Pick and write out variable 1 (major variable) in order

In this example since we don't have a sequential variable, write out the major variable, in this example, it's the name of the preschoolers. Major variables are usually the names.

Chris	Soph	Daniel	Rachel	Mike

Step 2: Identify and pick out variable 2 and variable 3

From the question we can deduce the other two variables are the *type of bike and colour* of the bike.

Variable 2 – Bike type (bicycle or tricycle)
Variable 3 – Bike colour (red, blue or green)

Step 3: Input clues (or facts)

Considering clue 4 Mike and Chris do not have tricycles, therefore have bicycles. From clue 5 Daniel has a blue bike.

Chris	Soph	Daniel	Rachel	Mike
Bicycle	???	???	???	Bicycle
green	???	Blue	???	green

From clue 1, there are 3 tricycles and the rest are bicycles. This means that Soph, Daniel and Rachel have tricycles.

Chris	Soph	Daniel	Rachel	Mike
Bicycle	Tricycle	Tricycle	Tricycle	Bicycle
green	???	Blue	???	green

Revisiting clue 5, where Daniel is the only one with a blue bike

Chris	Soph	Daniel	Rachel	Mike
Bicycle	Tricycle	Tricycle	Tricycle	Bicycle
green	Red	Blue	Red	green

Option D is the Correct Answer, since Sophie has a red tricycle.

I strongly recommend you practice a lot of logical problems and master the table method. The key skills for mastering this technique include

- Deducing the variables to work with.
- Inferring based on clues provided in the question
- Eliminating options efficiently

#59. Logical Puzzles – Drawing Tables for Complex Problems

Complex logical puzzle problems tend to confuse you by introducing elements that make it a little more difficult to deduce the three variables you need to solve the problem. Let's look at an example:

Five friends aged 18, 17, 16, 15 and 19 are going to a music event. Francis, India, Georgia, Anna and Chloe, wore skirts and t-shirts of different colours: blue, green, burgundy, yellow and red.

Francis wore a green skirt. Her shirt was neither red nor blue.

Anna wore a red skirt

No two girls wore a shirt and skirt of the same colour

India wore a burgundy t-shirt. The colour of her skirt was the same colour as the colour of Francis' t-shirt

Which of the following is True?

A. *India wore a red skirt*

B. *Anna wore a red t-shirt*

C. *Chloe wore a blue or burgundy skirt*

D. *Anna wore a yellow t-shirt*

This problem is tricky because you might have been caught out to use their age, name and outfit colour as the three variables. But if you look at the clues, you will notice that there is no mention of their ages. Additionally, colour is split into two sub-variables. This should prompt you to realise that age is irrelevant to solve the problem. Therefore, the three variables you will work with will be as follows:

Variable 1 (major variable) – Names

Varibale 2 – Colour of skirt

Variable 3 - Colour of t-shirt.

Once we have identified the variable we are working with, then you can continue with the table method as normal (answer C is the correct answer). If you are unsure what variables to use, another tip is to review the answer options, in our example there is no mention of their ages so it's irrelevant.

#60. Logical Puzzles – Recognise Weakest Formats.

Logical puzzles can be presented in text, table or graphs. During practice try to recognise which of the three formats is your weakest and practice more of this than the other types. Remember, the key to improving is prioritising weak areas.

#61. Logical Puzzles – Leverage Negative Clues and Double Clues

Some parts of the questions may consist of negative clues. These do not inform us anything exactly, but it gives us a chance to eliminate a possibility. Sentences like "P is not the mother of Q" or "B is not a hill-station" are negative information. Another helpful type of clue are double clues, sentences like "P wore the same colour as Q". Pay extra attention to these type of clues as they help narrow things down further: Be efficient in your approach by targeting clues that will give you the most amount of information for the time spent. Avoid clues which open up more possibilities until you have used all your options.

#62. Logical Puzzles – Only Deduce What you Need

Only work out what you need to pick the correct answer, stop at the point where you can validate or disprove each answer option. Pick answer and move on.

#63. Logical Puzzles- Master the Process of Elimination

In the worked through example provided in strategy #57 we employed elimination to pick the correct answer without necessarily finishing the grid. Practice and master this before test day. Remember that with each answer option you can rule out, your chances of picking the right answer increases.

#64. Drawing Conclusion – Develop an eye for Spotting Question-type

Another type of question you can expect in the DM subtest are ones where you have to draw conclusion from two or more given premises. You are given a text with multiple premises followed by five statements, and asked if each statement logically follows from the text, in which you answer 'Yes', or answer 'No' if they do not follow. Drawing conclusion problems are easy to spot because, ***they are one of two question-types where you have to drag-and-drop***. Following the text, you should expect to see five separate statements. Each statement will have a grey box next to it, which is where you will be dragging the 'Yes' or 'No' answer boxes. I strongly recommend you look out for this, it will prompt you to realise two things – firstly, question might be time consuming so you might want to deploy triage. Secondly, you might have to deal with a syllogism or interpreting information. Thus, ensure you act appropriately before attempting the question. Depending on the strategy you choose to adopt, you may want to flag and skip these questions and come back to them later (triage) or adopt the appropriate strategy to solve the problem.

#65. Solving Syllogisms with Venn Diagrams – Know the Basics

Let's look at the following statement:

Michael is a British citizen

It is a simple statement that tells you Michael is British. Now look at another standalone statement:

All British citizens are smart

When you combine both statements, what does it tell you? Since ALL British citizens are smart and Michael is a British citizen, then we can deduce that **Michael is smart**. This set of three statements makes up an argument, defined as a single comprehensive act of thought consisting of three propositions – two *premises* and a *conclusion*.

	Michael is a British citizen	← **Premise 1**
Argument	**All British citizens are smart**	← **Premise 2**
	Michael is smart	← **Conclusion**

A *premise* is a basic proposition that supports a conclusion and upon the truth of which an argument is based. For our above argument to hold, you have to believe each premise is true. Even if you don't think all British citizens are smart, you have to consider this is valid for the sake of the argument, only then can you reach the conclusion. The *conclusion* is the third proposition of an argument which gives a judgement based on the support of the two previous propositions. In other words, we can reach a conclusion based on two premises given in an argument. We must always assume a given premise is true, even if it doesn't make any sense. For example, if you had a premise that stated 'all cats are dog' you will have to consider this to be valid in order to reach a conclusion.

Now that you understand the elements of an argument, let's look at the types of premises.

	Positive	**Negative**
Universal	All A are B	No A are B
Partial	Some A are B	Some A are not B

One categorisation of premises is in term of *universal* or *partial* statements. Universal means applies to all and Partial means applies to a specific people or things. Another categorisation of premises is in terms of *Positive* (affirms something) or *Negative statements* (negates something). When we look at premises there are 4 types:

1. ***Universal Positive****:* A statement like <u>All A are B</u> is universal because it talks about ALL of A and it is a positive statement (no use of words like No or Not). Examples: All British citizens are smart, All British citizens are dumb, etc.

2. ***Universal Negative****:* A statement like <u>No A are B</u> is universal negative because it applies to ALL of A <u>not</u> being B, therefore A and B are disjoint sets. Examples: No British citizen is smart, No British citizen is dumb.

3. ***Partial Positive****:* A statement like <u>Some A are B </u> is positive but unlike universal, we are only talking about some of A not all A. Examples: Some

British citizens are smart, Some British citizens are dumb, Some British citizens are black.

4. ***Partial Negative***: *A statement like* <u>*Some A are not B*</u> *is a negative partial statement because we are talking about some of A being disjointed from B. Examples: Some British citizens are not smart, Not every British citizen is smart.*

All four types are important to understand because statements or premises in syllogism questions fall under one of these. So let's look at each one and try to understand them more using venn diagrams.

If you are unfamiliar with venn diagrams or may need a brush up on the topic. I recommend learning the basics before continue reading. A great place to start will be with old GCSE maths textbooks, if you've lost them, then consider online resources like the BBC bitesize. They have great tutorials to teach venn diagram basics, its important that you understand how to convert text-to-venn.

<u>All A are B</u> (Universal Positive Premise)

This means that all of set A are contained within set B. In other words, set A is a subset of Set B. This can be expressed as two possibilities when drawing a venn diagram.

Please note: In the exam you'll be given enough information to know which venn diagram to draw, for example if a problem said "All A are B but Not all

B are A, then this will rule out the possibility of venn 2.

Possibility 1: Where A is a proper subtest of B

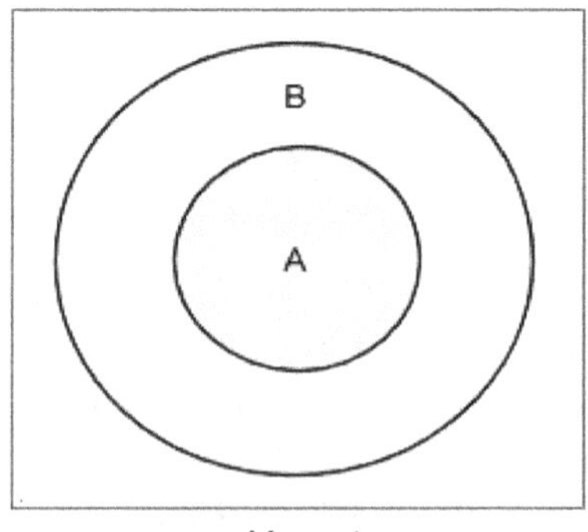

Venn 1

The given venn above shows Set A fully contained in Set B, so Set A is a *proper* subtest of B where B has got at least one extra element that's not A.

Possibility 2: There is another possibility for all of set A to be within set B is where **A and B** are equal:

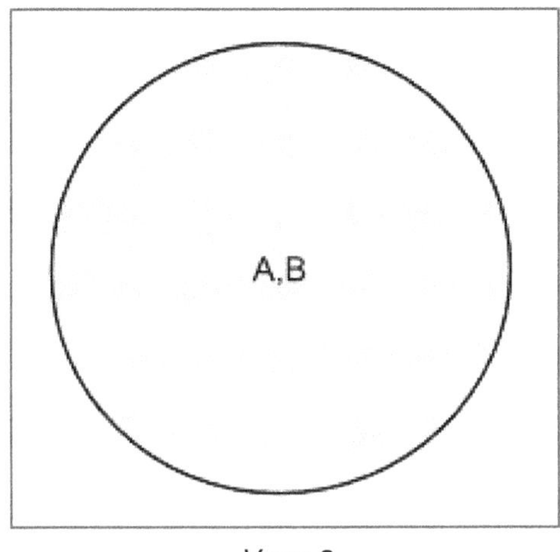

Venn 2

In this venn, A and B are shown to be equal. In other words, the '**All A are B**' rule still stands, the only difference is that we can't infer that there are some elements in set B that are not in Set A. The second venn diagram is an example of Set A being an improper subtest of B. Please note that 'All A are B' is different from 'All B are A' in the sense that 'All B are A' will be drawn so that the smaller subtest B is enclosed in the larger subtest A (thus making B a proper subtest of A).

<u>No A are B</u> (Universal Negative Premise)

This is the simplest to understand, since no A are B, Set A and Set B are disjointed, in others there is no overlap. Thus, **no element in A can be in B and vice versa** - we can go further by then saying that 'No A are B' is the same as 'No B are A'.

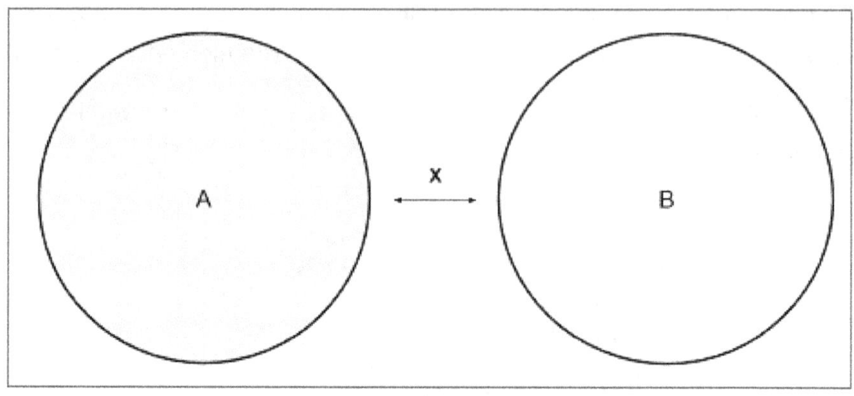

Venn 3

<u>Some A are B</u> (Partial Positive Premise)

In order to explain this type of premise, I want to start off by asking you a question. Consider the premise below:

Some women love dogs

What can we infer from the statement?

 A. *Some women love dogs and some women do not love dogs*

 B. *A few women love dogs*

 C. *At least one and possibly all women love dogs*

 D. *Not all women love dogs*

If you picked option A or D, then I strongly recommend you spend time working on your understanding of the meaning of qualifiers (see strategy #76). If you picked option B, then spend some time working on how to evaluate extreme language (strategy #17) - all three options are wrong. We cannot infer that there are women who do not love dogs unless given more information. As a standalone statement, we can only infer that <u>at least one and possibly all women love dogs</u> (therefore option C is the correct answer). Think about it, consider this statement "some students that bought this book are taking the UCAT", this doesn't mean that there are "students that bought this book who are not taking the UCAT", nor can we infer that "not every student that bought this book is taking the UCAT", we can only infer that "one and possibly all students that bought this book are taking the UCAT". No matter how bizarre or illogical a statement might be, you cannot infer beyond this scope e.g. "some cats are dogs" means "one and possibly all cats are dogs". Let's look at another premise:

Some cats are lions

Which of the following inferences are correct?

A.   *Some lions are cats*

B.   *Some cats are not lions*

C.   *At least one and possibly all cats are lions*

D.   *At least one and possibly all lions are cats*

E.   *Not every cat is a lion*

To solve this let's breakdown the meaning of the statement "some cats are lions" - the statement means "at least one and possibly all cats are lions" (option C). If we break this up, we can infer that it is possible that "at least one cat is a lion" and "all cats are lions". Therefore, we can infer that "some lions are cats" (option A) i.e. "at least one and possibly all lions are cats" (Option D). Therefore, Option A, C and D are correct. To help with your understanding of this, let's look at possible venn diagrams to express **Some A are B** (in other words at least one and possibly all of A are B):

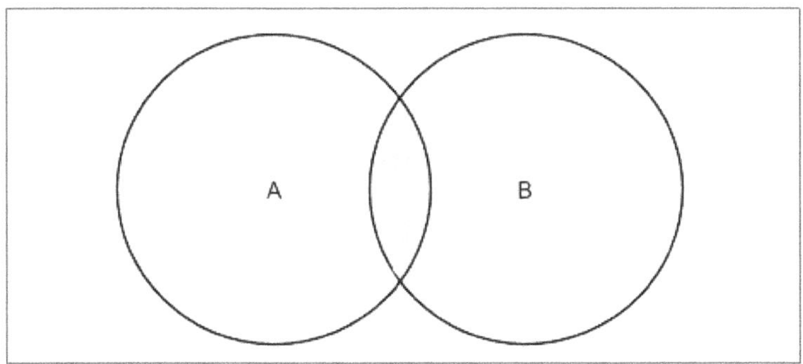

Venn 4

The above venn diagram is a possibility when expressing some A are B, where the <u>intersection must include at least one element that is in both set A and set B</u>. In this figure, there are elements that are only in A and elements that are only in B.

Possibility 2: Another possibility is where both set A and set B are equal. It helps to think about the meaning of *some*. For instance, the premise we covered earlier that stated "some women love dogs" means "one and possibly all women love dogs". Just because the premise says some women love dogs, we cannot infer that some women do not love dogs, but possibly all women love dogs. Hence the possibility of the venn diagram below where set A equals set B.

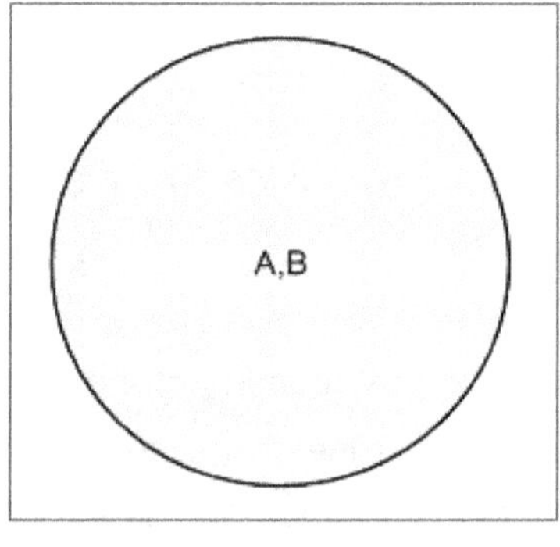

Venn 5

Possibility 3: Another possibility for Some A are B, is when set A is a proper subtest of set A. Since *one and possibly all of A is B*, then we can draw a venn that shows the entire set A enclosed with B, where B has an extra element:

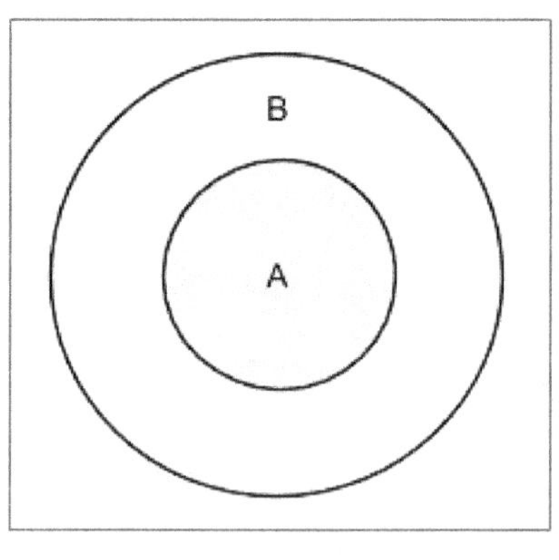

Venn 6

Possibility 4: The final possibility is the reverse where set B is a proper subtest of set A. For instance, in the premise we covered earlier that stated

"Some cats are lions" we deduced that we can infer "Some lions are cats" by breaking down the meaning of *some* in the context of the first premise. Therefore, the venn below applies where B (lion) is the smaller circle in the venn.

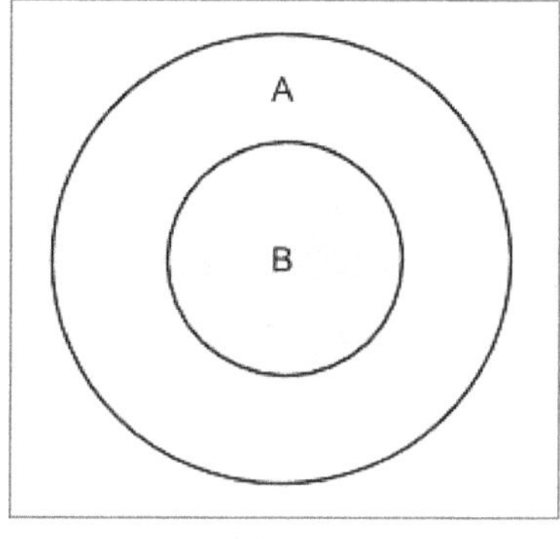

Venn 7

The thing to remember is that *Some A are B* is the same as *Some B are A.*

Important: *These are the four possibilities when dealing with Some A are B. The UCAT usually set problems that will help you narrow down which venn diagram to use. For example, "Not all A are B" will rule out Venn 5 and 6, then depending on the information in the passage you will know whether it is appropriate to use either venn 4 or venn 7 when drawing out your venn.*

<u>Some A are not B</u> (Partial Negative Premise)

Consider the premise below:

Some students are not intelligent

Which of the following can we infer?

> A.   *At least one student is not intelligent*
>
> B.   *Some students are intelligent*
>
> C.   *Possibly all students are not intelligent*
>
> D.   *A few students are not intelligent*

To solve this let's breakdown the meaning of the statement: we understand 'some' means 'at least one and possibly all'. Therefore, we can rephrase the premise as "at least one and possibly all students are not intelligent". Therefore, we can infer option A and C. Think about it this way; consider this statement "some students that took the UCAT did not buy this book", we cannot infer there are some students that took the UCAT that bought this book without more information. As a standalone statement we can only infer that "<u>one and possibly all students that took the UCAT didn't buy this book</u>". If we go back to the question: just because some students are not intelligent this doesn't mean we can infer that there are students that are intelligent, we do not have enough information to deduce this, so option B and D are wrong. To help with your understanding of this, let's look at possible venn diagrams to express **Some A are not B** (in other words at least one and possibly all of A are not B):

Possibility 1: The below venn diagram is a possibility when expressing some A are not B, where an area of A that is not <u>intersecting with B must include at least one element that is in only A.</u>

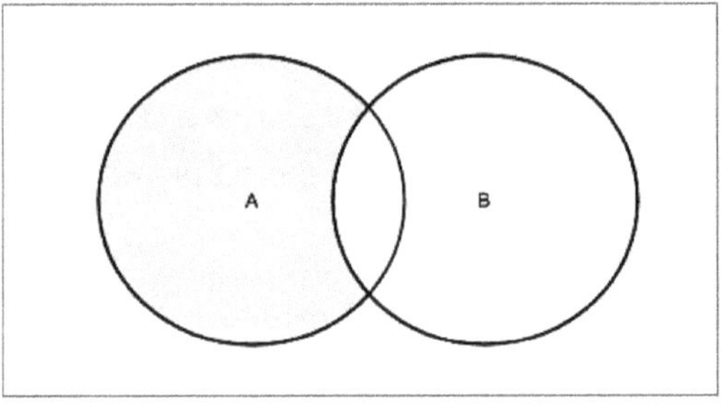

Venn 8

Possibility 2: Another venn possibility to express some A are not B, is when A is disjointed from Set B. This makes sense when you consider the meaning of Some A not B - "At least one and possibly <u>all</u> of set A is not Set B". We have;

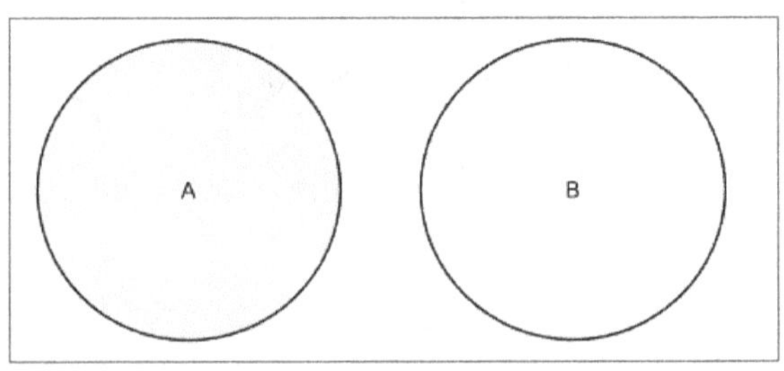

Venn 9

Possibility 3: Another possibility is for B to be a proper subtest of A where elements outside of Set B are enclosed within Set A.

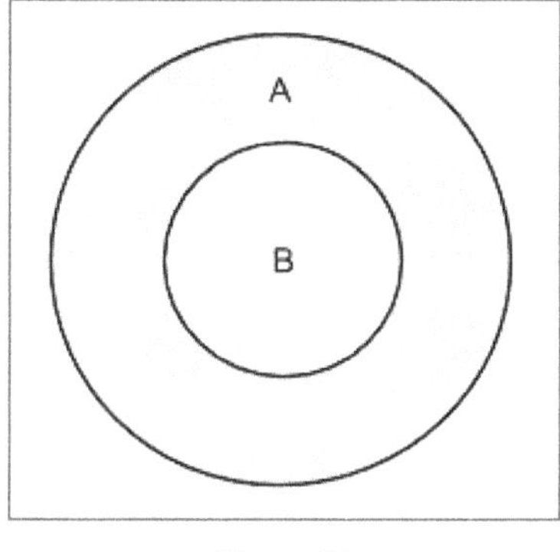

Venn 10

Syllogism problems in the UCAT tend to use partial negative premises in the paragraph, though most cases the questions may give you enough information to decide which venn to use. For example: "Some A are not B, and All B are A". This should prompt you to draw venn 10 instead of either venn 8 or 9.

#66. Syllogism with Venn – Applying Basics to Positive Conclusions

This strategy assumes you are familiar with the content in strategy #65 and can draw basic venn diagrams. Let's look at a simple syllogism to help with applying the key concepts covered earlier:

Some Fishes are vegan. All vegans are mammals

*Place 'Yes' if the conclusion follows. Place '**No**' if the conclusion does not follow:*

A.   *All fishes are mammals*

B.   *Some fishes are mammals*

C.   *Some vegans are mammals*

D.   All fishes are vegan

You can choose to re-read the statement multiple times to work out which conclusions are valid. However, you may want to consider drawing a venn diagram to depict the information.

Step 1: Consider all possibilities for each premise

This should be done mentally, think of all the possible ways each premise could be expressed as a venn.

Premise 1: Some fishes are vegan (positive)

Remember from strategy #65, there are four possibilities when dealing with a *partial positive* premise (Some A are B):

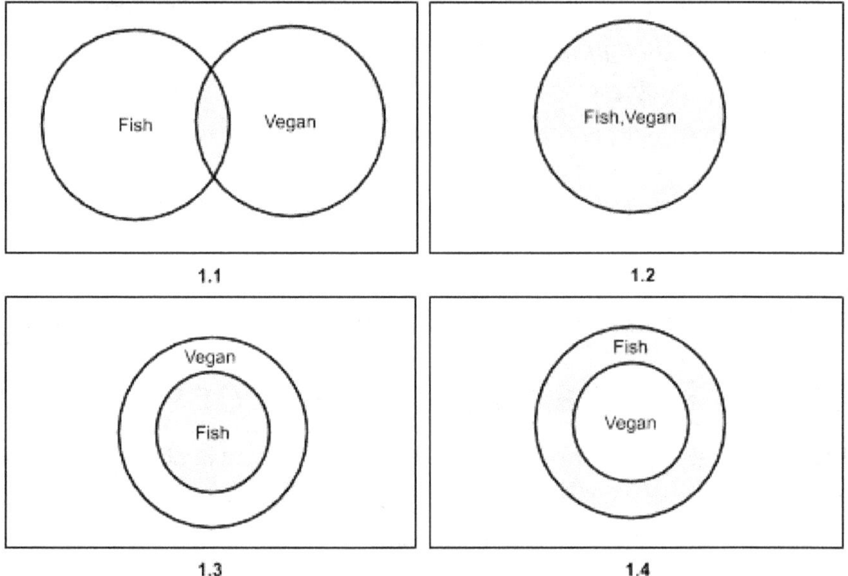

Premise 2: All vegans are mammals (positive)

Remember from strategy #65, there are two possibilities when dealing with a universal *positive premise* (All A are B):

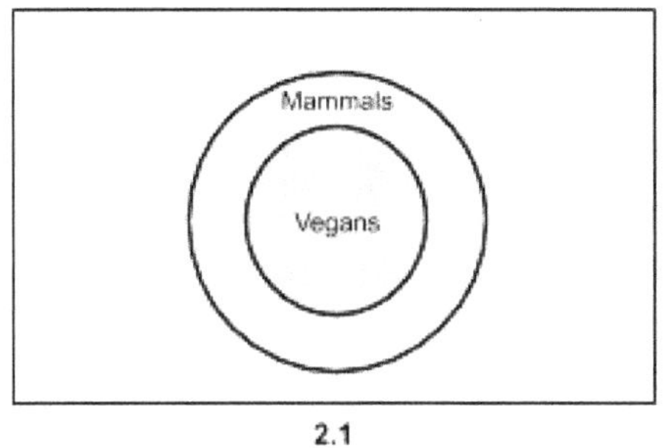

2.1

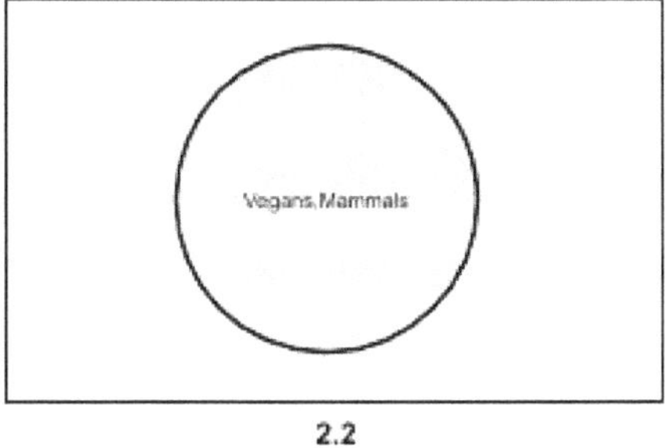

2.2

Now that we have laid out all the possibilities based on the two premises provided in the text. We now need to combine them. Unfortunately, there are multiple possibilities, and this will take up a lot of time to deduce. See the table below showing all the possible combinations of both premises combining their venn diagrams.

Venn Possibilities	1.1	1.2	1.3	1.4
2.1	1.1: 2.1	1.2: 2.1	1.3:2.1	1.4:2.1
2.2	1.1: 2.2	1.2: 2.2	1.3: 2.2	1.4: 2.2

As you can see from the table there are at least 8 different possibilities when you combine the venn diagrams for both premises. Moreover, for a **conclusion to be VALID, it must follow for every possible venn combination of possibilities.** For example, consider the statement _all fishes are mammals_, if we combine venn 1.2 and 2.1 this conclusion seems possible. Since vegans are a proper subtest of mammals (venn 2.1) and its possible for the fish set and vegan sets to be equal (venn 1.2); we can combine both venns to get 1.2: 2.1 where fishes and vegans are a proper subtest of mammals (see below):

253

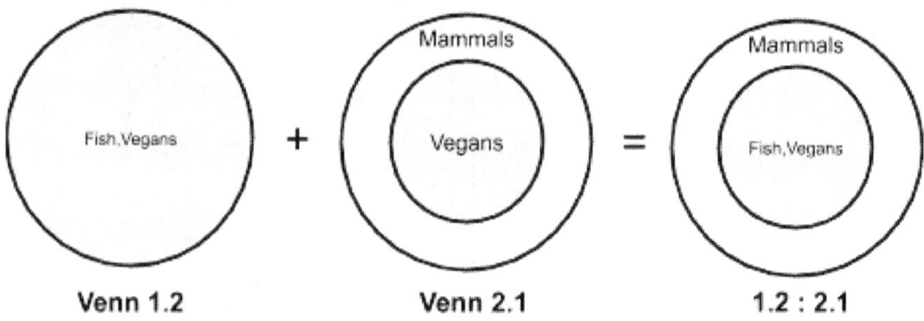

Venn 1.2	**Venn 2.1**	**1.2 : 2.1**

However, if you look at another combination say venn 1.1 and venn 2.2 the statement does not follow. Instead we get a partial overlap of fishes with the "vegans equal mammas" set. Since we are able to identify a possibility where all fishes are mammals **does not follow, then the statement is invalid** (see below)

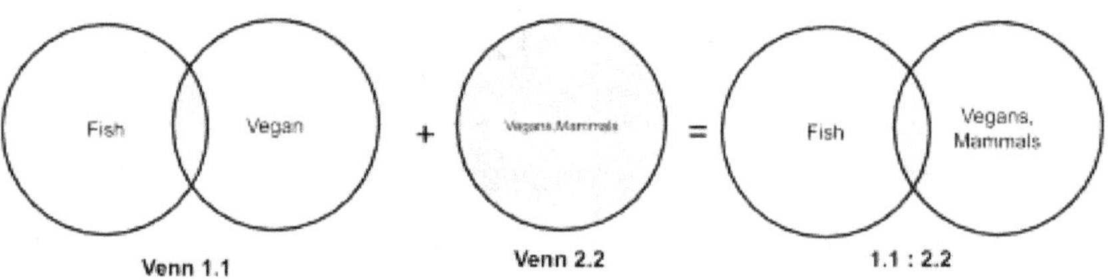

Venn 1.1	**Venn 2.2**	**1.1 : 2.2**

This method of solving syllogisms is time consuming as you will have to evaluate each possible venn combination to check if a conclusion holds. In the UCAT you won't have time, so will need a quicker strategy. The best approach is one that many of us are taught at schools, where you only draw and evaluate the **minimum overlap venn diagram**.

Step 2: Draw a minimum overlap venn diagram

The minimum overlap venn diagram is one that **combines the minimal venn possibility of one premise with the minimal venn possibility of the other**. Consider the second premise, *all vegans are mammals, there are two possibilities* - where vegans is a proper subtest of mammals or where vegans and mammals are equal.

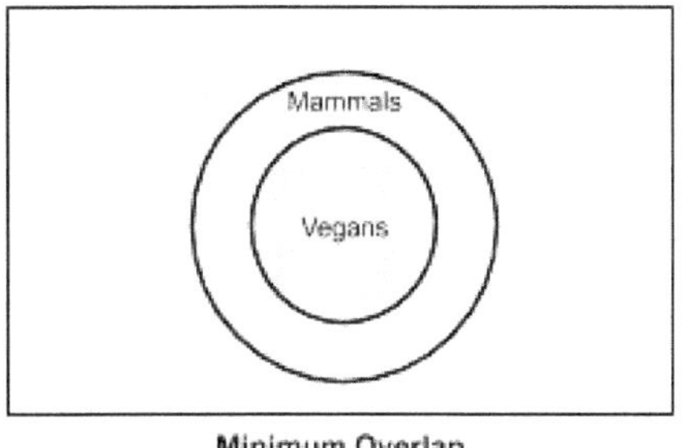
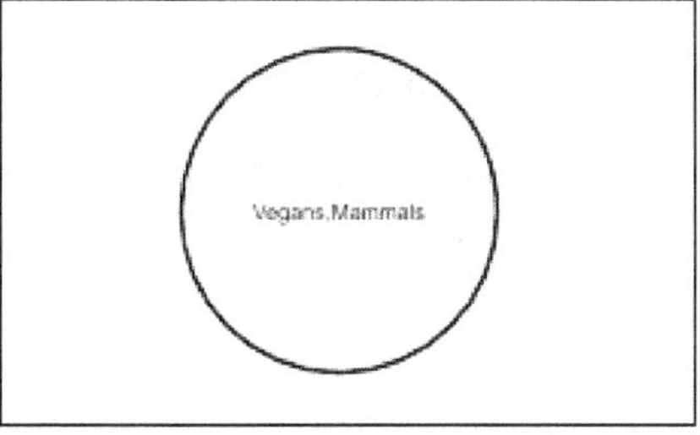

Minimum Overlap	Maximum Overlap

Out of the two venn possibilities, the one where vegans are a proper subtest of mammals is the minimal representation of the premise, because vegan is enclosed in mammals, where we presume mammals have other elements that are not vegan, thus making it the <u>minimal overlap possibility</u>.

Now consider the first premise *some fishes are vegan* with four different possibilities, which of the four venn diagrams would you say shows the minimal venn possibility of the premise? It would be venn 1.1, where there is a small overlap between fishes and vegans.

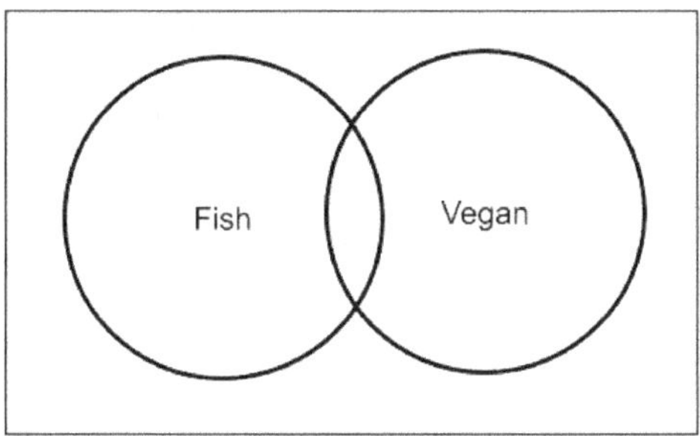

MINIMAL POSSIBILITY

Now that we have identified the minimal venn possibilities for each premise, let's combine them:

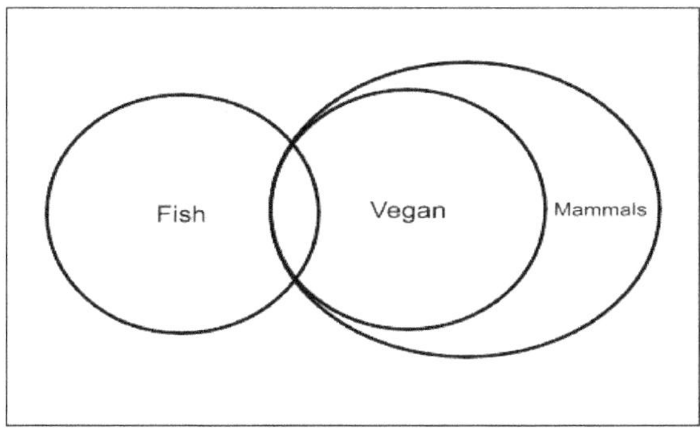

The venn above is the minimum overlap for the given premises to hold valid. If a **conclusion does not show in this minimum venn diagram, then it cannot be valid.**

Step 3: Use minimum possibility Venn Diagram to evaluate conclusions

Place 'Yes' if the conclusion follows. Place 'No' if the conclusion does not follow:

All fishes are mammals: This conclusion doesn't follow since there is only a small overlap between mammals and fish. Therefore, No.

Some fishes are mammals: This conclusion follows since there is an overlap between fishes and mammals. Therefore, Yes.

Some vegans are mammals: This follows since vegans is fully enclosed in Mammals. Remember that *some* means "at least one and possibly all". Therefore, Yes

All the fishes are vegan: This doesn't follow since fishes are not fully enclosed in vegans. Therefore, No

When dealing with positive conclusions you can draw conclusions by solely looking at the minimum overlap venn diagram. However, when dealing with negative conclusions, you may have to consider other possibilities, we dive into this in strategy #67.

#67. Syllogism with Venn – Applying Basics to Negative Conclusions

This strategy assumes you are familiar with advice on strategy #65 and. #66. When dealing with a negative conclusion you have to explore other possibilities beyond the minimum overlap venn diagram. Let's go through a similar example to the one in #66 to explain:

All fishes are vegan. No mammals are fishes

Place 'Yes' if the conclusion follows. Place 'No' if the conclusion does not follow:

A.   Some vegans are mammals

B.   No vegans are mammals

C.   All mammals are vegans

D.   Some mammals are not vegan

Start off as normal by thinking of all the possibilities for each premise:

Premise 1: All fishes are vegan (Positive)

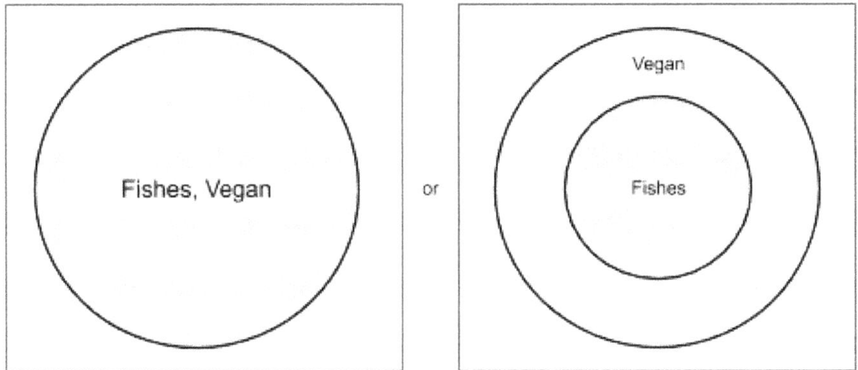

Premise 2: No mammals are fishes (Negative)

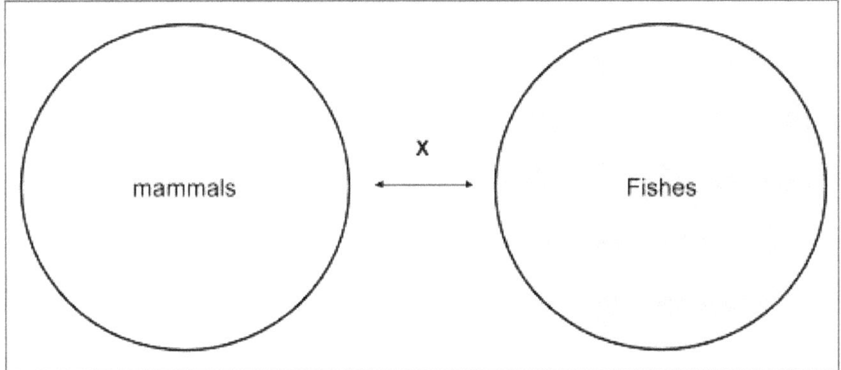

Please note: the 'x' in the venn diagram for premise 2 shows that there is no relationship between mammals and fishes, and under no circumstances must they overlap when drawing conclusions.

By thinking about the different possibilities mentally, we can construct a minimum overlap venn diagram to help evaluate the conclusions, we have:

257

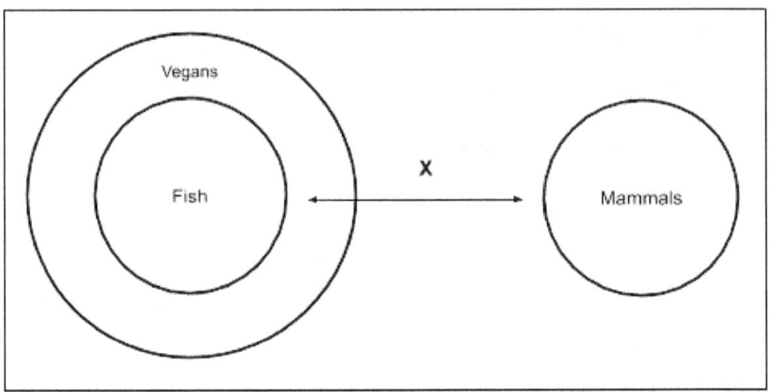

With our minimum overlap venn diagram completed, let's evaluate the conclusions:

A. Some vegans are mammals: This is a <u>positive</u> conclusion, so we can deduce directly from the minimum overlap venn diagram. This conclusion does not follow (since vegans does <u>not</u> overlap with mammals).

B. No vegans are mammals: This is a <u>negative</u> conclusion, so we have to explore beyond the minimum overlap venn diagram. Is it possible for ALL vegans to be mammals without contradicting the given premises? If you re-read the question and re-position the minimum overlay, the venn below is a possibility:

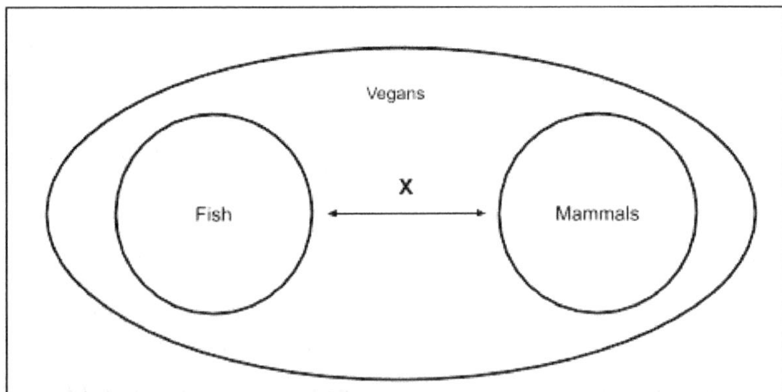

You can see from the new venn, that it is possible for mammals to be vegans without contradicting the given premise "<u>all fishes are vegan</u>. <u>No mammals are fishes</u>". Since we have recognised possibility, then it doesn't follow. Therefore, the conclusion no vegans are mammals does <u>not</u> follow.

Important: *When presented with a positive conclusion (e.g. Option A), the statement* **must show in the minimum overlap venn for it to be valid**. *When presented with a negative conclusion, you have to* **explore the possibility of the opposite without contradicting the given premises**. *If the opposite is possible, then the conclusion is NOT valid. For example, if a conclusion states "No A are B" then explore if it's possible for "All A are B". If this is possible without contradicting the given premises, then "No A are B" is invalid.*

C. All mammals are vegans: This is a <u>positive</u> conclusion, so we can deduce directly from our minimum overlap venn diagram. We can see there is no overlap; conclusion does <u>not</u> follow.

D. Some mammals are not vegan: This is another <u>negative</u> conclusion, so we have to explore beyond the minimum overlap venn diagram. If you take another look at the venn we drew earlier to solve conclusion (B):

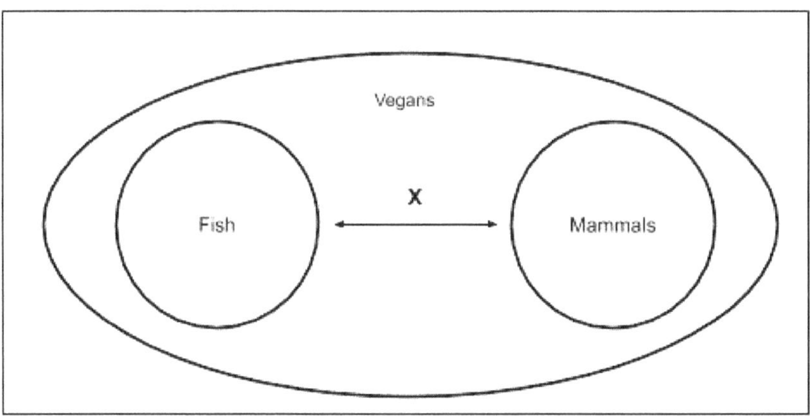

We can deduce that it is possible for "at least one or all of mammals" to be vegan without contradicting the given premises *"All fishes are vegan. No mammals are fishes"*. Therefore, the conclusion that Some mammals are not vegan does <u>not</u> follow.

Positive statements are as easy as interpreting the minimum overlap venn diagram, whilst negative conclusion require you to think of the other possibilities that do not contradict the given premises, reread the question

#68. Syllogism with Venn – Changing Text to Venn

Now that we have looked at how to apply venn diagrams in evaluating positive and negative conclusions. Let's take a look at commonly used words or phrases used in the exam and how they could translate into venn diagrams:

- "At least some A are B" = **"Some A are B".** Ignore 'At least' because it is the same thing when drawing a minimal overlap venn diagram. For example; *at least some buses are cars*:

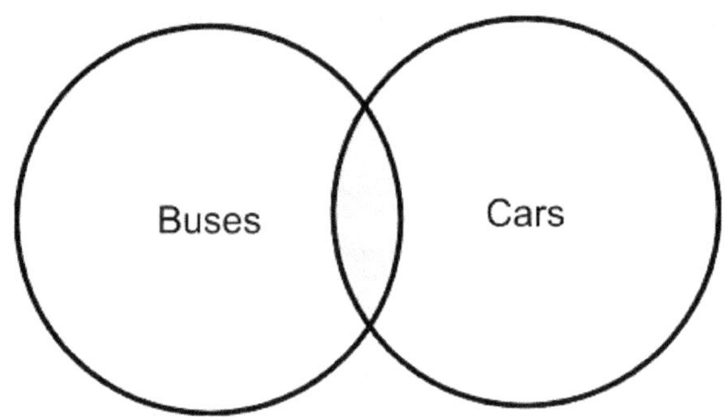

-
- "Not all A are B" e.g. Not all buses are cars,

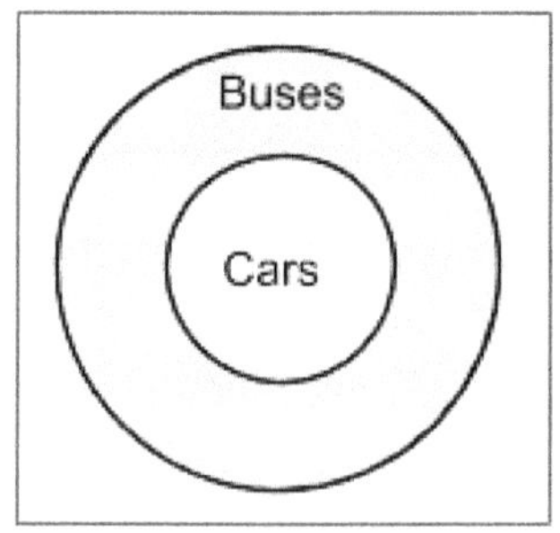

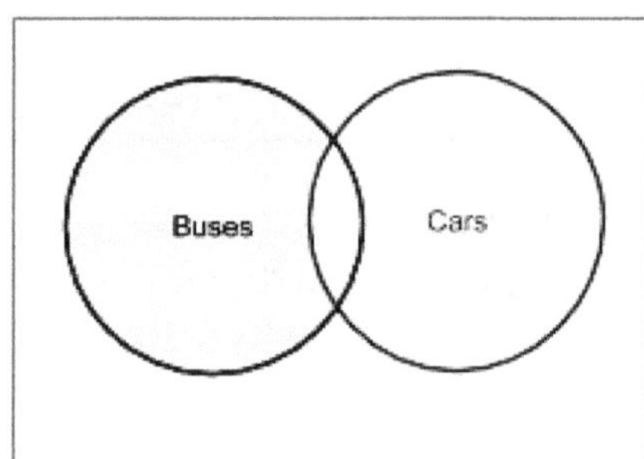

The examples we covered in strategy #66 and 67 were problems with 2 premises. In the exam you will be provided with about 3 -4 premises from which you must construct a minimal overlap venn (see strategy #69).

Nonetheless, I have provided common words used for the different types of premises covered ins strategy #65.

- Universal Positive words (All A are B) - *All, Each, Every, Only. E.g Only buses are cars*

- Universal Negative words (No A are B) – *No, None, Never, No one, All not. E.g. No none bus is a car.*

- Partial Positive words (Some A are B) – Some, Most, Many, Few, Only a few, Most of, Almost, Almost all. E.g. a few buses are cars

For most syllogism problems in the UCAT, expect a sentence or two where it may be easier to convert the information to venn. Practice translating text to venn and keep an eye out for these commonly used words and phrases.

#69. Syllogism with Venn – Applying Basics to Confusing Text Problems

This strategy assumes you are familiar with advice in strategy #65 - #68. Positive and negative premises in the UCAT can sometimes be presented in a way that is confusing in the exam. Thus this makes it difficult to recognise the type of venn diagram to draw.

Let's consider an example:

Not all people at the Met Gala were celebrities, but all the celebrities that attended were actors and at least some celebrities were not musicians.

*Place 'Yes' if the conclusion follows. Place '**No**' if the conclusion does not follow:*

A. *Some musicians at the Met Gala were celebrities*

B. *Some actors at the Met Gala were both celebrities and musicians*

C. *All the actors at the Met Gala were celebrities or musicians*

D.   *Not all actors at the Met Gala who were celebrities were*
       musicians

When drawing your minimal overlap venn. Start with the positive statements and link other statements to the venn. In this problem we know that all celebrities that attended the Met Gala were actors, therefore:

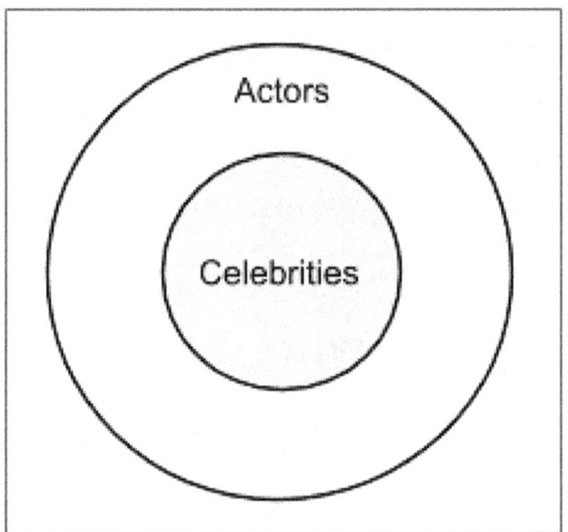

Now that we have established the positive premise what other rules surround it's elements, i.e. actors or celebrities? The text says at least some celebrities were not musicians. Remember from strategy #68 we established "at least some" is another way of just saying "some". Therefore, all we are left with is "some celebrities were not musicians". Therefore, we have:

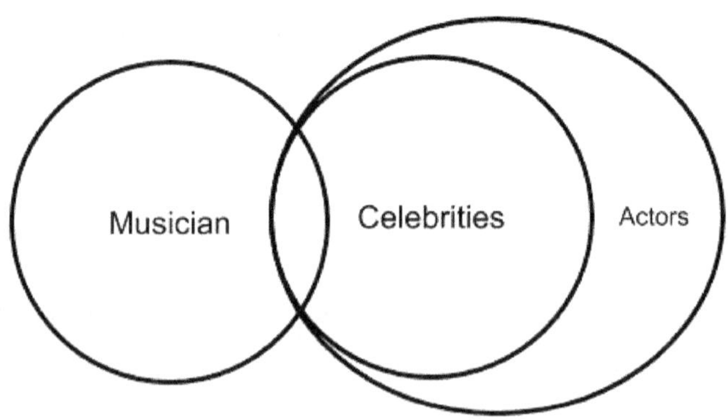

The final part of the says that "not all people at the met gala were celebrities". Now this is where some students get confused. We understand that this can be rephrased as "some but not all people at the Met Gala are not celebrities". However, considering the context of the question we can have:

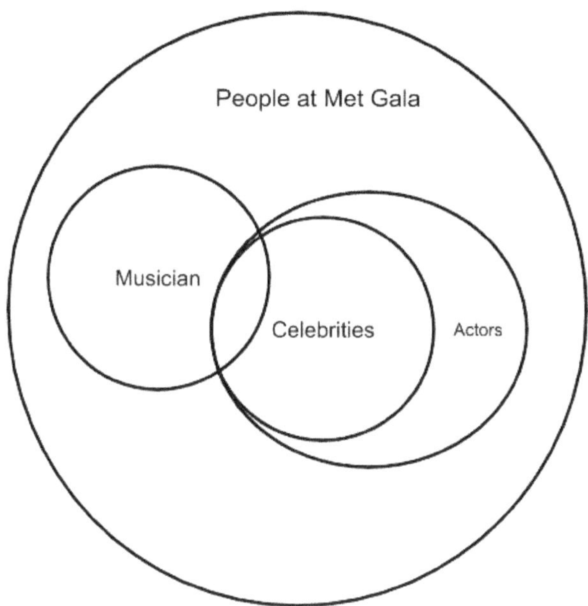

By making celebrities a subset of "people at the met gala", the premise "not all people at the met gala were celebrities" still stands. Now that we have drawn our venn, let's go through the conclusions.

A. Some musicians at the Met Gala were celebrities: This is a positive conclusion so no need to look beyond the venn. From the venn diagram we can see that this follows.

B. Some actors at the Met Gala were both celebrities and musicians: This is another positive statement, we can see from the venn diagram this conclusion follows.

C. All the actors at the Met Gala were celebrities or musicians: This is a positive statement and does not follow as we can see from the venn diagram.

D. Not all actors at the Met Gala who were celebrities were musicians:
This is a negative statement, so we may have to possibly explore beyond the venn. The opposite of this would be _All actors who were celebrities were musicians_. _We can see this does not follow from the minimum overlap venn above,_ so "not all actors who are celebrities were musicians" does follow.

#70. Syllogism with Venn – Start with Positive statements when drawing Venn

The Venn method for solving syllogism is one of three methods in this guide (see strategy #72 and #75). Though extremely beneficial be sure to start with the positive premises when drawing out your venn especially if the passage is a mix of negative and positive premises. Also, be open to using other methods and picking the one that is most appropriate to help you interpret the information provided more accurately.

If you are given a negative premise and a negative conclusion, be sure to double check you have enough information to draw if the conclusion is valid or not. Sometimes examiners include conclusions where you "cannot tell" if there valid based on the information in the passage. Therefore select "No".

#71. Solving Syllogisms with Venn – Guessing Strategy

Guessing should always be used as a last resort. However, if you find yourself in a sticky situation where you either do not have time or have no clue whether a conclusion follows or not. Here is a guessing strategy recommended by a contributor that scored 840 in the DM section. I tested it myself and it's a pretty good guessing approach:

Conclusion Type	Answer	Examples
Universal Positive	Most likely does NOT follow. Pick NO.	All A are B

Partial Positive	Most does follow. Pick Yes	Some A are B
Universal Negative	Most likely does NOT follow. Pick NO.	No A are B
Partial Negative	Most likely does follow. Pick Yes	Not all A are B

This is based on the same logic that we use when evaluating extreme language in the Verbal Reasoning subtest (strategy #19), where extreme claims are most likely incorrect, and softer claims are most likely correct.

#72. Solving Syllogisms with the Rule Grid Method - Basics

The Rule grid method is another method for solving syllogisms and interpreting information questions, it is great for getting your head around some of the most complex syllogisms you can find in the exam. It works by defining the relationship between two items either by 0 (non-existent), 50 (partial) or 100 (universal). For example, consider the premise "All dogs are cats" we can write this out as follows:

$$\text{Dogs} \xrightarrow{\text{100}} \text{Cats}$$

This make sense, since all dogs are cats, then we expect the rule to be universal (i.e. 100).

Let's look at another premise, "Some dogs are cats". This on the other hand will be partial "50" with an arrow pointing from dogs to cat.

$$\text{Dogs} \xrightarrow{\text{50}} \text{Cats}$$

Now let's look at a more than one premise, consider "Some dogs are cats. All cats are lions". This will follow as:

265

$$\textbf{Dogs} \xrightarrow{\textbf{50/100}} \textbf{Cats} \xrightarrow{\textbf{100}} \textbf{Lion}$$

Consider the premise, "Not all dogs are cats. At least some cats are lions". This would also follow a similar layout, except the meaning of the arrows will be different:

$$\textbf{Dogs} \xrightarrow{\textbf{50}} \textbf{Cats} \xrightarrow{\textbf{50}} \textbf{Lion}$$

Similar to the venn method you are using a diagrammatic approach to solving syllogism problems. Let's look at the same problem covered in strategy #66:

Some Fishes are vegan. All vegans are mammals

*Place 'Yes' if the conclusion follows. Place '**No**' if the conclusion does not follow:*

- A. *All fishes are mammals*

- B. *Some fishes are mammals*

- C. *Some vegans are mammals*

- D. *All fishes are vegan*

Step 1: Construct your rule grid

$$\textbf{Fishes} \xrightarrow{\textbf{50}} \textbf{Vegans} \xrightarrow{\textbf{100}} \textbf{Mammals}$$

Step 2: Evaluate conclusions

A. All Fishes are mammals

The goal is to get from point A (in this case Fish) to point B (Mammals) without contradicting the conclusion. So as we move from Fishes to Vegans we come to a contradiction, since "Some" fishes (i.e. partial) are vegans. Therefore, the conclusion "all fishes…" cannot follow.

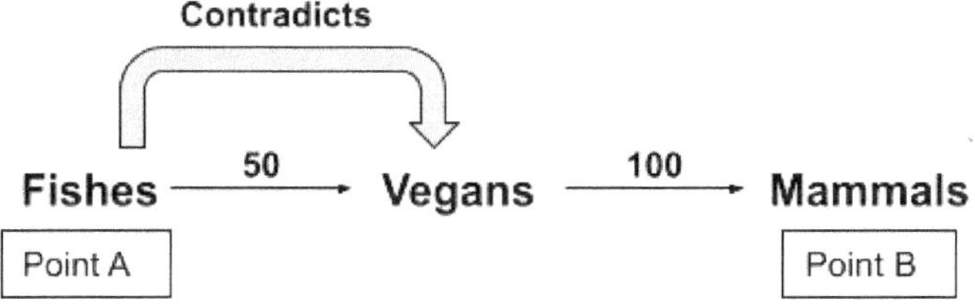

For conclusion to follow all fishes must be vegan (i.e 100) and all vegans must mammals (i.e. 100)

B. Some Fishes are mammals

Same as before, we will try to go from point A (Fish) to B (Mammals) without any contradiction. Starting at fishes, we can move to vegan since some fishes are vegan, then we can also move along to mammals since all vegans are mammals, therefore the conclusion follows:

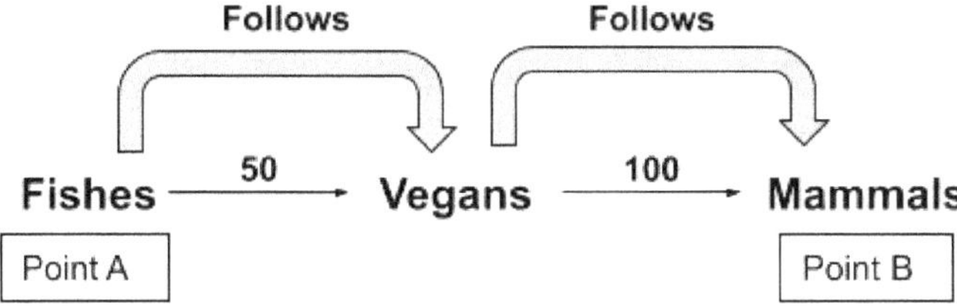

C. Some vegans are mammals

Starting at vegans we can move to mammals since the statement doesn't

not contradict. Therefore, conclusion follows

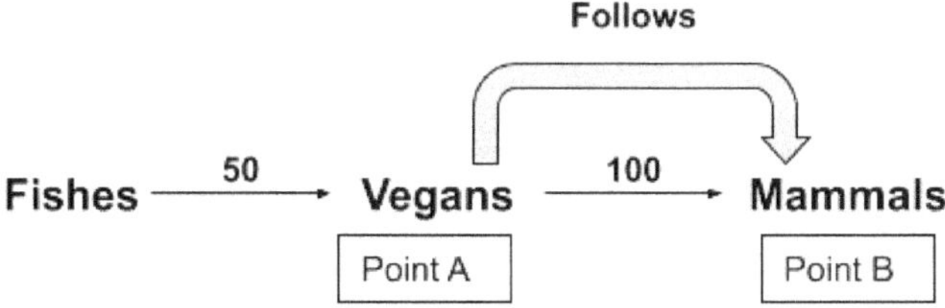

D. All fishes are vegan

Starting at fishes, we cannot move to vegan since it contradicts. Therefore, the conclusion does not follow.

267

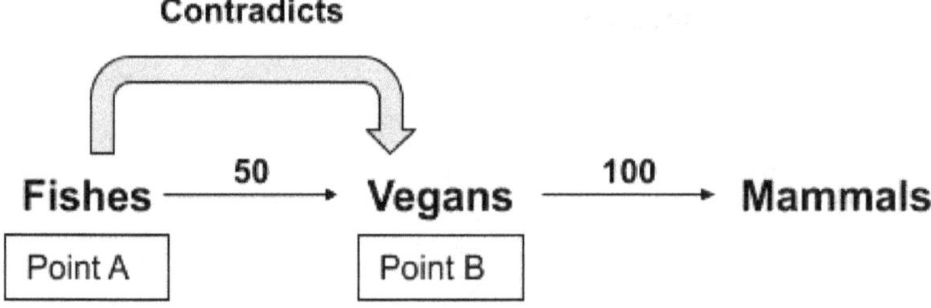

#73. Solving Syllogisms with Rule Grid Method – Making Inference

This strategy assumes that you are familiar with the basics in strategy #72. Making inference with the rule grid method follows the basic principle that if **Some A is B,** then we can infer of **Some of B is A**. Same as if **All A is B** then **Some B is A**.

To help explain this, let's attempt the problem in strategy #69 using the rule grid method:

Not all people at the Met Gala were celebrities but all the celebrities that attended were actors and at least some celebrities were not musicians.

*Place 'Yes' if the conclusion follows. Place '**No**' if the conclusion does not follow:*

A.   *Some musicians at the Met Gala were celebrities*

B.   *Some actors at the Met Gala were both celebrities and musicians*

C.   *All the actors at the Met Gala were celebrities or musicians*

D.   *Not all actors at the Met Gala who were celebrities were musicians*

The rule grid will be as follows

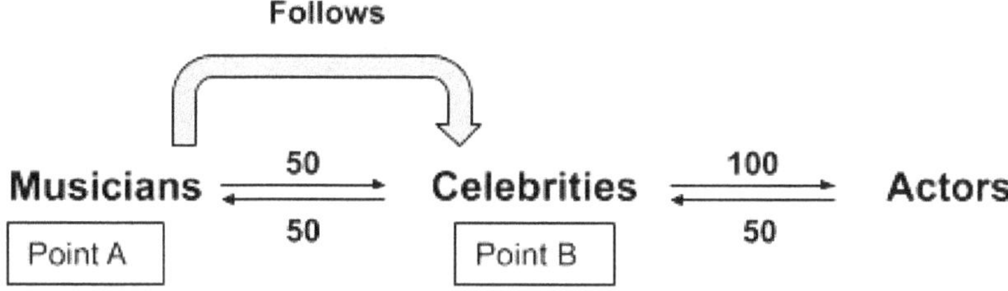

Since all celebrities were actors we can infer some actors were celebrities. (i.e. 50 from right to left). Also, the text says "at least some celebrities were not musicians", this indicates a partial relationship between celebrities and musicians in both directions.

A. Some musicians at the Met Gala were celebrities

This follows as it does not contradict the rule grid when we move from point A (musician) to celebrities (point B).

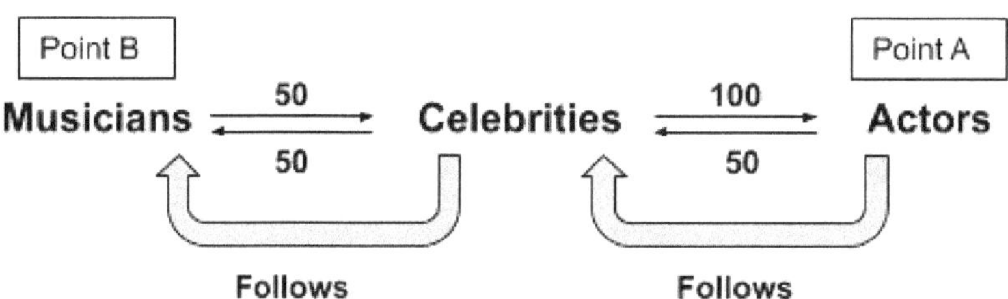

B. Some actors are the Met Gala were both celebrities and musicians

This follows as it does not contradict the rule grid when we move from point A (actors) to musician (point B).

C. All the actors at the Met Gala were celebrities or musicians

This does not follow since some actors are celebrities and so it contradicts with the conclusion. This means we are unable to move from actors to celebrities and are therefore unable to move from celebrities to musicians.

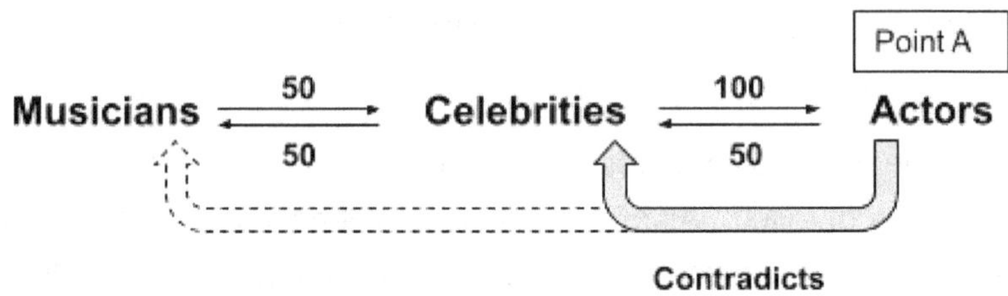

D. Not all actors at the Met Gala who were celebrities were musicians:

This follows because we can partially move from point A. to point B without contradiction. Therefore, conclusion follows.

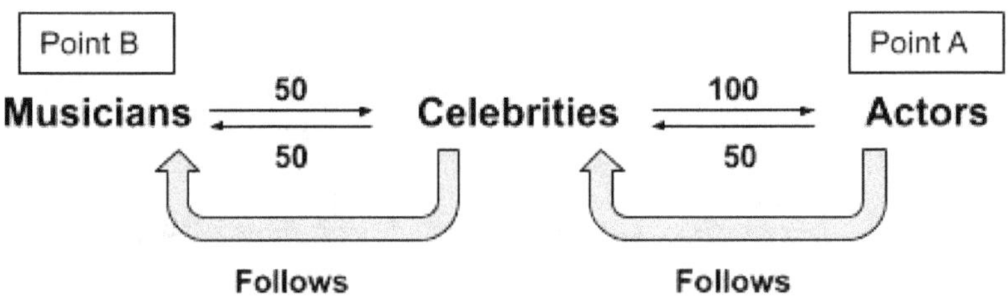

#74. Solving Syllogisms with Rule Grid Method – Exception Problems

Let's apply the rule grid method to solving exception problems. Consider the question below:

In the Jones family, not all family members are males, however, all males in the family are six feet tall except for Patrick and Daniel.

*Place 'Yes' if the conclusion follows. Place '**No**' if the conclusion does not follow:*

A.   *Some of the males in the Jones family are 6 feet tall*

B.   *If Michael is a family member, he is 6 feet tall*

C.   *If a 6 feet tall male is a member of the family, he is neither Patrick nor Daniel*

Let's construct our rule grid:

The question includes an exception rule, where all males are 6 feet EXCEPT Patrick and Daniel, we can express this in our rule grid as follows:

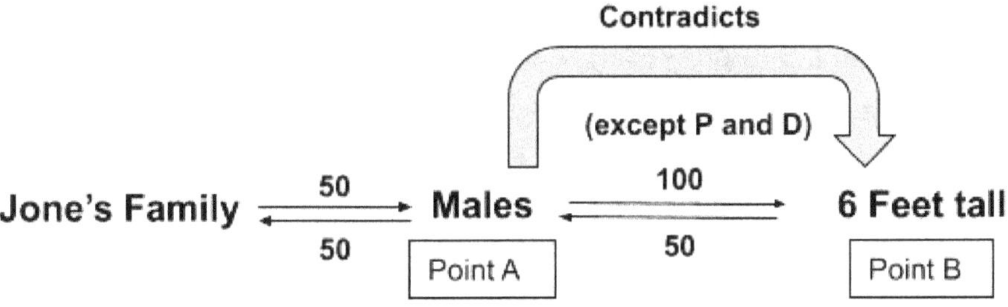

Now let's work through each conclusion and determine whether they follow or not:

A. Some of the male in the Jone's Family are 6 feet tall

This does not follow since there is an exception rule when you move from males to 6 feet tall – a scenario where Patrick and Daniel are not 6 feet tall.

B. If Michael is a man in the family, he is 6 feet tall

This follows, since Michael is not Patrick nor Daniel. We can move from Males to 6 feet tall.

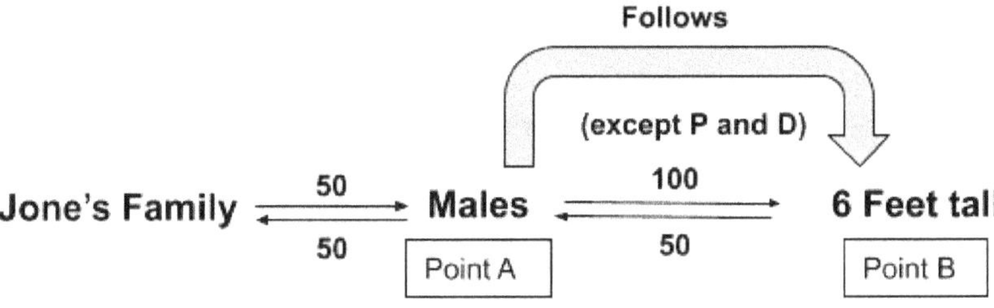

C. If a 6 feet tall male is a member of the family, he is neither Patrick nor Daniel

This is straightforward, of course it must follow since we know all male members are 6 feet tall except Patrick and Daniel.

D. Patrick and Daniel are members of the Jones family that are either more than 6 feet tall or less than 6 feet tall.

This follows, since they are not 6 feet tall. They can either be more than or less than 6 feet.

You can see in the worked through example, we didn't use our grid to answer all the questions. I strongly recommend to practice rephrasing and validating the text and using methods like the venn method or rule grid method to only help visualise the information. Never rely solely on one method! They will always be tricky questions in the exam. Consider the conclusion below:

Not all family members of the Jones who are 6 feet tall are males:

This does not follow since we do not have enough information from the text to conclude. Therefore, our rule grid won't help in this case. You would have had to go over the text again to see if you find any information on non-male members of the Jones family.

#75. Solving Syllogisms with Non-Venn Methods – Reading & Rephrasing

The best way to approach syllogism is to focus on relationships, instead of trying to rationalise what you are reading and who or what the items are, focus on the links between them and pay attention to key qualifying words, (see strategy #76). As these can give you important hints about relationships between items. Always read over information carefully and more than once. Sometimes it helps saying things over in your head or out loud or rephrasing them, for instance "if some dogs are cats then that means….". Think about each conclusion in turn and decide if it follows.

#76. Solving Syllogisms– Understand the Meaning of Qualifiers

There are a number of key qualifiers used in the UCAT when it comes to syllogism problems – they influence the meaning of the statement and thus

influence whether a conclusion is valid or not. Understanding the meaning of each word is crucial when dealing with syllogism:

'**ALL**' means whole quantity; 100%. E.g. "Every"

'**SOME**' means at least one and possibly all. This is the qualifier that catches most students out. For example, if a statement said "some men love going to the movies", we cannot automatically infer that there are also "some men that do not love going to the movies", rather you should interpret is as "some men love going to the movies and possibly all men love going to the movies", unless the text provides information that suggests otherwise, you cannot infer that there are men who do not like going movies.

'**NONE**' means by no amount; zero.

'**ONLY**' means no one else or nothing more besides; solely.

"**NOT ALL**" – means some but not all (i.e. at least one)

#77. Solving Syllogism – Never Make Assumptions

Making an inference involves using what is explicitly mentioned in the statement to make a logical deduction about what is not. It is possible to mistakenly make reasonable assumptions that are wrong. Only use the information presented in the text. The wording of texts give insight into the type of relationships between two items. A conclusion only follows if you are certain there is a logical process from the information in the text to that particular statement. If something is *likely* to have happened and the statement says something *must* have happened, then it does not follow.

#78. Syllogism – Know the type of Conclusions to Expect

By developing an eye for spotting the type of conclusions, you reduce the likelihood of falling for invalid statements. Let's go over the main types used and strategies to help spot them:

1. Directly stated: These are the easiest conclusions to spot as they either rephrase the given text or directly contradict it. With practice you should be able to spot them. Always read the given text at least once and deduce the direct conclusions on your own before viewing the list of statements. This way it is easier to spot them.

2. Not enough information: These are similar to 'Can't Tell' options in the verbal reasoning subtest. Examiners can include statements that you cannot confirm or deny their validity without more information. Therefore, they do not follow. These can be hard to recognise since examiners tend to include elements of truth, and without realising it you end up making an assumption. The good news is that examiners never include more than one in a series of conclusions. In most cases, not all, they tend to be the one of the last two statements, so when reading them make sure to mentally check you are not making any assumptions.

3. Inference: This is the most common type of conclusion and they vary in difficulty. They require you to determine the validity of a statement based on information not directly stated in the text. This requires a lot of practice and understanding some of the key rules of logic. A great way to help with deciphering these types is to adopt strategies like the venn method (#65), rule grid (#72) and re-reading/rephrasing (#75). If this is a real difficulty for you, then consider guessing strategies (#71). Expect statements where you have extra information outside of the text (hypothetical statements). In these cases, you have to consider the rule within the text to make an inference. However, there is a risk you may not have enough information for the statement to follow, so be aware of this.

#79. Syllogism – Beware of Examiner Tricks

Examiners can't try to trick you into making an assumption and picking the wrong answer. There are many ways they can do this when it comes to syllogism problems. Here a few helpful tips to reduce the likelihood of falling victim to them:

Read negative statements carefully: The text may provide a premise that is negative. Be sure to understand the relationship between the items and what can be inferred from the statement. Always read negative premises carefully and more than once.

Focus on qualifiers and relationships: Pay attention to what is happening between the items in a statement. The wording of a statement gives clues as to what logical process to take in order for you to make a conclusion. It helps to rephrase the text. For example, "Some students at St Johns School are not tall" can be mentally rephrased "at least one but not all student are tall".

Be careful of reverse statements and exceptions: A true statement one-way doesn't mean its valid if you reverse it. Always look out for reverse statements and evaluate the given text accordingly. Also be aware of exceptions. For example, a text might say "All boys at St Johns School are tall except Pete and John", then you may be given a conclusion that states, "some boys at St Johns are tall". This doesn't follow since we have an exception (i.e. Pete and John).

Watch out for distractors and extra information: There may be conclusions that are confusing that may need further validation. You may find yourself going back and forth to the text multiple times. Many of the times, these conclusions do not follow. Rather than spending too long to evaluate them, cut your losses, pick 'No' and move on. Extra information is often a sign that a conclusion that doesn't follow. Always double check before selecting answer, remember the text may include a rule that can be applied to select the correct answer.

#80. Interpreting Information – Identify Weakest sub-type and Practise loads

Another type of question you can expect in the DM subtest are ones where you have to interpret the meaning of data, these are usually in the form of graphs and charts. Other times they may be textual that require you to do a bit of Maths to pick the correct answer. Similar to syllogism problems, they can be drag-and-drop questions where you have to place Yes or No next to the conclusions provided. During practice identify the type of graphs or charts that confuse you and expose yourself to more data in the same format and interpret them. For example, if you struggle with interpreting scatter plots, look online for more scatter plots to decipher, if you can find Maths problems to solve, that would even be better.

#81. Interpreting Information – Start with the Title of the Graph or Chart

When analysing graphs and charts, it is important to determine quite quickly what the diagram is displaying and why such information is pertinent to the context of the question. Be aware that more than one type of graph can be used to represent a single set of data in the UCAT. Start by reading the title of the diagram before diving into specifics. The title is usually either above or below the diagram, they are brief but informative, and provides a bit of context about the data.

#82. Interpreting Information – Read the labels (X and Y axes)

Read the axes of the graphs in order to determine which type of data is being represented. The x-axis is the independent variable, or that which can be changed. The y-axis is the dependent variable, or that which depends on the independent variable. For example, on a graph of the height of rose plants during a period of six weeks, the x-axis would have the weeks, whereas the y-axis would have the height.

#83. Interpreting Information – Never overlook the Key or Legend

Look at the key, which typically is in a box next to the graph or chart. It will explain symbols and colours used in the graph or chart. It is common for students to skip this. However, it is used to identify the number of categories present in a graph. Make sure to read and understand it before reading the question.

#84. Interpreting Information – Read important Points on the Graph

Always keep an eye out for the most important points. These are peaks, lows, turning points and intersection points. At these points, take a mental note of the numbers on the x and y-axes and try to determine what they mean, use this to help in defining the general trend.

#85. Interpreting Information – Define General Trend

This builds on strategy #84. Determine the general trend of a graph or chart. Look for the bar or point with the highest and lowest peaks. For a line graph and a scatter plot, look at the slope of the line. If the line is pointing to the upper right corner, then the slope is positive. If the line is pointing to the lower right corner, then the slope is negative. Look for data points that do not seem to fit the general trend. Not all sets of data display a perfect trend. Examine such points and make a mental note. If there is one bar, dot or part of the line that is out of place, then this may not be significant enough to affect the entire conclusion.

#86. Interpreting Information – Focus on what you need to interpret

The graphs and charts in the exam will have a lot of information, after reading the question only focus on the data you need to interpret. Pay attention to words in the answer options, like "average", "maximum/minimum", "increase/decrease" and "rise/fall" that can help with selecting the most appropriate answer.

#87. Interpreting Information – Read and understand the Stem & Options

Do not go straight to the question as it is likely you have missed necessary information - you will need to return to answer the question anyway. Make sure you understand the data and stem before jumping to the answer options, thus reducing the likelihood of matching corresponding aspects that look similar. For single-option questions, make sure to also read all of the answer options before picking an appropriate answer.

#88. Interpreting Information – Validate Conclusions

Always double check the data provided supports a given statement. However, some answer options might contain partially true information, where one part seems correct, but another part is wrong. Be careful not to waste too much time trying to validate the incorrect aspect. They tend to be wrong, so depending on the question-type, either eliminate option or select No.

#89. Interpreting Information – Beware of examiner tricks

Always take note of the questions you answer incorrectly due to you falling for examiner tricks. Pay attention to question types, phrases or words that arise repeatedly in these questions. This will help you eliminate the trick answer options faster, and so you are less likely to fall for them in the live test.

#90. Interpreting Information – Practice Non-Graphical Question-types

Some interpreting information questions are textual and will consist of text-based mathematical information that will either require a calculation to reach a numerical answer or will require the interpretation of the meaning of mathematical information to select an applicable statement. I strongly recommend to practise these questions during preparation.

#91. Interpreting Information –Draw or Write out Information

It can be helpful to draw out the information for text-based questions. Some interpreting information questions are disguised as venn or logical puzzle problems. If possible, draw out information to help with solving the problem. For more on logical puzzles see strategies #50 - #63, and venn diagrams see strategies #100 - #105.

#92. Evaluating Arguments – The Basics

In the exam you'll be given a certain proposition, followed by four arguments as answer options. When you are evaluating arguments in the DM subtest, it's important to understand that you are **not picking the option that is "politically correct"; instead the goal is to select the option with the strongest argument whether you agree or not.** The key to doing well in this question type is being able to eliminate **weak arguments while setting aside your personal belief.** Before we dive into strategies, let's go over the fundamental concepts of evaluating an argument:

What is an argument?
An argument is a claim or a set of claims with reasons and evidence offered as support. An argument consists of three things:

- **Claim** - the position being argued.
- **Reason** - why the claim should be valid.

- **Evidence** - the examples, statistics or facts to back up the claim.

What makes a strong argument?

A strong argument is solely based upon reasons, facts and figures that can be proven without reasonable doubts. They tend to address all areas of the proposition and rely on little to zero assumption.

What makes a Weak argument?

Weak arguments are not backed by proven opinions or facts. Most times, the argument for a particular topic is watery, irrelevant or largely based on assumption (lacking evidence).

#93. Evaluating Arguments – Points for Analysis

You will analyse the logic of each answer option by evaluating both the use of evidence and the logical connections. When reading an argument, consider the following:

- what evidence is given?
- what logical deduction are made?
- what assumptions (likely not stated) are made?
- does the argument address all areas of the proposition?

Also evaluate the reasoning and structure of the argument. Look for transition words to show the logical connections (e.g. *however, thus, therefore, evidently, hence, in conclusion*). Then evaluate the following:

- Identify the argument's claims, reason, evidence and underlying assumptions. Evaluate their quality.
- What leaps are being made from one point of logic to another?

#94. Evaluating Arguments – Eliminate on First Reading

There are some arguments that you will be able to eliminate on the first read, they include:

- **Irrelevant arguments:** Such arguments are out of context with regard to the given proposition so you will be able to spot them easily.

- **Simple assertions:** These arguments are related to the given subject but do not give any evidence/reason to believe it. In other words, they are neither strongly favourable nor strongly against the given statement.

- **Vague/ambiguous arguments:** As the name says itself, these arguments are unclear and do not state the evidence explicitly. Even if the argument is contextual, you are unable to extract a clear meaning/message from this kind of argument.

#95. Evaluating Arguments – Use the FEARS mnemonic (Strength Analysis)

When evaluating an argument, a good mnemonic which you can use as a checklist to help determine its strength is FEARS, which stands: **Factual**, **Entirety**, **Assumption**, **Relevancy** and **Sensible**, see explanations below:

- **Factual** – is the argument based on facts rather than opinion? Strong arguments use facts or statistics to back claims.

- **Entirety** – is the argument addressing the whole question, not only one aspect of it? Strong arguments address all areas of the statement.

- **Assumption** - is the evidence based on assumptions? Strong arguments use zero to little assumptions.

- **Relevancy** – is the argument directly addressing the statement? Strong arguments directly address the proposition

- **Sensible** – is the argument generally sensible and reasonable to deduce? Strong arguments make sense and are sensible deductions.

With enough practice, this will become second nature. However, when you are torn between two statements, mentally going through the acronym can prove helpful in comparing and picking the right answer.

#96. Venn Diagrams – Brush up on the Basics

A Venn diagram is a diagram that shows all possible logical relations between a finite collection of different sets. In the Decision-Making subtest you may be presented with the following question-types:

- **Type 1**: These are questions where you are given a passage which you can interpret into a venn diagram.

- **Type 2**: These are questions that can be solved by drawing a venn diagram.

- **Type 3**: These are questions where you are provided with a set of statements and set of different venn diagrams in which you pick the venn that best represents them.

During practice, identify rusty areas and work on them, start simple then work up to complex problems. Use the below bullet points as a guide during additional study (source: AQA GCSE Maths Specification):

- Construct a Venn diagram to classify outcomes and calculate probabilities. Use set notation to describe a set of numbers or objects.

- Construct Venn Diagrams from information given and extract information from a Venn Diagram. E.g. In a survey of 30 students, 15 have a dog and 23 have a cat. How many have both, if 4 students do not have either?

- Construct Venn diagrams to solve more complex probability problems (where the structure for diagrams may not be given).

#97. Venn Diagrams - Develop an Approach for each question-type

We discussed the types of venn questions you can expect in the Decision Making subtest in strategy #96. Be sure to develop and hone your approach for dealing with each question-type. Also pay attention to the number of diagrams and variables in a problem, some questions may have two, others may have three. It's Important to recognise if this influences your ability to solve the problem correctly and on time. Here are some great tips to ensure you pick an approach that improves both accuracy and speed:

- **Read questions carefully:** Pay close attention to wording and what is being asked in the question.
- **Use shortcuts when possible**: Only do as much working out as you need.
- **Always review all answer options before picking answer**
- **Don't get overwhelmed by problems with a lot of information**: You may not need all the information that is provided in the question.

#98. Probabilistic Reasoning – Brush up on Core Concepts

Probability is the study of how likely things are to happen. We express probabilities either as fractions, decimals, or percentages. This is because they always fall between 0 and 1, where 0 represents total impossibility and 1 represents total certainty. In the Decision Making subtest, you will be typically given a scenario and a question to validate, you will be given four answer options. Two of the options will agree with the question and offer an explanation as to why they agree. The other two will disagree and have an explanation. Thus, you need to pick the correct response to the question and why it is the correct response.

During practice identify areas you need to refresh on, start simple then work up to complex problems, use the below bullet points as a guide during additional study (Source: AQA GCSE Maths Specification):

- Record, describe and analyse the frequency of outcomes of probability experiments using tables and frequency trees.

- Apply ideas of randomness, fairness and equally likely events to calculate expected outcomes of multiple future experiments.

- Relate relative expected frequencies to theoretical probability using appropriate language and the 0 to 1 probability scale.

- Apply the property that the probabilities of an exhaustive set of outcomes sum to 1

- Apply the property that the probabilities of an exhaustive set of mutually exclusive events sum to 1

- Construct theoretical possibility spaces for single and combined experiments with equally likely outcomes and use these to calculate theoretical probabilities

- Calculate the probability of independent and dependent combined events, including the use of tree diagrams and other representations, while understanding the underlying assumptions.

#99. Probabilistic Reasoning - Develop an Approach

Having a systematic approach to solving probability questions in the exam can be very effective. When presented with a problem, make sure to read the stem and question quickly. If possible, try to answer the question in your head before looking at the answer options. If necessary, draw out a table or diagram during calculations. Once you have decided whether you are picking Yes or No, review the options, keep in mind that just because an answer is true doesn't mean it is relevant (therefore it might be wrong due to lack of relevancy). Here are some great tips to ensure you pick an approach that improves both accuracy and speed:

- **Read Stem and Questions carefully**
- **Pay close attention to proportion and order during calculations**
- **Always read all answer choices before picking answer:** it is important to note that just because an option is true, doesn't mean it is relevant.
- **Master the elimination strategy:** Narrow down choices by recognising incorrect statements
- **Keep an eye out for common examiner tricks**

Additional Strategies

Have a Timing contingency plan (see Strategy #48)

Have a Question Triage Strategy (See Strategy #47)

Have a Flagging Strategy (See Strategy #41)

Use Keyboard Shortcuts (See Strategy #42)

QUANTITATIVE REASONING

TIPS, TACTICS AND STRATEGIES TO IMPROVE YOUR UCAT QUANTITATIVE REASONING SCORE

#100. Take note of the Question Length and Approach Accordingly

You may have noticed that questions in the QR subtest come in different formats – text, tabular or graphical. Before test day, develop a systematic approach to answering each type. How you approach graphical questions will most likely be different from how you approach text questions. So, you want to make sure you develop an approach for each type before test day. For example; for short text questions you may want to read the stem before reading the question. However, for long text questions you may want to read the question before the stem, so you know what information to focus on. During prep have an approach for each question format in the exam (use the table below as a guide):

Format	Types	Definitions
Text	Short Text	These are text problems that are less than 200 words
	Long Text	These are text problems longer than 200 words
Tabular	Simple or Familiar	These are simple tables, with 2 or less variables
	Complex/ Multiple/Unfamiliar	These are tables with more than 2 variables or tables that you are unfamiliar with.
Graphs	Familiar	These are graphs that you are familiar with
	Unfamiliar / Complex	These are graph problems that you are not familiar with.

#101. Memorise the Formulas for Commonly Tested Concepts

Understanding and applying certain numerical concepts is required in the QR subtest. It helps having a handful of useful formulas at your fingertips that you can apply to answer some problems quickly and accurately. Here are some of the most commonly tested topics in the exam. Try to memorise and practice some formulas to save time:

- Calculating averages
- Calculating speed, distance and time
- Proportions and ratios
- Percentages and percentage change
- Income tax
- Percentage change
- Basic geometry - area, perimeter, circumference and volume of 3D shapes.

#102. Practice Reading Graphical and Statistical Data

There are a lot of graphs, charts, and tables that will be covered on the test. You should practise analysing one-variable data in bar graphs, histograms and line graphs—as well as two-variable data in scatter plots and two-way tables. In other words, **you should be fluent in reading these various representations of data.** You should be able to describe overall patterns, identify positive and negative trends and finally be able to distinguish between linear and exponential growth. Statistical data crosses over with graphical analysis and also explores concepts in averages such as mean, median and mode. In the UCAT, you can expect to interpret charts and graphs to extract the mean, median or mode from a set of statistical data, then be required to use figures in some capacity to solve a problem.

Examiners want to know that you understand maths thoroughly enough to use it in real-world settings and be able to draw conclusions about what they imply. All questions in the subtest are in real-world scenarios and can be in textual, tabular or graphical form.

#103. Master solving Linear and Exponential Model Problems

At GCSE level you may have been familiar with functions such as **linear, quadratic and exponential**. These mathematical models form the basis of UCAT quantitative reasoning questions, and this can either be in the form of text, table or graph. You should practise analysing and drawing conclusions with regards to the above functions. In the UCAT, problems will typically follow the linear or exponential model:

Linear Model

A good example of linear growth is **simple interest**. This is where you earn interest on your principal, each period, but not on any interest that has been added since that first deposit. This is modelled by the function: A=P(1+rt). P is the principal, *r* is the interest rate, and *t* is the amount of time interest has been accruing. I strongly recommend **learning this formula by heart as it can help save some time on problems that follow a linear model**.

Exponential Model

An important example of exponential growth is **compound interest**. This is where you earn interest on the interest you've previously earned. This is modelled by the function: $A = P(1 + \frac{r}{n})^{nt}$, where P is the principal, r is the interest rate (typically annual), n is the number of times the interest compounds per period (typically a year), and t is the amount of time that has passed since the principal began accruing interest. I strongly recommend **learning this formula by heart as it can help save some time when you spot an exponential problem.** However, be sure to read questions carefully when dealing with exponential problems. For example, the stated rate of change may not be the same as the rate of change over time.

This is typical of compound interest: You might take a loan at 9%, but if it compounds monthly, you're really taking a loan at $A = P(1 + \frac{0.09}{12})^{12} - 1 = 9.38\%$ at the end of the year. On the other hand, you might make a deposit that accrues interest at a rate of 5%, but if it compounds quarterly, so you're really getting $A = P(1 + \frac{0.05}{4})^4 - 1 = 5.095\%$ at the end of the year.

Both models can come in any form - popular examples include taxes, money and rate, schedules and train time. You are expected to be able to work through problems mathematically by recognising the model you need to solve them. You should always consider the units involved, if there happens to be a shift of units (from feet to miles, or minutes to seconds), you should account for that as you calculate. Always keep track of the practical meaning of variables (e.g. income, price, speed, distance, weight, etc.). You're going to be analysing real values with variables so don't forget what each variable represents and be sure you understand how a change in one variable or quantity affects another.

#104. Skim Questions Intelligently

This builds on strategy #100, depending on your approach, it may be good idea to skim through the question quickly to understand the 'type' of data included before reading in-depth and assimilating the entire data provided. So that when you read the question, you will be able to quickly determine where to find the relevant data you need to answer it. This approach will save you more time in the exam. With enough practice, you will be able to skim and draw out information very quickly under time pressure. Make sure to do the following during skimming:

- **Focus on the relevant information** – begin by narrowing down only the information you need, and then briefly skim through the data while ignoring the redundant details.
- **Pay attention to the units** – the question may refer to units that are different to those presented in the table/graph.
- **Notice any additional information** – such information can be provided in the headline, under the table/graph, or in an asterisk.

#105. Eyeballing - Inspect & Estimate whenever possible

You will be surprised by the amount of questions in the test you can answer correctly by eyeballing i.e. looking at data and answer options without any calculations. This approach will save you a lot of time in the exam, I recommend this approach for **problems that require one step calculations**. For example, if the answer options are close together in value you may be more suitable to work precisely to figure out the exact answer. However, if there is a large difference between the options, it may be suitable to use eyeballing and estimation to pick the correct answer. Estimating is great to use when there a huge difference in the answer options or they are well spaced out. For example, if the answers are to the nearest thousands, and the data is given to the nearest ten, you can round the data to the nearest hundred. Another great time to estimate is to look for trigger words like 'approximate' or 'estimate' in the question. In order to sharpen your estimation skills, try to practice solving several questions without performing the complete calculation and instead look for shortcuts and rely on estimations. Through practice, using these techniques will gradually become more and more natural.

Eyeballing doesn't necessarily mean doing no calculations, rather you do fewer calculations by inspecting and estimating when possible.

#106. Problem-Solving: Adopting the Six-Step Framework in the Exam

The six-step framework provides a good basis that can be used to solve a majority of problems in the QR subtest, it is as follows:

Step 1: What is the question format?

This builds on strategy #100 where you recognise the length of the question and act appropriately. You may choose to either deploy triage or attempt the problem.

Step 2: What Information is provided?

Skim question and take note of key numbers and variables. You must pay attention to the units and other metrics that could influence final answer.

Step 3: What Information do I need?

Decide which bits of information are useful. Start to think about which type of maths might be used to solve the problem. Also think about the form the answer will take. Is it asking for money, time or distance for example? Does the answer have to be a whole number? Will the answer have any units?

Step 4: What Information don't I need?

It is important to decide as quickly as possible if there is any information which does not need to be taken into account when working out the answer

Step 5: What maths can I do?

This is where you begin to tackle the problem. Look for a way into the problem. For example, if there is a percentage or ratio included, this is usually a good place to start. Some problems might require multiple topics to solve them, keep an eye of for this as well.

Step 6: Is my solution correct?

There are checks that should always be done after arriving to a solution. Think about whether your answer seems reasonable. Is it possible to check the answer you got? Small errors can lead to incorrect answers. Check any working out, even if it was done on a calculator. Can you check the answer backwards too? Work backwards and see whether the answer agrees with what you were told in the question. For example, in a question on ratio, the total amount is given at the start. Check that any answers add up to this total amount. Check no answers have been rounded until the very end as rounding too early can lead to the final answers being incorrect.

#107. Convert Problems into Algebraic Equations

There are some word problems in the UCAT where it may be easier to translate into algebraic equations to solve them. This approach will make the questions clearer to solve especially when you are dealing with problems that require two or more calculation steps.

Monica is a scientist studying the production of antibodies by two white blood cells. She noticed that Type A cell produced 20% more antibodies than Type B cell. Based on Monica's observation, if Type A cell produced 144 antibodies, how many did the Type B cell produced?

A. 118

B. 120

C. 129

D. 163

Let's try to think about this problem in terms of x. If type A produced 20% more antibodies than type B, we can write this as an expression:

x + 0.2x = Number of antibodies produced by type A ; thus

1.2x = Number of antibodies produced by type A

where, **x is the number of antibodies produced by type B cells**.

The problem tells us that Type A produced 144 antibodies. Since we know that 1.2x is equal to the number of antibodies produced by Type A, we can write the following equation:

1.2x = 144

Now, all we have to do is divide both sides by 1.2 to find the number of antibodies produced by type B cells.

$x = 144/1.2 \longrightarrow x = 120$ (option B)

#108. P.I.N method – Plug in Answer Options

Sometimes you may find yourself confronted with a problem that you may think will take too long to solve. And other times, you may be given so many different variables in a single problem that you want to make absolutely sure you have the correct solution. When this happens, starting from the answer options can often help get you to the right answer quicker. The basic idea of plugging in numbers (P.I.N) is that you use the answer options in place of variables or unknowns in your problem. **This technique works well when dealing with word problems in which you are presented with several variables and can create an equation to solve it**. If you have managed to rule out some of the options through logical deductions, then hopefully you will only have to plug in a few of the options. Never systematically work through the options, start with the option that you instinctively think might be correct, then proceed to you next best guess. In the word problem in strategy #107, you could have eyeballed the options and used common sense to eliminate option A and option D, then input both 120 and 129 as x into the equation "1.2x = 144" to see if either balances the equation.

#109. Even and Odd Arithmetic Rules (Elimination Strategy)

An odd number is a number that is not a multiple of two, and an even number is an integer that is a multiple of two. In the UCAT, the key to tackling certain problem quickly could lie in recalling a few logical facts about even/odd integers, here are some of them:An **even number** can only be formed by the sum of either 2 odd numbers (odd + odd = even), or 2 even numbers (even + even = even).

- An **odd number** can only be formed by the sum of an odd and even number (odd + even = odd, or even + odd = odd).
- An **even number** can only be formed by multiplication in three ways: even·odd, odd·even, and even·even.
- An **odd number** can only be formed by multiplication in one way: odd·odd = odd.

even	+	even	=	even
odd	+	odd	=	even
odd	+	even	=	odd
even	−	even	=	even
odd	−	odd	=	even
even	−	odd	=	odd
odd	−	even	=	odd
even	x	even	=	even
odd	x	odd	=	odd
odd	x	even	=	even

You can save some valuable time in the exam by using this logic to eliminate answer options based on them being odd or even numbers. With a problem in the exam where the final calculation requires you to multiply two odd numbers, you can immediately eliminate any even number in the answer options **since multiplying an odd number by another odd number will always result to an odd number**. This can be applied to when adding or subtracting numbers during calculation in the exam.

This strategy can also be used as an eyeballing technique when you know the numbers you are working with and how you intend to arrive at answer.

#110. Recognise Easy, Medium & Hard Questions

The main difficulty in the QR section is timing, you have on average 40 seconds to find the answer to each question. Given that the exam is sprinkled with questions of varying levels of difficulty, practice developing an eye for recognising easy, medium and hard questions. It does require some practice to identify at a glance whether a question is easy or not. However, with enough practice it will become second nature. Use this strategy to deploy question triage. One triage strategy is to go through questions systematically but pick out the easy ones to ensure that they get done accurately. Once you have done the easier questions, then go back to the medium/hard questions and address them until you run out of time.

Easy/Simple	One-step calculations or questions that can be solved by eyeballing.
Medium	Two-step calculations or questions that can be solved quickly by using a bit of logic and elimination.
Hard/Complex	Multi-step calculations that are time consuming, or questions that include a lot of text/data to read

#111. Give yourself time limits (based on the Difficulty of the Question)

It is important that you maintain a good pace in this section. A great strategy is to give yourself time limits based on the question's level of difficulty. One strategy is to aim to complete easy questions in 15 – 20 seconds, medium questions in 30- 40 seconds and hard questions in 40-60 seconds. The idea is that by spending less time on the easy questions, you can spend a little longer on the more difficult ones. Force yourself to move onto another question once you have overstepped the target time allocated. In cases where you have completed the calculation and didn't arrive to any of the answer options, make an educated guess and move on. DO NOT re-solve!

#112. Set time markers to monitor Pace

A great strategy to monitor your time is to give yourself time markers to help determine whether you are on track to finish or not. For example, you should have done the 18th question in the first 12 minutes. If you are behind, then you make a conscious effort to speed things up. Avoid monitoring how long you spend on each individual question. This is a waste of time as you will lose valuable time looking at the timer, plus some questions will be easier than others and therefore take less time. Here is a rough time marker guide you can use for the QR subtest (I have included a time margin to allow for time to review flagged questions):

Question No.	Time (minutes into test)
Question 9	6 minutes
Question 18	10 minutes
Question 27	17 minutes

#113. Percentages: Income Tax, Tariff and VAT

I strongly recommend doing additional practice solving tax problems. They are very common in the UCAT. Spending extra time on this concept will build on your ability to solve percentage change problems quicker. You will be able to digest data more easily and reach solutions quickly. For example, you could be given a banding table showing the total tax paid on annual taxable income and be asked to calculate the income tax of a person on a given income. Trickier questions might ask you to work out what percentage of their taxable income a person pays in tax. Alternatively, you may be given the amount of tax paid and be asked to work out a person's income. The same reasoning applies to VAT/tariff questions where you may be required to calculate the VAT or work out the original cost of goods. Expect hard questions that require multiple steps to arrive at final answer.

#114. Percentages: Simple Interest & Compound Interest

This builds on strategy #102 where you gain familiarity with linear and exponential functions. In the UCAT, questions can take any form, expect to calculate interest or work out new balance over a given time period. Other money questions that follow the same reasoning include borrowing, savings, investing, appreciation and depreciation.

#115. Percentage Change: Revenue & Discounts

Get comfortable solving percentage change in the context of profits and loss, as well as reductions/increments on the price of goods and services. Expect these calculations in tax problems (#113) and interest (#114) as well. Remember when calculating percentage change it is the amount something has changed as a percentage of its original value; thus the formula goes as follows:

$$P.C = \frac{finalvalue - initalvalue}{intialvalue} X100$$

Alternatively,

$$P.C = \left(\frac{Finalvalue}{Intialvalue} - 1\right) X100$$

Never divide by the new value (i.e. final value), when calculating percentage change, you always divide by the old or initial value. It is important to remember the above formula as it won't be provided in the exam.

#116. Percentages: When Appropriate use Equations to set up calculations

Practice creating linear equations to solve percentage problems in the UCAT. This can prove beneficial when you are dealing with questions that present multiple data that relate to each other.

Example: What is 35% of 80

X = 0.35 x 80

Example: 15% of what number is 4

0.15x = 4

Example: What percent of 350 is 70

$$\frac{x(350)}{100} = 70$$

Example: A pair of trousers has been reduced by 40% and now costs £50. How much did it cost originally?

0.6x = 50

Example: A new car is bought for $50,000. Every year it depreciates by 12.5%. Calculate how much it is worth after two years.

$x = 0.875^2 (50{,}000)$

#117. Percentages: Mental Shortcuts to Finding Percentages (Easy)

It is helpful to get into the habit of doing calculations mentally without the use of a calculator. There are some shortcuts you can use to **finding percentages** in one-step that can help on test day. Here are key concepts to practise:

Finding 100%

To calculate 100% of a number, it stays the same - nothing changes. For example: 100% of £160 is £160.

Finding 50%

To calculate 50% of a number, find half (i.e. divide by 2). For example: 50% of £160 is £80.

Finding 25%

To calculate 25% of a number, find half (50%) then half of that. For example: 25% of £160 is £40. (i.e. divide by 4).

Finding 10%

To calculate 10% of a number, you move the decimal point 1 position to the left. For example: 10% of 160 is £16 (i.e. divide by 10)

Finding 1%

To calculate 1% of a number, you move the decimal point 2 positions to the left. For example: 1% of 160 is £1.60 (i.e. divide by 100)

#118. Percentages: Mental Shortcuts to Finding Percentages (Intermediate)

This builds on strategy #117, where you have to mentally calculate percentages for numbers that are not so straightforward and may require two-step calculations. Here are some key concepts you should practise:

Finding 75%

Find half. Then half of that. Then add them together.

Why? Because half = 50%, half of that is 25%. Adding them together gives: **50% + 25% = 75%.** For example, 75% of £24 is £18 (i.e £12 + £6)

Finding 5%

Find 10% then halve it.

Why? Because dividing by 10 is the same as finding a tenth, which happens to be 10%. Half of 10% is 5%.

For example: 5% of £50 = £2.50 (10% of 50 is 5. Now halve it to get 2.5).

Finding 20%

Find 10% then double it.

Why? Because dividing by 10 gives you a tenth, which is 10%. Doubling 10% gives you 20%.

For example: 20% of £9 = £1.80 (10% of 9 is 0.9. Now double it to get 1.8).

#119. Percentages: Mental Shortcut to Finding Percentages (Advanced)

You have now covered both easy (#117) and Intermediate (#118) shortcuts to finding percentages. Build on them and practice more difficult percentage changes (expect these harder calculations in the exam). See examples below:

Finding 21%

Find 20% then add 1%

For example: 21% of 240 = (48 + 2.4) = 50.4

Finding 42%

Find 40% then add 2%

For example: 42% of £48 = (19.2 + 0.96) = £20.16

Finding 93%

Find 90% then add 3%

For example: 93% of 55 = [(55-5.5) + 1.65] = 49.5 +1.65 = 51.15

Finding 56%

Find 60% then minus 4%

For example: 56% of 112 = [(11.2 x6) − (4 x 1.12)] = 67.2- 4.48 = 62.72

Alternatively, you can find 50% and add 5% and 1% (56+ 5.6 +1.12)

Finding 37%

Find 40% then minus 3%

For example: 37% of $47 = [(4.7 x4) − (3 x 0.47)] = 18.8 − 1.41 = $17.39

Alternatively, you can find 30% and add 5% and 2%

#120. Fast Mental Trick to Save a ton of time when calculating Percentages.

Finding percentages can be calculated mentally a lot quicker with the multiplication method Use this trick to work through easy percentage calculations. Here are some examples:

Example: 30% of 50

If you adopt the reasoning in strategies #117 and #118 then you could solve this problem by finding 10% and tripling it which is 15. Good! However, you can solve this a lot quicker with basic multiplication. At school you were most likely taught the following in order to solve the above problem:

$$\frac{30}{100} x \ 50 = 15$$

Where the zeros cancel each other out and you end up with 3 x 5, which is

equal to 15. **When dealing with percentages that are multiples of 10 (e.g. 10%, 20%, 30% and so on) you can use simply cancel out the zeros and multiply them together.** Let's look at some examples:

40% of 120
4 x 12 = 48

20% of 80
2 x 8= 16

60% of 180
6 x 18 = 108

You can use the same reasoning when calculating percentages for numbers **without a zero on the end.**

30% of 34
3 x 3.4 = 10.2

70% of 63
7 x 6.3 = 44.1

#121. Percentages: Practice using Mental maths in Multi-step problems

You will find that percentage change questions in the UCAT are usually 3-4 step calculations. Therefore, using the mental shortcuts could prove beneficial and save you a bit of time. Let's look at a percentage change problem:

Annual Taxable Income Bracket	Tax Rate
£0 – £8,950	10%
£8,950 – £35,950	15%
£35,950 -£85,950	25%
£85,950 - £125,950	28.5%

Sandra has an annual income of £28,950. What is her income after tax, to the nearest £?

A.   £21,712

B.   £23,341

C.   £25,055

D.   £24,240

Step 1 - Mental calculation (subtraction)
28,950 – 8,950 = 20,000

Step 2 – Mental shortcut (see strategy #117)
15% of 20,000 = (2000+ 1000) = £3000

Step 3 – Mental calculation (addition)
3000 + 895 (10% of 8950) = £3895

Step 4 – Use onscreen calculator
28950 – 3895 = £25,055

Work through percentage questions in UCAT books and online courses and force yourself to some of the calculation steps mentally without a calculator.

When solving multiple-step calculations, keep track of your reasoning by writing down the solution to one of the steps on a piece of paper. In the live

#122. Percentages: Using Onscreen Calculator (Beginner, No Function)

A simple onscreen calculator will be made available to use in the quantitative reasoning subtest. If used correctly can save time in the exam. A great strategy when using the onscreen calculator is to **use shortcuts and minimise the maths when possible**. For example, if you need to work out the new price of a £3.00 item at 20% discount, it is quicker to calculate 80% of £3, rather than calculating 20% then taking that number away from £3. You are essentially reducing the number of steps to solve the problem – this is an example of the multiplier method and it helpful when inputting digits in

the calculator. Use the onscreen calculator to work through the following examples:

Example: Monica invests £134 into her savings account with interest paid at 1.9% per annum into the same account. Calculate her new balance after 12 months.

Solution:

Monica's bank balance will be increased by 1.9%

Therefore, the new balance is 101.9% of the initial amount (100% + 1.9%) thus, the multiplier is 1.019.

New balance: 134 x 1.019 = £136.54 *(input [134 x 1.019] in calculator)*

Example: All Game consoles are reduced by 40% on Christmas Eve and then a further 20% on Boxing Day. Play Station consoles usually cost £140. What is the percentage discount on price on Boxing Day?

Solution:

Christmas Eve: The sale price of the console is reduced by 40%, so the reduced price is therefore 60% of the original amount = 0.6 x 140 = 84
(Remember: you can use the mental maths trick in strategy #120 – where 60% of 140 = 6 x 14 = 84)

Boxing Day: The console has a further 20% discount that's therefore 80% of £84 = 8 x 8.4 = £67.20 [type in 8 x 8.4 in calculator]

Percentage discount = $\frac{67.20 - 140}{140}$ x 100 = -52 (therefore 52% discount)

Example: An electrical retail company pays \$100 for a blender. During a summer sale, the company offers a 20% discount on the normal marked price of the product. The company is still making a 10% profit during the sale. What is the marked price before the discount is applied?

Solution:

Find out what the sale price of the blender is to make 10% profit for the company:

10% profit = 10% of 100, that is 1.10 x \$100

Sale price = \$110 *(easily solved with mental maths)*

The sale price of the blender was the original amount which has been reduced by 20%. We can construct an algebraic equation (strategy #107).

0.8x = \$110

Where *x* is the marked price before discount

Therefore, x = 110/0.8 = \$137.50 *[input 110 ÷ 0.8 in calculator]*

The key thing to take from this is that you shouldn't be too reliant on the onscreen calculator, use mental maths when possible.

#123. Percentages: Using Onscreen Calculator (Intermediate, using the Percentage Function)

The key to inprinting functions on the UCAT calculator is that you have to work from **right to left.** Let's see some examples to explain before looking at a UCAT problem.

Example: 22.5% of 1575

[You could work it out mentally by doubling 10% (157.5 x 2) then adding 2.5% (15.75 x 2.5)] – but for most students this will be time consuming.

Instead you could use the percentage function on the onscreen calculator. Always start from **right to left, where the percentage button is the last function used**, see below:

Step 1 - Type in **1575**
Step 2- Press the **multiply function** button (x)
Step 3 – Type **22.5** then press the **percentage** function button (%) – screen will change to 0.225.
Step 4 – Press **equal** button (=)
Answer (displayed on screen) = 354.375

Let's look at another example, try to do this one with the onscreen calculator simulator on the blog, visit www.themedicblog.co.uk/ucat-calculator:

Example: 15.8% of 1674

Step 1- Type in **1674**
Step 2 – Press **multiply function** button (x)
Step 3 – Type **15.8**, then press the **percentage** function button (%) – screen will change to 0.158
Step 4 – Press **equal** button (=)
Answer = 264.49

Now let's look at a few percentage problems and use the percentage function to solve them. Try to solve them on your own using only the onscreen calculator before looking at the solution.

A London Deli offers 30% off their baguettes after 3pm. A chicken baguette originally costs £3.50, a ham baguette costs £2.50 and a falafel baguette costs £4. Customers have the option to double up for an additional £1.

Question 1: If a customer bought a falafel baguette at 4.30pm, how much would it cost?

A. £1.85

B. £3.25

C. £2.40

D. £2.80

Solution:

Simplify question - since its after 4pm customer will get 30% off. The questions can be simply paraphrased as '70% of £4.00'.

Step 1 - Type in **4**

Step 2 - Press the **multiply function** button (x)

Step 3 – Type **70** then press the **percentage** function button (%) – <u>screen will change to 0.7000000</u>.

Step 4 – Press **equal** button (=)

Answer (displayed on screen) = 2.8000000 (£2.80)

Question 2: *If a customer bought a falafel baguette at 2pm and a double chicken baguette at 5.15pm, how much did the customer spend on the day?*

    A.   *£7.15*

    B.   *£6.95*

    C.   *£7.35*

    D.   *£8.00*

Solution:

Simplify the question by paraphrasing it mentally:

Total spend = Normal price of Falafel + 30% off double chicken

Total Spent = £4 + [70% x (£4.50)]

Working from right to left:

Step 1 – Type in **4.50**

Step 2 – Press **multiply function** button (x)

Step 3 – Type 70 then press the percentage function (%) – <u>screen will change to 0.7000000</u>

Step 4 – Press Equal button (Answer = 3.15)

Step 5 – Press the **addition function** (+) then press 4

 Step 7 - Press equal button (=)

Answer (displayed on screen) = <u>7.15</u>

Important tip: *it will become apparent later why I'm explaining the percentage function, however it may be more time efficient in the exam to skip step 1 to step 3 (i.e. using the percentage function) and simply **multiply 0.7 by 4.5** to get 70% of £4.5. We have:*

Step 1 – Type in **4.50**
Step 2 – Press **multiply button** (x), then type 0.70
Step 3 – Press Equal button (Answer = 3.15)
Step 4 – Press the **addition button** (+), then **press 4**
Step 5 - Press equal button (=)
Answer (displayed on screen) = <u>7.15</u>

The percentage function is great to use when you have difficult **percentage problems (like percentages with a decimal point)** or when you have **many percentages to calculate in a single problem**:

Question 3 : *One of the falafel baguettes was reduced by 20% of its original price as it had been out all morning. A customer buys it at 2.00 pm and came back to return it at 4.30 pm because it didn't taste right. The deli apologised and offered him another baguette with an extra 22.5% discount. The customer buys the double falafel baguette instead and store refunds the difference. How much does he get back?*

    A.   *40p*

    B.   *49p*

    C.   *82p*

    D.   *55p*

Solution:

Sale 1: 80% of normal falafel baguette
Sale 2: 77.5% of (70% of price of double falafel)

Start with sales 2 as it looks more complicated:
Step 1 – Type in **5** (price of double falafel)
Step 2 – Press **multiply function** button (x) then type 0.7
Step 3 – Press **Equal button** (Answer = 3.5)
Step 4 – Press **multiply function** button (x)

Step 5 – Type **77.5,** then press the **percentage** function button

Step 6 - Press equal button (=)

Answer (displayed on screen) = 2.71 (jot it down on whiteboard)

Sale 1 can be deduced by mental maths by finding 80%: of normal falafel price (i.e. 100% - 20%) $\rightarrow$ 4 – (2 x 0.4) = 3.20

Difference = 3.20 – 2.71 = 0.49

#124. Percentages: Using Onscreen Calculator (Advanced; Using the Memory Function)

The onscreen calculator has four main functions. It has a percentage function (which we've discussed – strategy #123), memory function, square root function and the positive/negative function. The memory function is another helpful function when dealing with percentages. It allows you save a number temporarily which is useful for problems that have multiple steps. When you press "**M+**" – short for Memory Sum – the calculator will save the number currently on the screen. This memory lasts while you perform other functions, and even if you press "ON/C" – short for "ON or Clear" button to start a new calculation. To erase the memory without affecting the current calculation, press 'M-' button then the "MRC" button.

Storing a number

To store a number on screen for later use in calculations, hit "M+". An M will appear to the left of the display to show that an answer's been stored. The Memory Sum (M+) also adds to memory register tally (see below). See an example below:

5	Tally = 5
5　4	Tally = 9
5　4　3	Tally = 12

Using a stored number

To display the number saved in memory, press "MRC". Pressing this button once recalls the number. After recalling a number, you can perform any regular operation on it. You can also recall a number mid-operation, such entering "2 + MRC =." Note that until you store a new value, the memory continues to keep its original value even after recall.

Modifying the memory

You can perform simple operations on a stored number without recalling it by using the "M+" and "M-" keys. Press "M+" to add the displayed value to the existing number in memory. Press "M-" to subtract the displayed value from the number in memory. To subtract in the opposite direction, recall the memory first, subtract with the regular minus key and then store the result. You can also press "M-" without anything in memory to store the negative of the currently displayed number. Take a look at the examples provided, try to solve them using the memory function before looking at the solution.

Example: What is the sum of 10% of £2.45, 20% of £5.67 and 12.9% of £4.87?

Solution:

You could easily just use the multiplication function on the calculator and jot down each percentage change before adding them up . However, it is time efficient to use the memory function. Think of the memory **function as an alternative way to write down a number you may need later**.

Tip: start with the complicated calculation: in this case would be 12.9% of £4.87

Step 1 – Type in **4.87**
Step 2 – Press **multiply function** button (x)
Step 3 – Type **12.9,** then press the percentage function (%) – <u>screen will change to 0.129</u>
Step 4 – Press Equal button (Answer = 0.6282300)
Step 5 – Press **M+** (this will add 0.62832300 to the memory; M will appear on the left)
Step 6 – Type 5.67
Step 7 – Press multiply button (x), then 0.2 then equal (=)

Step 8 – Press **M+** (this will add 1.134 to memory register)

Step 9 - Type 2.45

Step 10 - Press **multiply function** button (x), then 0.1 then equal (=)

Step 11 - Press **M+** (this will add 0.245 to memory register)

Step 12 - Press **MRC** (to recall register total = 2.0072300)

Example: What is 33.5% of £5.40 deduct 5.8% of £4.80?

Solution

Step 1 – Solve 33.5% of 5.40

Type **5.40** then **multiply** function button (x) then **33.5** then the **percentage function** button and **equal** button.

Step 2 – Add answer to memory

Press **M+** button to the save number on screen to memory register. M should appear on the left of the screen.

Step 3 – Solve 5.8% of 4

Clear screen (pressing the ON/C button) to avoid confusion. Type **4** then **multiply** function button (x) then **5.8** then the **percentage function** button and **equal** button.

Step 4 – Deduct answer from memory register

Press **M-** button to deduct the number on screen from memory register.

Step 5 – Recall Memory Register

Press **MRC** button to recall the number in the memory register. **Remember that pressing M- then MRC will clear the memory so after step 4 press the ON/C button to clear screen before pressing MRC to recall memory register).**

Answer (displayed on screen) = 1.53 (Rounded up to 2 decimal place)

Example: A customer buys the following items from the supermarket: 3 toothpastes (£1.00 each), 2 toothbrushes (£1.50 each) and 2 reduced shower gels (30% OFF original price of £2.99). He later comes back to return one of the shower gels. How much did he spend on the day?

From the problem you can deduce that we need to deduct 1 of the reduced shower gels from the total spend. Thus, it makes sense to start with the total spent on shower gels.

Step 1 – Calculate total spent on 1 shower gel.
Type **2.99,** then **multiply** button then **0.7** then **equal** button.

Step 2 – Save total spent on 1 shower gel in memory (because we will come back to it later to deduct it)
Press **M+** button to the save the number on screen to the memory register. M should appear on the left of the screen.

Step 3 – calculate amount spent on 2 shower gels
This will be the number on screen (price of 1 shower gel) multiplied by 2 therefore: **multiply** button, then **2** then **equal** button.

Step 4 – Add remaining items
We can use a bit of mental maths when adding the remaining items:
Number on screen (4.186) + 6 then **equal**

Step 5 – Deduct price of 1 shower gel
Number on screen (10.186) **minus** the number in memory (Press **MRC**) then **equal**

Answer (displayed on screen) = £8.09 (rounded)

#125. Know when to use the onscreen calculator versus mental maths

Don't use the UCAT calculator for simple maths that would be quicker to solve mentally Not only is it simpler to solve things like (4x5)or (2400/2) without going through the calculator, but it also cuts down on entry errors (i.e. accidentally typing in 2400/3) that could affect your answer. Learn mental maths tricks to work out things like (548 + 346) or (23 x 45) instantly.
 Be careful not to rely too heavily on the onscreen calculator. For instance, say you had a complicated question that required three steps of calculation to derive the answer. I would recommend only using the calculator for one of the three calculation steps if you can. You can lose time inputting numbers on the calculator, so limit its use during practice.

313

#126. Percentages: Build yourself up during practice

The level of maths required in the percentage problems is relatively simple – they just require multiple steps, and when you add the time pressure it can feel difficult. Practice as much as you can, If you feel rusty on a topic start with 1-step problems then work your way up to 3 step problems. Additionally, build your mental maths skill and onscreen calculator skills. Many of the questions are of similar nature, so recognise difficulties that you encounter in reasoning as you build your skills up.

#127. Percentage Change: Beware of Examiner Tricks

In some questions you may be asked to calculate percentage increase or decrease. Always remember that the percentage calculated is in relation to the starting point. For example, if the sales of a product were \$320 in 2018 and were \$400 in 2019 then the percentage increase between 2018 and 2019, was 25% (i.e. 80/320) and not 20% (i.e. 80/320). You can be sure that both 20% and 25% will be provided in the answer options. Another common trick is to trick candidates with problems where there are multiple percentages being applied. For example, the price of a £120 stereo was reduced by 20% on Christmas eve and then a further 40% by Boxing day. This is not a 60% discount on the original price. When rushing these can all be easily missed.

#128. Mental Maths Trick – Multiply any two-digit number by 11

Let's begin with one of the easiest mental maths tricks – how to multiply, in your head, any two-digit number by eleven. It's very easy once you know the secret. Consider the problem:

$$23 X 11$$

To solve this problem, simply add the digits, 2 + 3 = <u>5</u>, put the 5 between the 2 and the 3, and there is your answer: 2<u>5</u>3.

Now you try, **solve 35 x 11** without writing anything down or using a calculator. Use a calculator to check answer.

One more. Without writing anything down or using a calculator, **solve 81 x 11**. Did you get it?

Now before you get ahead of yourself, I have only shown you half of what you need to know. Suppose the problem is

$$75X11$$

Although $7 + 5 = 12$, the answer is NOT 7125. As before, the 2 goes between the numbers, but the 1 needs to be added to the 7 to get the correct answer - 825. Think of the problem this way:

$$1725825$$

Here is another example. **Solve 99 x 11**. Since $9 + 9 = 18$. The answer is 1089. Without writing anything down or using a calculator **solve 39 x 11?** Did you get it? Take a moment to practice a few times.

You can use this method to multiply three-digit numbers. For instance, consider the problem **314 x 11**, the answer will still begin with 3 and end with 4. Since $3 + 1 = 4$, and $1 + 4 = 5$, the answer is 3454.

Okay let's look at a UCAT type scenario and see how we can apply this concept. Imagine a problem where you had to calculate the new price of a $31 item with a 10% increase. Instead of "whipping" out the calculator, you should be able to work out the new price instantly.

The new price will be 110% of the item price = 1.1 x 31

Don't get confused or put off by the decimal point (ignore it for now) to get:

$$11X31$$

Simply add the digits, $3 + 1 = 4$, put the 4 between the 3 and the 1 and your answer is 341.

Now bring back the decimal point to give $34.1.

#129. Mental Maths Trick – Squaring a two-digit number that end in 5

Here is another trick. As you know, the square of a number is a number multiplied by itself. For example, the square of 6 is 6 x 6 = 36. Later (strategy # 137) I will share a simple method that will enable you square any two-digit or three-digit number (strategy #138). This method is especially simple when the number ends in 5. To square a two-digit number that ends in 5, you need to remember only two things:

1. The answer <u>begins</u> by multiplying the first digit by the next higher digit.
2. The answer <u>ends</u> in 25

For example, to square the number 45, we simply multiply the first digit (4) by the next higher digit (5), then attach 25. Since 4 x 5 = 20, the answer is 2025. Easy right? How about the square of 85? Since 8 x 9 = 72, we can immediately deduce that 85^2 = 7225.

We can use this same trick when multiplying two-digit numbers with the same first digit, and second digits sum to 10. The answer begins the same way that it did before (the first digit multiplied by the next higher digit), followed by the product of the second digits. For example, let's try 82 x 88. (both numbers begin with 8, and the last digits sum to 2 + 8 = 10). Since 8 x 9 = 72, and 2 x 8 = 16, the answer is 7216.

Now let's take look at another problem, try 35 x 35 – without using a calculator? Did you get? Take a moment to practice a few times.

#130. Mental Maths Trick – Two-Digit Addition

My assumption is that you know how to add and subtract one-digit numbers. The skills that you require here will be needed for larger addition problems, as well as virtually all multiplication problems in later strategies. Most of us are taught to do maths on paper from right to left and that's fine for maths on paper. But if you want to do mental maths in your head (even faster than you can on paper), then it is better to work from **left to right**. When you compute the answer from right to left, you generate the answer backwards.

Also, if you want to estimate your answer, it's more important to know that your answer is "a little over 1700" than to know that your answer "ends in 4". Thus, by working from left to right , you begin with the most significant digits of your problem. If you are used to working from right to left, then you may need to change for the exam. With practice you will find that it is the most natural and efficient way to do mental maths. The fundamental principle of mental arithmetic is to simplify your problem by breaking it into smaller, more manageable parts. The easiest two-digit addition problems are those that do not require you to carry any numbers (when the first digits sum to 9 or below). For example, 47+ 32. We can solve this by working from left to right by breaking it down into something more manageable, 47 + 30 + 2. After adding 30, you have the simpler problem 77 + 2, which equals 79. Let's look at another problem, solve 43 + 26. Think of the problem this way:

$$43 + 20 = 63 + 6 = 69$$

Now let's try a calculation that requires you carry a number: **67 + 28**. Adding from left to right, you can simplify the problem by adding 67 + 20 = 87; then 87 + 8 = 95.

$$67 + 20 = 87 + 8 = 95$$

Now try **84 + 57**. Try it on your own mentally calculating from left to right. Use a calculator to check your answer. If carrying numbers trips you up a bit, don't worry. This will take some time to getting used to. With practice,

you can begin to train your mind until it comes automatically. Try another problem for practice, 68 + 45. How did you do? If you would like to try your hands at some additional problems, ask a friend or family member to test you.

#131. Mental Maths Trick – Three-Digit Addition

The strategy for adding three-digit numbers is the same as for adding two-digit numbers; you add from the left to right. After each step, you arrive at a new (and simpler) addition problem. Let's try the problem: 538 + 327. Starting with 538, we add 300, then add 20, then add 7. After adding 300 (538 + 300 = 838), the problem becomes 838 + 27. After adding 20 (838 +

20 = 858), the problem simplifies to 858 + 7 = 865. All mental addition problems can be done by this method. The goal is to keep simplifying the problem until you are just adding a one-digit number. Notice that 538 + 327 requires you to hold on to six digits in your head, whereas 838 + 27 and 858 + 7 require only five and four digits respectively. As you simplify the problem the problem gets easier! Try to solve 623 + 159 in your mind. Going from left to right, after adding the hundreds (623 + 100 = 723), you were left with 723 + 59. Next you should have added the tens (723 + 50 = 773), simplifying the problem to 773 + 9, which you then summed to get 782.

When doing these problems mentally, do not try to see the numbers in your mind – try to hear them. When first doing these problems, practice them out loud. Reinforcing yourself verbally will help you learn the mental method more quickly.

Three-digit problems really do not get much harder than the following: **858 + 634**. Going from left to right, after adding the hundreds (858 + 600 = 1400), you were left with 1458 + 34. Next you should have added the tens (1458 + 30 = 1488), simplifying the problem to 1488 + 4, which you then summed to get 1492. Let's try another one for practice: **759 + 496**. This addition problem is a little more difficult since it requires you to carry numbers in all three steps. However, with this particular problem you have the option of using an alternative method. I am sure you will agree that it is lot easier to add 500 to 759 than it is to add 496, so try adding 500 and subtracting the difference:

$$759 + 500 - 4$$

So far, we have broken up the second number to add to the first one. It doesn't matter which number you choose to break up, but it's good to be consistent. That way, your mind will never have to waste time deciding which way to go if the second number happens to be a lot simpler than the first.

#132. Mental Maths Trick – Two-Digit Subtraction

When subtracting two-digit numbers, your goal is to simplify the problem so that you are reduced to subtracting (or adding) one-digit number, let's begin with a very simple subtraction problem: 86 – 25, this can be viewed as:

$$86 - 20 - 5$$

After each step, you arrive at a new and easier subtraction problem. Here, we first subtract 20 (86 − 20 = 66), then we subtract 5 to reach the simpler problem 66 − 5 for the final answer of 61. Of course, subtraction problems are considerably easier when there is no borrowing (<u>which occurs when a larger digit is being subtracted from a smaller one</u>). But the good news is that "hard" subtraction problems can be turned into "easy" addition problems. For example, **86 − 29**. There are two different ways to solve this problem mentally.

1. First subtract 20, then subtract 9

$$86 - 20 - 9$$

But for this problem, I would prefer the following strategy:

2. First subtract 30, then add back 1

$$86 - 30 + 1$$

Look at it like this: since you **subtracted too much from 86 (30 − i.e. 1 too much) you add it back to reach 57**.

Here is the rule for deciding which method to use: **if a two- digit subtraction problem will require borrowing, then round the second number up (to a multiple of ten). Subtract the rounded number then add back the difference**. For example, 54 − 28 would require borrowing (since 8 is greater than 4), so round up 28 up to 30, solve 54 − 30 = 24, then add back 2 to get 26 as your final answer. Now try your head at **81 − 37** without a computer or writing anything down, how did you do? Since 7 is greater than 1, we rounded up 37 to 40, subtract it from 81 (81 − 40 = 41), then add back the difference of 3 to arrive at the final answer. With just a bit of practice, you will become comfortable working subtraction problems both ways. Just use the rule earlier to decide which method will work better. For more practice ask a friend or family member to test you.

#133. Mental Maths Trick – Three-Digit Subtraction

Now let's start with a three-digit problem: **958 – 417.** This problem doesn't require you to borrow any numbers over since every digit in the second number (417) is less than the first number (958), so you should not find it too hard. Simply break it down and subtract one digit at a time, simplifying as you go: 958 – 400 = 558 – 10 = 548 – 7 = <u>541</u>. Now let's try another problem mentally, solve **874 – 762.** Since all the digit of 762 are less than 874, we subtracted 700 (874 – 700 = 174), then subtracted 60 (174 – 60 = 114); then subtracted 2 to arrive at the final answer. Now let's try a subtraction problem that requires you to borrow: **747 – 598**: At first glance it looks pretty tough, but if you subtract 747 - 600 = 147, then if add back 2, you reach your final answer of 147 + 2 = 149.

$$747 - 600 + 2$$

Now try one yourself: **853 – 692** without using a calculator or writing anything down. Did you first subtract 700 from 853? If so, did you get 853 – 700 = 153? Since you subtract by 8 too much, did you add back 8 to reach 161. Now, the examples so far have been a bit easier because you were subtracting numbers close to a multiple of 100. But what about other problems, like **725 - 468**. If you subtract one digit at a time your mental sequence would look like this:

$$725 - 400 = 325 - 60 = 265 - 8 = 257$$

This method mentally might take some readers a bit of time. But wouldn't it be easier to round up the second number to 500?

$$725 - 500 = 225 + ?? = ??$$

Subtracting 500 is easy; 725 – 500 = 225. But you would have subtracted too much. The trick is to figure out how exactly how much too much. At first glance, that answer is far from obvious. To find it, you have to know how far 468 is far from 500. The answer can be found using complements, a nifty technique that will make many three-digit problems a lot easier to do.

Using Complements:

To teach complements, let's start with a test, how far from 100 are each of these numbers?

5768492179

Here are the answers:

$\underline{5}7 + \underline{4}3 = 100$
$\underline{6}8 + \underline{3}2 = 100$
$\underline{4}9 + \underline{5}1 = 100$
$\underline{2}1 + \underline{7}9 = 100$
$\underline{7}9 + \underline{2}1 = 100$

Notice that for each pair of numbers that add to 100: the first digits (one the left – underlined) add to 9 and the last digits (on the right - not underlined) add to 10. We say that 43 is the complement of 57, 32 is the complement of 68, and so on. Now find the complement of these two-digit numbers:

3759934408

To find the complement of 37, first figure out what you need to add to 3 in order to get 9 (the answer is 6). Then figure out what you need add to 7 to get 10 (the answer is 3). Hence 63 is the complement of 37. Use this reasoning to calculate the complements of the other numbers in your head. Notice like everything else we have done so far the complements are determined from left-to-right. As we have seen, the first digit adds to 9, and the second digits add to 10 (an exception to the rule occurs in numbers ending in 0 – e.g., 30 + 70 = 100 – but those complements are simple). What do complements have to do with mental subtraction? Well, they allow you convert difficult subtraction problems into simple straightforward addition problems. Let's consider the last subtraction problem: 725 – 468. To begin you subtracted 500 instead of 468 to arrive at 225 (725 -500 = 225). But then, having subtracted too much, you needed to figure out how much to add back. Using complements gives you the answer in a flash. How far is 468 from 500? The same distance as 68 from 100. If you find the complement of 68 using the method shown earlier, you will arrive at 32. Add 32 to 225, and you will arrive at 257, your final answer.

Try another three-digit subtraction problem: solve **821 – 259.** To compute, mentally subtract 300 from 821 to arrive at 521, then add back the complement of 59, which is 41, to arrive at 562, our final answer. Here is another problem for you to solve: **645 – 372.** How did it go? You would have subtracted 400 to arrive at 245 then added 28 (compliment of 72). Your mental sequence would look something like this:

$$645 - 400 = 245 + 20 = 265 + 8 = 273$$

Subtracting a three-digit number from a four-digit number is not much harder, as the next problem illustrates: solve 1246 – 579. By rounding up the second number to 600 and subtracting from 1246, leaving 646, then add back the complement of 79, which is 21. Your final answer is 646 + 21 = 667.

#134. Mental Maths Trick – 2-BY-1 Multiplication

For this technique you will learn how to quickly multiply in your head one-digit numbers by two-digit numbers. However, there is one small prerequisite for mastering this strategy – you need to know your **multiplication tables from 1 to ten**. All readers should be fine with this skill, however, there may be some multiplication calculations that may take you a bit longer than normal. For me it's 7 x 8, which is 56, for some reason (unknown to me) I have to think about it. You want to almost think automatically when doing any one-digit multiplication. For those of you who need to shake the cobweb loose, check out the multiplication table we have provided on the blog at www.themedicblog.co.uk/multiplication-table. Ask a friend to randomly ask you questions and see which ones you can answer automatically. Any multiplication that you can't answer right away or need to use another multiplication to work it out (for example to work out 6 x 7, you mentally think 6 x 6 = 36 + 6), take note of these slow points and learn them until it becomes automatic. If you worked your way through strategies #70 to #73, you would have got into the habit of adding and subtracting from left-to-right.

You'll see that multiplication becomes a lot easier when you do the same and think from left to right (fr one thing you start to say your answer aloud before you have finished the calculation). Let's tackle our first problem: **42 X 7.** First, break up 42 (40 +2), multiply 40 x 7 = 280 (note that 40 x 7 is just like 4 x 7, with a friendly zero attached). Next, multiply 2 x 7 = 14. Then add 280 plus 14 (use left-to-right method – refer to strategies #70 and #71) to arrive at 294. Let's try another example: **48 x 4.** You should first break down the problem into small multiplication tasks that you can perform mentally with ease. Since 48 = 40 + 8, multiply 40 x 4 = 160, then add 8 x 4 = 32. The answer is 192.

Here are two more problems that you should be able to solve fairly quickly: **62 x 3** and **71 x 9**. Try doing them in your head before checking answers. These two examples are especially simple because the numbers being added essentially do not overlap at all. Another easy type of multiplication problem involves numbers that begin with five. When the five is multiplied by an even digit, the first product will be a multiple of 100, which makes the resulting addition problem easy. For example, solve **58 x 4.** How did you find it? Notice how much easier this problem is to do from left to right. Try your hands on another one: **87 x 5.** Again, easy right! It takes far less time to calculate "400 + 35" mentally than it does to type on the onscreen calculator "**87** x **5** then **=**".

Let's look at a problem that is a little harder: solve **38 x 9.** As usual, we break the problem down into easier problems. Multiply 30 x 9 plus 8 x 9, giving you 270 + 72. The addition problem is slightly harder because it involves carrying a number. The mental sequence here would be 270 + 70 = 340 + 2 = 342. With practice, you will become more adept at juggling problems like these in your head, and those that require you to carry over will almost be as easy as those that don't. Try solving **67 x 8** mentally without a calculator.

Rounding up:

You saw in strategies #72 and #73 how useful rounding up can be when it comes to subtraction. The same goes for multiplication, especially when you're multiplying numbers that end in eight or nine. Let's take the problem **69 x 6.** If calculated in the usual way, where you would add 360 + 54 to arrive at final answer.

However, it is easier to round the 69 up to 70 and subtract 6 (420 - 6). Try another one: **78 X 9**: it is easier to round 78 up to 80 (80 x 9 = 720) and subtract 18. The subtraction method works well for numbers that are one or two digits away from a multiple of 10. It doesn't work so well when you need to round up more than two digits because the subtraction portion of the problem gets difficult. I strongly recommend practicing more 2-by-1 multiplication problems. If you would like to practice more, make up your own questions. Calculate them mentally, then check your answer with a calculator. Once you feel confident that you can perform these problems rapidly in your head, you are ready to move to the strategy #135.

#135. Mental Maths Trick – 3-BY-1 Multiplication

Now that you know how to do 2-by-1 multiplication problems in your head (strategy #134), you will find that multiplying three digits by a single digit is not much more difficult. You can get started with the following 3-by-1 problem (which is really just a 2-by-1 problem in disguise): **320 x 7.** Was it easy for you? If this problem gave you trouble then you might want to review the material in strategy #130 to #134. First, break down 320 (300 + 20), then multiply 300 x 7 = 2100. Next, multiply 20 x 7 = 140. Finally, add 2100 plus 140 = 2240. Let's try another 3-by-1 problem similar to the one you did, except we have replaced the 0 with a 6 so you have another step to perform: solve **326 x 7.** In this case, you simply add the product of 6 x 7, which you already know to be 42, to the first sum of 2240. Since you do not need to carry any numbers, it's easy to add 42 to 2240 to arrive at 2282.

In solving this and other 3-by-1 multiplication problems, the difficult part may be holding in memory the first sum (in this case, 2240) while doing the next multiplication problem (in this case, 6 x 7). There is no magic secret to remembering that first number, but with practice I guarantee you will improve your concentration, and holding on to numbers while performing other functions will get easier. Let's try another problem: **647 x 4.** This will be 600 x 4 = 2400. Next multiply 40 x 4 = 160. Then add 2400 + 160 = 2560. Finally, 2560 + 28 = 2588. Even if the numbers are large, the process is just as simple. For example: **987 x 9.** This can be solved by multiplying 900 x 9 = 8100, then adding 720 (8 x 9) = 8820. Then, 8820 + 63 (7 x 9) = 8883.

In strategy #134 we saw that problems involving numbers that begin with five are sometimes especially easy to solve. The same is true for 3-by-1 problems: Let's try to solve **563 x 6.** This is 3000 + 360 + 18 = 3378. Notice that whenever the first product is a multiple of 1000, the resulting addition problem is no problem at all. This is because you do not have to carry any numbers and the thousand-digit does not change. If you were solving the problem above in the exam, you should be able to eliminate and quickly pick an answer that began with three thousand with confidence (tip: **knowing the first digit of a problem is enough to sometimes to pick an answer option in the exam**). Try the same approach in solving the next problem, where the multiplier is a 5: solve **663 x 5** in your head. How did you do? You would have multiplied 5 by 600, then added the product of 60 x 5, then finally added the product of 3 x5 to get your final answer.

Let's escalate things by trying a couple problems that require some carrying. Solve **184 x 7, 684 x 9, 376 x 4** and **648 x 9**? How did it go? The first of these problems are easy enough to compute mentally. The difficult part comes in holding the preliminary answer in your head while computing the final answer. In the case of the last problem, it is easy to hold 5400 + 360 = 5760, but you may have to repeat 5760 to yourself several times while you multiply 8 x 9 = 72. Then add 5760 + 72. Sometimes at this stage I will start to say my answer aloud before finishing. With practice you will improve your concentration, and holding on to numbers while performing other functions will get easier.

The next two problem require you to carry two numbers each, so they may take you longer than those you have do done so far. But with practice you will get faster: solve **489 x 7.** When you are first tackling this problem, repeat the answers to each part out loud as you compute the rest. In the above problem, for example, start by saying, "twenty-eight hundred plus five hundred and sixty", a couple of times out loud to reinforce the two numbers in memory while you add them together. Repeat the answer – "thirty-three hundred sixty"- several times while you multiply 9 x 7 = 63. Then repeat "thirty - three hundred sixty plus sixty-three" aloud until you compute the final answer of 3423. If you are thinking fast enough to recognise that adding 60 + 63 will require you to carry a 1, you can begin to mould the final answer a split second – "thirty-four hundred and…twenty-three". Try solving **224 x 9** in your head.

Let's end this section on 3-by-1 multiplication problems with some special problems you can do in a flash because they require one addition step instead of two: Let's solve **511 x 7.** This can be solved by breaking down 511 (500 + 11), so 500 x 7 = 3500, plus the product of 11 x 7 = 77. Thus, the final answer is 3577. In general, if the product of the last two digits of the first number (11) and multiplier (3) is known to you without having to calculate it (in this case 11 x 3 = 33), you will get to final answer much more quickly. Let's look at another problem: **925 x 8.** This problem can be solved a lot quicker by adding 200 to 7200 (7200 + 200) = 7400. These special problems are common in the UCAT, so keep an eye out for them, they are disguised but you will be able to spot them with practice. For example, a percentage change problem where one of the calculation steps required you to figure out the sum of three items bought at £4.25 each – this is effectively, 425 x 3, which will be 1200 + 75 = 1275. Bring back the decimal points to give £12.75. Give this technique a go with the following problems: **975 x 4** and **312 x 9.** Set exercises to reinforce learning, I assure you that doing mental calculations is just like riding a bicycle or typing. It might seem impossible at first, but once you have mastered it, you will never forget it.

#136. Mental Maths Trick – 2-BY-2 Multiplication

Multiplying two-digit numbers is something you may often have to do in the UCAT. When multiplying two-digit numbers, you can use different methods to arrive at the same answer. We will look at the different approaches, I encourage you to try each method and pick the one you find easiest:

The Addition Method

To use the addition method to multiply any two-digit numbers, all you need to do is perform two 2-by-1 multiplication problems (for 2-by-1 mental multiplication refer to strategy #134) and add the results together. For example: **46 x 42.** Here, you break up 42 in 40 and 2, two numbers that are easy to multiply. Then you multiply 40 x 46 (which is just 4 x 46 with a 0 attached, or 1840). Then you multiply 2 x 46 = 92. Finally, you add 1840 + 92 = 1932. Basically, **you break down one of the two-digit numbers (in this case 42 = 40 + 2) and multiply each component to the other two-digit number** – therefore, (40 x 46) + (2 x 46). Attempt the same problem but this time break down 46 instead of 42. How did you do? The catch with the second way (breaking down 46) is that multiplying 6 x 42 is harder to do than multiplying 2 x 46, as in the first approach. Moreover adding 1680 + 252 is more difficult than adding 1840 + 92. So how do you decide which number to break up? I try to choose the number that will produce the easier addition problem. In most cases – but not all – **you will want to break up the number with the smallest last digit** because it usually produces a smaller second number for you to add.

Now try your hands on the following problems: **48 x 73** and **81 x 59.** How did you do? The second problem illustrates why numbers that end in 1 are especially attractive to break up. If both numbers end in the same digit, you should break up the larger number. For example: **84 x 34** would be easier solved as **(80 x 34) + (4 x 34)** = 2720 + 136 = 2856. If one number is significantly much larger than the other, it often pays to break up the larger number, even if it has a larger last digit. You will see what I mean when you try the following problem: **74 x 13.** Solve this both ways and compare. Did you find breaking 74 easier than breaking up 13? I did.

The next problem is a real challenge the first time you try it: solve **89 x 72** in your head, looking back at the problem if necessary. If you have to start over a couple times, that's okay. If you got the right answer the first or second time, pat yourself on the back. 2-by-2 multiplication problems really do not get tougher than this. If you did not get the answer right away, do not worry. I'll share other strategies for dealing with problems like this.

The Subtraction Method

The subtraction method comes in handy when one of the numbers you want to multiply ends in 8 or 9. The following problem illustrates what I mean: **59 x 17**. Although most people find the addition easier than subtracting, it is usually easier to subtract a small number than add a big number. If we had done this problem by the addition method, we would have added 850 + 153 = 1003.

Instead with the subtraction method you treat 59 as 60 − 1, then multiply 60 x 17 = 1020. But you multiplied by too much. How much? By 1 x 17, or 17 too much. So subtract 17 from 1020 to arrive at 1003. Now try again the challenging problem at the end of addition method: **89 x 72.** Use the subtraction method, wasn't it a lot easier? You would have solved (90 x 72) = 6480 − 72 = 6408. Now, here's a problem where one number ends in 8: **88 x 23.** In this case, you should treat 88 as 90 − 2, then multiply 90 x 23 = 2070. But you multiplied too much. How much? By 2 x 23, or 46 too much, So subtract 46 from 2070 to arrive at 2024, the final answer. Not only do I use the subtraction method with numbers that end in 8 or 9, but I also for numbers in the high 90s because 100 is such a convenient number to multiply. For example, multiply **96 x 73**. This is a lot easier when you break up 96 to 100 - 4.

When the subtraction component of a multiplication problem requires you to borrow number, using complements (as learned in strategy #133) can help you arrive at the answer more quickly. Consider the earlier problem 96 x 73. Breaking down 96 into 100 − 4, you would arrive at 7300 − 292, it's easier to round 292 to 300, so you end up with 7300 − 300 = 7000. However, you deduced too much. By how much? 8 too much (the complement), so you add it back = 7000 + 8 = 7008 (for more on using complements check out strategy #133). There's another way to use complements that saves more time when doing subtractions. Consider the problem 340 − 78. Common sense tells you the answer is in the 200s. If you do the difference between 40 and 78, which is 38. Then take the complement of 38, which is 62. The final answer is 262.

Let's try a problem: **88 x 76**, where you would end up 6840 - 152. There are two ways to perform the subtraction component. The "long" way where you would subtract 200 and add back 48. The "short" way is to use common sense and realise that answer will be 66 hundred and *something*. To determine *something,* we subtract 52 − 40 = 12 and find the complement of 12, which is 88. Hence the answer is 6688.

Let's try another problem: **67 x 59.** Again, you would end up with 4020 − 67. You can see the answer will be 3900 and *something*: Because 67 − 20 = 47, the complement 53 means that the answer is 3953. As you may have realised, you can use this method with any subtraction problem in the UCAT that requires you to borrow a number, not just part of a multiplication problem.

The Factoring Method

The factoring method involves no addition or subtraction at all. You use it when one of the numbers in a two-digit multiplication can be factored into one-digit numbers.

To factor a number means to break it down into one-digit numbers that, when multiplied together, give the original number. For example, the number 24 can be factored into 8 x 3 or 6 x 4. It can also be factored in to 12 x 2, but we prefer to use only single-digit factors. Here are some examples of factored numbers:

42 = 7 x 6

63 = 9 x 7

84 = 7 x 6 x 2. or 7 x 4 x 3

To see how factoring makes multiplication easier, consider the following problem: **46 x 42**. Previously we have solved this problem by multiplying 46 x 40 and 46 x 2 and adding the products together. To use the factoring method, treat 42 as 7 x 6 and begin by multiplying 46 x 7, which is 322. Then multiply 322 by 6 for the final answer of 1932. You already know how to do 2-by-1 and 3-by-1 multiplication from strategy #134 and #135 respectively, so this should not be too hard:

$$46x42 = 46x(7x6) = (46x7)x6 = 322x6 = 1932$$

Of course, this problem could also have been solved by reversing the factors of 42:

$$46x42 = 46x(7x6) = (46x7)x6 = 322x6 = 1932$$

In this case, it is easier to multiply 322 x 6 than it is to multiply 276 x 7. In most cases, I like to use the larger factor in solving the initial 2-by-1 problem and to reserve the smaller factor for the 3-by-1 component of the problem.

Factoring results in a 2-by-2 multiplication problem being simplified to an easier 3-by-1 (or sometimes 2-by-1) multiplication problem. The advantage of the factoring method in mental calculations is you do not have to hold much in memory. Let's look at another example, **75 x 63**:

$$75x63 = 75x(9x7) = (75x9)x7 = 675x7 = 4725$$

As before, you simplify this 2-by-2 problem by factoring 63 into 9 x 7 and then multiplying 75 by these factors. Alternatively, you could split 75 into its factors:

$$63x75 = 63x(5x5x3) = (63x5)x5x3 = 315x5x3 = 1575x3 = 4725$$

Try to solve the following method mentally: **57 x 24** using the factoring method. Compare this approach to the addition method. With the addition method, you would have to perform two 2-by-1 problems and then add. With the factoring method, you have just two multiplication problems: a 2-by-1 and a 3-by-1, and then you are done. The factoring method is usually easier on your memory.

Remember that challenging multiplication problem earlier in the addition method: 89 x 72. We tackled it easily enough with the subtraction method, but factoring works even faster:

$$89x72 = 89x9x8 = 801x8 = 6408$$

The problem is especially easy because of the 0 in the middle of 801. Our next example illustrates that it sometimes pays to factor the numbers in the order that exploits this situation. Let's look at two ways of mentally calculating **67 x 42**:

$$67x42 = 67x7x6 = 469x6 = 2814$$

$$67x42 = 67x6x7 = 402x7 = 2814$$

Ordinarily, you should factor 42 into 7 x 6, as in the first example, following the rule of using the larger factor first. But the problem is easier to solve if you factor 42 into 6 x 7 because it creates a number with a 0 in the centre, which is easier to multiply (consider such numbers as *friendly products*). Try to look for friendly products to solve the **43 x 56** mentally. Did you find it? When using the factoring method, it pays to find friendly products whenever you can.

Earlier in the book (strategy #128) you learned how easy it is to multiply numbers by 11. It usually pays to use the factoring method when one of the numbers is a multiple of 11, as seen in the examples below:

$$52x33 = 52x11x3 = 572x3 = 1716$$

$$83x66 = 83x11x6 = 913x6 = 5478$$

You now have all the basic skills you need to be a fast mental calculator when multiplying 2-by-2 problems. All you need is more practice.

#137 Mental Maths Trick – Squaring two-digit Numbers

Squaring numbers in your head is one of the easiest mental calculations you can do. The first step is to figure out the distance from the number you're squaring to the nearest multiple of ten (also called the absolute value). For example, let's consider 23^2, the nearest multiple of 10 to 23 is 20, and the distance between 23 and 20 is 3. To square a number, you subtract and add the absolute value from the original number to obtain two numbers (20 and 26) then multiply them together (20 x 26 = 520), then add the square of the absolute value $(520 + 3^2)$. Thus, the square of 23 is 529. Let's look at another example: calculate 13^2, the absolute value of 13 is 3, so therefore we will multiply 16 (13 + 3) and 10 (13 - 3), then add 3^2:

$$13^2 = 16x10 = 160 + 3^2 = 169$$

Let's examine another problem 77^2, you can work this out the same way by finding the absolute value, which is 3 (since the nearest multiple of 10 is 80):

$$77^2 = 80x74 = 5920 + 3^2 = 5929$$

Now try to calculate 56^2 and 96^2 in your head. Use a calculator to check. Squaring numbers that end in 5 is even easier, since the absolute value is always 5, the numbers to be multiplied will both end in multiples of 10. Hence, the multiplication and the addition are especially simple. Work out 85^2 and 35^2 in your head. Also check out strategy #129 for more on squaring two-digit numbers that end with 5 and set exercises to reinforce learning.

331

#138 Mental Maths Trick – Squaring three-digit Numbers

This strategy assumes you have already mastered how to square two-digit numbers (see strategy #137). Just as you square two-digit numbers by finding the distance from the nearest multiple of 10, to square three-digit numbers, you find the distance from the number you're squaring to the nearest multiple of 100. Take 193^2:

$$193^2 = 200x186 = 37{,}200 + 7^2 = 37{,}249$$

By using the above method, you've transformed a 3-by-3 multiplication problem into a far simpler 3-by-1 problem. After all, 200 x 186 is just 2 x 186 = 372 with two zeros attached. Now all you have to add is $7^2 = 49$ to arrive at 37,249. Now try squaring 706 mentally and check your answer with a calculator.

Squaring a number that's further away from the a multiple of 100 is tougher. Try your hand at calculating 314^2 mentally. You would have done 300 x 328 = 98400 then added 14^2. If 14^2 = 196 comes to you in a flash (through memory or calculation), you're in good shape. Just as 98400 + 196 = 98,596. If you need more time to compute 14^2, repeat the number 98,400 to yourself a few times before you go on calculate 14^2 which is (18 x 10) + 4^2 = 196.

The further away you get from a multiple of 100, the more difficult squaring three-digit numbers becomes. Try 529^2 and 863^2. Take my words that as you become more familiar with two-digit squares, these three-digit problems get easier. Last exercise, try calculating 359^2 in your head. How did you find it? They don't get much harder than that! If you got that right first time take a bow!

#139. Mental Maths Trick – One-digit Division

Mental division is a particularly handy skill to have in the UCAT. You'll be confronted with many situations in the exam that calls on this skill. The ability to divide in your head can save you time in the test. With mental division, the left-to-right method of calculation comes into its own. The is the same method we all learned in school, so you will be doing what comes naturally.

The first step when dividing mentally is to figure out **how many digits will be in your answer**. To see what I mean try on the following problem for size:

$$179 \div 7$$

To solve this problem, we are looking for a number, Q, such that 7 times Q is 179. Now, since 179 lies between 7 x 10 = 70 and 7 x 100 = 700, Q must lie between 10 and 100, which means our answer must be a two-digit number. Knowing that, we first determine the largest multiple of 10 that can be multiplied by 7 whose answer is below 179. We know 7 x 20 = 140 and 7 x 30 -= 210, so our answer must be in the twenties. To figure out the second digit we subtract 179 − 140 = 39. Our problem has now been reduced to the division problem of 39 ÷ 7. Since 7 x 5 = 35, which is 4 away 39, we have the rest of our answer, namely 5 with a remainder of 4 , or 5 and $\frac{4}{7}$. Altogether we have our answer, 25 with a remainder of 4, or if you prefer $25\frac{4}{7}$.

Let's try similar division problem using the same method of mental computation:

$$675 \div 8$$

As before, since 675 falls between 8 x 10 = 80 and 8 x 100 = 800, your answer must be below 100 and therefore is a two-digit number. To divide 8 into 675, notice that 8 x 80 = 640 and 8 x 90 = 720. Therefore, your answer is *80 something*. But what is that "something"? To find out, subtract 640 from 675 for a remainder of 35. Since 8 x 4 = 32, the final answer is 84 with a remainder of 3, or $84\frac{3}{8}$.

Like most mental calculations, division can be thought of as a process of simplification. The more you calculate, the simpler the problem becomes. What began as $675 \div 8$ was simplified to a smaller problem $35 \div 8$. Now let's try a division problem that results in a three-digit answer: **$947 \div 4$.**

This time, your answer will have three digits because 947 falls between 4 x 100 = 400 and 4 x 1000 = 4000. Thus, we must first find the largest multiple of 100 that can be multiplied by 4 whose answer is below 947. Since 4 x 200 = 800, our answer is definitely in the 200s. Subtracting 800 from 947 gives us our new division problem, $147 \div 4$. Since 4 x 30 = 120, we can now say the number is "*two hundred and thirty something*". After subtracting 120 from 147, we compute $27 \div 4$ to obtain the rest of the answer: 6 with a remainder of 3, all together we have 236 with a remainder of 3, or $236\frac{3}{4}$. The process is just as easy as dividing a one-digit number into a four-digit number, as in our next example.

$$2196 \div 5$$

Here, the answer will be in hundreds because 2196 is between 5 x100 = 500 and 5 x 1000 = 5000. Since 5 x 400 = 2000, our answer is definitely in the 400s, and our problem as reduce to 196 divided by 5, which can be solved as in the previous examples to give $439\frac{1}{5}$.

Actually, there is a much easier way to solve the above problem. We can simplify our problem by doubling both numbers. Since 2196 x 2 = 4392, we have:

$$2196 \div 5 = 4392 \div 10 = 439.2$$

#140. Mental Maths Trick – Two-digit Division

This strategy assumes you already have mastered the art of dividing by a one-digit number (#139). Naturally, division problems are harder as the number you divide by gets larger. Fortunately, I'll share some techniques. To make your life easier in the test. Let's start with a relatively easy problem first:

$$597 \div 14$$

Since 597 lies between 14 x 10 and 14 x 100, the answer (also called a quotient) lies between 10 and 100. To determine the answer, you must look into how many times 14 goes into 590. Because 14 x 40 = 560, you now know that your answer is *forty something*. Next subtract 560 from 597, which is 37 and reduces your problem to dividing 14 into 37. Since 14 x 2 = 28, your answer is 42. Subtracting 28 from 37 leaves you with a remainder of 9. Therefore, your final answer is $42\frac{9}{14}$.

Let's look at another problem: **682 ÷ 23**. In this problem the answer is a two-digit number because 682 falls between 230 (23 x 10) and 2300 (23 x 100). To figure out the tens digit of the two-digit answer, you need to ask how many times 23 goes into 680. If you try 30, you'll see it's slightly too much, as 30 x 23 = 690. Now you know that the answer is *20 something*. Then subtract 23 x 20 = 460 from 682 to obtain 222. Since 23 x 9 = 207, the answer is 29, with a remainder of 222 − 207 = 15 (final answer is $29\frac{15}{23}$).

Now consider: **491 ÷ 62**. Since 491 is less than 62 x 10 = 620, your answer will simply be a one-digit number with a remainder. You might guess 8, but 62 x 8 = 496, which is a little high. Since 62 x 7 = 434, then the answer is 7 with a remainder of 491 − 434 = 57, or $7\frac{57}{62}$.

Actually, there's a nifty trick to make problems like this easier. Remember how you first tried multiplying 62 x 8, but found it came out a little high at 496? Well, that wasn't a wasted effort. Aside from knowing that the answer is 7, you can also compute the remainder will be 5 less than 62, the divisor. Since 62 − 5 = 57, your answer is $7\frac{57}{62}$. Now try 380 ÷ 39 using the shortcut we just learned. So 39 x 10 = 390, which is too high by 10. Hence the answer is 9 with a remainder of 39 − 10 = 29.

Your next challenge is to divide a two-digit number into a four-digit number: **3657** ÷ 54. Since 54 x 100 = 5400, you know your answer will be a two-digit number. To arrive at the first digit to your answer, you need to figure how many times 54 goes into 3657. Since 54 x 70 = 3780 is a little too high, you know your answer must be 60 something. Next, multiply 54 x 60 = 3240 and subtract 3657 − 3240 = 417. The problem is now simplified to 417 ÷ 54. Since 54 x 8 = 432 is a little too high, your last digit is 7 with a remainder $54 - 15 = 39$ (final answer is $67\frac{39}{54}$). Now try your hand at mentally solving problem with a three-digit answer: **9467 ÷ 13.** Use a calculator to check you answer.

Simplifying Division Problems:

If by this point, you're suffering from brain strain. I want to share with you a couple of tricks for simplifying certain mental division problems. These tricks are based on the principle of dividing both parts of the problem by a common factor. If both numbers in the problem are even numbers you can make the problem twice as easy by dividing each number by 2 before you begin. For example, **858 ÷ 16** has two even numbers, and diving each by 2 yields the much simpler problem of **429 ÷ 8.** Now try one for practice: **3618 ÷ 54.** Use a calculator to check your answer. If you're really alert you could divide both sides of the problem by 18 to arrive at an even simpler problem of **201 ÷ 3.** Watch out for situations like these that can be divided by 2 multiple times, such as **1652 ÷ 36 = 413 ÷ 9.** You may usually find it easier to divide the problem by 2 twice than to divide both numbers by 4. Next, when both numbers end in 0, you can divide each by 10:

$$580 \div 70 = 58 \div 17 = 8\frac{2}{7}$$

But if both numbers end in 5, <u>double them</u> and then <u>divide both by 10</u> to simplify the problem. For example: **475 ÷ 35**

$$475 \div 35 = 950 \div 70 = 95 \div 7 = 13\frac{4}{7}$$

Finally, if the divisor ends in 5 and the number you're dividing into ends in 0, multiply both by 2 and then divided by 10, just as you did above. Solve 890 x 45 mentally.

$$890 \div 45 = 1780 \div 90 = 178 \div 9 = 19\frac{7}{9}$$

#141. Memorize decimal equivalents of common fractions (Decimalization)

Converting fractions or percentages to decimals is a common scenario you may expect when solving problems in the QR subtest. In the case of one-digit fractions, most of them have special properties that make them easy to remember. Anytime you can reduce a fraction or simplify a percentage to one of following fractions, it is extremely beneficial to already know the decimal equivalent. Commit to learning the decimal equivalent of fractions from halves through to elevenths. This isn't as hard as it sounds. As you'll see below, most are easy to remember.

Chances are you already know the decimal equivalent of the following fractions:

$$\frac{1}{2} = .50 \quad \frac{1}{3} = .333\,.... \quad \frac{2}{3} = .666\,...$$

Likewise:

$$\frac{1}{4} = .25 \quad \frac{2}{4} = \frac{1}{2} = .50 \quad \frac{3}{4} = .75$$

The fifths are easy to remember:

$$\frac{1}{5} = .20 \quad \frac{2}{5} = .40 \quad \frac{3}{5} = .60 \quad \frac{4}{5} = .80$$

The sixths require memorising only 2 new answers:

$$\frac{1}{6} = .20 \quad \frac{2}{6} = \frac{1}{3} = .333\,... \quad \frac{3}{6} = \frac{1}{2} = .50 \quad \frac{4}{6} = \frac{2}{3} = .666\,... \quad \frac{5}{6} = .833\,...$$

I'll return to the seventh in a moment. The eighths are easy:

$$\frac{1}{8} = .125 \quad \frac{2}{8} = \frac{1}{4} = .25 \quad \frac{3}{8} = .375\,(3x\frac{1}{8} = 3x0.125 = .375)$$

$$\frac{4}{8} = \frac{1}{2} = .50. \quad \frac{5}{8} = .625\,(5x0.125) \quad \frac{6}{8} = \frac{3}{4} = .75 \quad \frac{7}{8} = 0.875\,(7x0.125)$$

The ninths have a magic all on their own:

$$\frac{1}{9} = .\overline{1} \quad \frac{2}{9} = .\overline{2} \quad \frac{3}{9} = .\overline{3} \quad \frac{4}{9} = .\overline{4}$$

$$\frac{5}{9}=.\overline{5}\ \frac{6}{9}=.\overline{6}\ \frac{7}{9}=.\overline{7}\ \frac{8}{9}=.\overline{8}$$

Where the bar indicates that the decimal repeats. For instance, $\frac{4}{9}=.\overline{4}=$ .444…

The tenths you already know:

$$\frac{1}{10}=.10\ \frac{2}{10}=.20\ \frac{3}{10}=.30$$

$$\frac{4}{10}=.40\ \frac{5}{10}=.50\ \frac{6}{10}=.60$$

$$\frac{7}{10}=.70\ \frac{8}{10}=.80\ \frac{9}{10}=.90$$

For the elevenths, if you remember that $\frac{1}{11}=.0909$, the rest is easy:

$$\frac{1}{11}=.0909\ \frac{2}{11}=.\overline{18}(2x.0909)\ \frac{3}{11}=.\overline{27}(3x.0909)$$

$$\frac{4}{11}=.\overline{36}\ \frac{5}{11}=.\overline{45}\ \frac{6}{11}=.\overline{54}\ \frac{7}{11}=.\overline{63}\ \frac{8}{11}=.\overline{72}\ \frac{9}{11}=.\overline{81}\ \frac{10}{11}=.\overline{90}$$

The sevenths are truly remarkable. Once you memorise $\frac{1}{7}=.\overline{142857}$, you can get all the other sevenths without having to compute them:

$$\frac{1}{7}=.\overline{142857}\ \frac{2}{7}=.\overline{285714}\ \frac{3}{7}=.\overline{428571}$$

$$\frac{4}{7}=.\overline{571428}\ \frac{5}{7}=.\overline{714285}\ \frac{6}{7}=.\overline{85714242}$$

In the exam you will have to calculate fractions, keep your eyes peeled for ways you can simplify fractions and covert them to decimals. If the denominator of the fraction is an even number, you can simplify the fraction by reducing it in half, even if the numerator is odd. For example:

$$\frac{9}{14}=\frac{4.5}{7}=.6\overline{428571}(4.5x.\overline{142857})$$

In the UCAT you would only need to work out 4.5 x 0.14 ($\frac{1}{7}$ rounded to 2 decimal places). Learning decimalization helps with converting quickly so you don't have to use the onscreen calculator.

When the divisor ends in 5, it almost always pays to double the problem then divide by 10, for example:

$$\frac{29}{45} = \frac{58}{90} = \frac{5.8}{9} = .6\overline{44}$$

Numbers that end in 25 or 75 should be multiplied by 4 before dividing by 100:

$$\frac{31}{25} = \frac{124}{100} = 1.24$$

$$\frac{62}{75} = \frac{248}{300} = \frac{2.48}{3} = .82\overline{66}$$

#142. Master the art of Guesstimation (Approximation Method)

In earlier strategies you've been perfecting mental techniques necessary to figure out the exact answers to maths problems. Often, however in the exam, knowing a ballpark estimate is enough to eliminate options and pick the correct answer. Some questions in the UCAT may ask for an estimate. Thus, mastering Guesstimation is a key, as it can save a ton of time in the exam especially when dealing with time consuming problems. We will look at Guesstimation methods for Addition, subtraction, division and multiplication. As usual, we will do all computation from left-to-right (see strategy #130 for more on the left-to-right method).

Addition Guesstimation

Guesstimation is a way to make your life easier in the exam when the numbers of a problem are not simple or are too long to remember. The trick is to round the original numbers up or down to the nearest thousands, hundreds or tens. For example, try to find the sum of 8,367 + 5819 in your head?

When guesstimating, you want to round the numbers first, so the earlier problem could be 8000 + 6000 to give 14,000. Notice how we rounded up the first number down to the nearest thousand and the second number up. Since, the exact answer is 14,186, our relative error is small.

If you want to be more exact, instead of rounding off to the nearest thousand, round off to the nearest hundred. So, mentally you would solve 8400 + 5800 to arrive at 14,200. The answer is only 14 off from the correct answer, an error of less than 0.1%. This is good Guesstimation! Try a five-digit addition problem, rounding to the nearest hundred: 46,187 + 19,378. By rounding to the nearest hundred, our answer will always be off by less than 100. If the answer is larger than 10,000 your guesstimate will be within 1% of the exact answer.

Subtraction Guesstimation

The way to guesstimate the answers to subtraction problems is the same – you round to the nearest thousand or hundreds digit, preferably the latter. For example, let's consider 8,367 - 5,819. You can either guesstimate by mentally solving 8000 – 6000, or by solving 8,400 – 5,800. You see that byrounding to the nearest thousand leaves you with an answer that quite a bit off the mark. By rounding to the second digit (hundreds, in the example), your answer will usually be within 3% of the exact answer. For this problem, this is only off by 52, a relative error of 2%. If you round the third digit, the relative error will usually be below 1%.

Division Guesstimation

The first, and most important step in guesstimating the answers to a division problem is to determine the magnitude of the answer. Let's look at an example: Solve **57,867 ÷ 6**. The first step is to round off the larger number to the nearest thousand and change the 57,867 to 58,000. By looking at the new problem (58,000 ÷ 6) you should be able to deduce that the answer will be less than 10,000 (6 x 10,000 = 60,000) and more than 9000 (6 x 9000= 54,000), so the answer is *nine thousand and something.* You can estimate what that *something* is by looking at the problem deeper, note that 58 divided by 6 is $9\frac{4}{6}$, in other words 58,000 divided by 6 is $9\frac{4}{6}$ *thousand.*

If you are on your toes you would have realised that dividing 4 by 6 gives you $\frac{4}{6} = \frac{2}{3} \approx 0.667$ (see decimalization strategy #141). Since you know the answer is 9,000 something, you're now in a position to guess 9,667. In fact, the actual answer is 9,645 – that's close enough to guess in a multiple-choice.

Division on this level is simple. But in the exam expect larger division problems. Let's say we want to compute the amount of money a football player earns a day if he makes £5 million per year. You would solve this by computing 5,000,000 ÷ 365. First you must determine the magnitude of the answer. Does the player earn thousands every day? Well, 365 x 1000 = 365,000, which is too low.

Does the player earn tens of thousands every day? Well, 365 x 10,000 = 3,650,000, and that's more like it – this tells you your answer is in the *ten thousands.* To guesstimate your answer, divide the first two digits (i.e. 50 by 36) and figure that's $1\frac{14}{36}$, or $1\frac{7}{18}$. Since 18 goes into 70 about 4 times, your guess is that the player earns about £14,000 per day. The exact answer is £13,698.63. Not a bad estimate.

Here is a crazy problem for you. How many seconds does it take light to get from the sun to the earth? Well, light travels at 186,282 miles per second, and the sun is (on average) 92,960,130 miles away. I doubt you're particularly eager to attempt this problem by hand. Fortunately, it's relatively simple to guesstimate an answer. First, simplify the problem to 93,000 ÷ 186. Dividing 930 by 186 yields 5 with no remainder so answer is 500. The exact answer is 499.02, so this is a respectable guesstimate.

Multiplication Guesstimation

You can use much of the same techniques to guesstimate your answers to multiplication problems. For example, consider 88 X 54 which you could approximate as 90 x 50 = 4500. Rounding up to the nearest multiple of 10 simplifies the problem considerably but you are still off by 252, or about 5%. You can do better if **round both numbers by the same amount, but in opposite directions**. That is, if you round 88 by *increasing* 2, you should also *decrease* 54 by 2: Thus, 90 x 52 = 4680.

341

Instead of a 1-by-1 multiplication problem, you now have a 2-by-1 multiplication problem, which should be easy enough for you to do. Your guesstimation is off by only 1.5%.

When you guesstimate the answer to multiplication problems by rounding the larger number up and the smaller number down, **your guesstimate will be a little low**. If you round the larger number down and the smaller number up so that the numbers closer together, **your guesstimate will be a little high**. The larger the amount by which you round up or down, the greater your guesstimate will be off from the exact answer. For example, consider **73 x 65**. This could be simplified as 70 x 68 = 4760. Since the numbers are closer together after you round them, your guesstimate is a little higher than the exact answer (4745). Consider another problem, **67 x 67**. This could be simplified as 70 x 64 = 4480, since the numbers are farther apart, the estimated answer is lower than the exact answer. You can see that this multiplication guesstimation method works quite well. Also notice that is problem is just 67^2 and that our approximation is just the first step of the squaring techniques (see strategy #137). You will observe that guesstimation is most accurate when the original numbers are close together. Try estimating a 3-by-2 multiplication problem: consider 728 x 63. By rounding 63 down to 60 and 728 up to 731, you create a 3-by-1 multiplication problem, which gives you 731 x 60 = 43,860. Which is 2004 off the exact answer, an error of 4.3% Now try guesstimating the following problem: 367 x 492. You can estimate this by rounding 492 up to 500 and

367 down to 359, your answer will be off by 1000. That's because the multiplication problem is larger and the size of rounding is larger, so the resulting estimate will be off by a greater amount. But the relative error is still under 1%.

#143. Spot Triggers to know when to Guesstimate (Precision vs Estimation)

This builds on strategy #142, where you approximate and use rounded figures to solve problems. In the UCAT, there are a few triggers you can spot to help you determine whether you should guesstimate or solve more precisely:

- **Analyse Answer options** – If the answer options are close together in value it may be more suitable to work precisely to figure out the exact answer. However, if there is large difference between the options, it may be suitable to use guesstimation to pick the correct answer.
- **Triggers used in Question** – Look out for where it is specified or implied in a question, words such as 'estimate', 'approximate' or 'rounding to the nearest…' in the question should trigger guesstimation.
- **Problem takes more than 3-steps to solve** – if you can determine before solving a problem it is time consuming, consider guesstimating to save a bit of time.

#144. Speed Distance and Time: Formula and Calculations

Often found in text format, this question-type is one many students become easily familiar with, so don't get nervous if you don't know how to approach it. *Speed* is a measure of how quickly an object moves from one place to another. It is equal to the *distance* travelled divided by the *time*. It is possible to find any of these three values using the formula below:

$$Speed = \frac{Distance}{Time}$$

The above formula can be rearranged to solve Distance and Time. As seen below:

$$Time = \frac{Distance}{Speed}$$

$$Distance = Speed X Time$$

An easy way to remember the formulae is to put distance, speed and time (or the letters D, S and T) into a triangle as seen below:

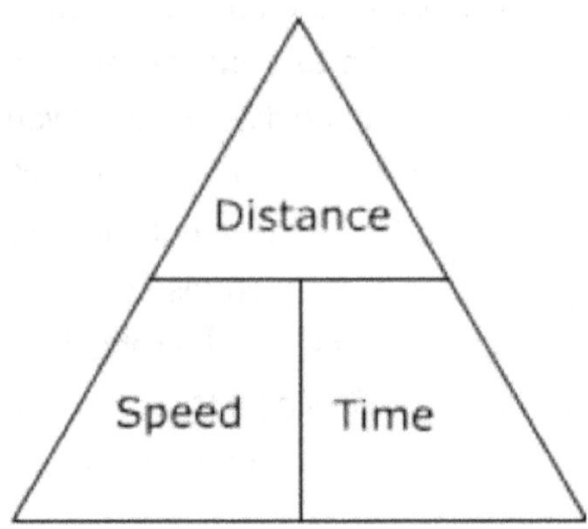

The way to use this triangle is as follows: take your finger and cover up the letter which represents the thing that you're trying to calculate. Then, the triangle will tell you what to do with the other two quantities to get the value you want. For example, if we want to calculate the speed, then we construct this triangle and cover up the speed (since that's what we want). Then, we see that what's left over is "distance over time", or in other words, distance divided by time will give us the speed.

Calculating Speed

These are common in the quantitative reasoning subtest. However, never expect problems to be straight forward. Many times, examiners provide the distance and time in different units which will require additional steps to solve the problem. Other times, you'll need to solve for the average speed, that will have multiple parts before getting the final answer. For example:

Michael walks uphill to university for 45 minutes at just 8 km/hr. He then travelled back home along the same route downhill at a speed of 24 km/hr. What is the average speed for the entire trip?

Solution: Correct Answer is 12 km/hr. Be sure in the exam to expect an option with 16 km/hr to catch some students out.

A helpful tip is to glance at the answer options to double check the units. For example, if the answers are in m/s but you've been given the distance in kilometres and time in hours then you know you need to do a conversion as an additional step.

Questions can also be presented in a graphical format where you are provided with a distance-time graph and asked to work out the speed where the gradient of the line is equal to the speed of the object. When dealing with graphs, be sure to double check the unit of axis. For example, expect examiners to have answer options in km/hr but the axis on the graph are different, e.g. are in Km (y-xis) and minutes (x-axis).

Calculating Distance

These problems are not as common as calculating speed, but it has come up in past UCAT tests. Make sure to double check units, questions can present information in one unit but answer options are in another. You may be presented with a speed-time graph where the question may ask you to deduce the distance covered. Using geometry, the distance covered can be calculated by **finding the area under the line**. In the above diagram, that would be the *area of the triangle* + *area of the square*. Be sure to double check the unit of the graph's axis is the same as answer options.

Calculating time

This is also common in the quantitative reasoning subtest. You may need to derive the time. Same as the above skills, double check the unit of the answer options before solving problem.

#145. Speed Distance and Time: Speed Conversion Shortcut (km/hr to m/s)

Unit conversion is at the core of difficult speed, distance and time problems. Converting units is not difficult. It's just that they can be easily missed and calculations can be time-consuming at times. If you can master this skill and are able to do conversions quickly, you should find all problems in relation to this topic pretty easy. Common conversion scenarios you can expect to do in the exam:

- Converting kilometres (km) to metres (m) and vice versa

- Converting hours (hr) to minutes (mins) and vice versa

- Converting hours (hr) to seconds (sec) and vice versa

- Converting minutes (mins) to seconds (sec) and vice versa

- Converting km/hr to m/s and vice versa

- Converting m/sec to Km/hr and vice versa

Learning some helpful shortcuts can save time when moving from one unit of speed to another. For example, converting speed from **km/h** to **m/s** is a simple as multiplying by $\frac{5}{18}$. Whilst converting from **m/s** to **km/hr** is as simple as multiplying the number by $\frac{18}{5}$. For example, 36 km/hr is $36 \times \frac{5}{18} = 10$ m/s.

#146. Speed Distance and Time: Determining Acceleration

Acceleration is the rate of change in *speed* in a given *time*. It can be calculated by dividing the change in speed by the time taken for the change.

$$Acceleration = \frac{Change\,in\,Speed}{Given\,Time}$$

Expect questions in the graphical format, where you are given a speed-time graph and may be asked deduce the acceleration. This will be the **gradient of the line in the graph**. More difficult problems may have multiple parts before arriving to final answer. Always be sure to check units as well.

#147. Fractions, Ratio & Proportion: Calculating Ratios

Ratios are usually shown as two or more numbers separated with a colon, for example 8:5 or 1:4 or 3:2:1. While it's easy enough to work out a ratio, it's rarely so straightforward in the UCAT, especially when time-consuming problems require you to deduce the numbers you need to work with. In the exam, expect ratio problems where you have to do multiple calculations before arriving to the two numbers needed to create the ratio. Some cases you may be given a table and be asked to deduce a ratio based on a specific scenario. During practice, try to work out with format of ratio problems you seem to struggle with, then assess you process by recognising the underlying reason to why you struggle with this, consider the following:

- Recognising the information needed to calculate ratio

- Ratio is the wrong way around

- Simplifying ratios

- Scaling Ratios

- Ratios in Geometry

- Ratio in Mixtures

- Converting fractions or percentages to ratios

- Finding the unknown value of something based on the ratio provided

- Finding the total value of the group using the ratio provided

- Sharing of a total amount based on the ratio provided

These are the most common scenarios that come up in the exam when dealing with ratio problems. If you are fine with the above skills, practice complex problems where you have to derive the values you need to create a ratio. It never gets harder than that in the exam. Here are a few tips to help when calculating ratios in the UCAT:

- **Use Cross-Multiplication Method when possible**: One of the ways that ratios are particularly useful is that they enable us to work out new and unknown quantities based on an existing (known) ratio. For example, there are four rings and seven bracelets in the jewellery box. If this ratio were maintained, how many rings would there be if there were 28 bracelets?

- **Calculate the factor (size) when applicable**: Using the example earlier, if the increase in number of bracelets (28/7 = 4) and to then multiply the number of rings by that same number (4 x 4 = 16).

- **Make sure you are reading the ratio the right way**. For example, a ratio of 2 pink bracelets to 6 red bracelets should be expressed 2:6 not 6:2. The first item in the sentence comes first.

- **Be careful with reading the wording**. For example, people often make mistakes with questions such as "Bob has eight dogs and four cats. Calculate the ratio of dogs to pets." It can be tempting to say the ratio is 8:4, but that would be incorrect because the question asks for the ratio of dogs to *pets*. Therefore, you need to calculate the total number of animals (8+4 = 12), so the correct ratio is therefore 8:12 (or 2:3).

- **Don't be put off by units or decimals**. The principles remain the same whether they apply to whole numbers, fractions, £ or m^2, but do ensure you note the units in your calculations, and where possible convert them to the same units. For example, if you have a ratio of 500g to 0.75kg, then convert both sides to either grams or kilos.

#148. Fractions, Ratio & Proportion: Calculating fractions

Expect to regularly work with fractions when solving problems in the UCAT. It is an important numeracy skill. In the exam expect to perform the following:

- Multiplying fractions
- Dividing fractions
- Simplifying fractions
- Adding Fractions
- Subtracting fractions
- Converting fractions to Ration or Percentages.

These are the common skills you can expect in the exam. Use it as a rough guide to help recognise weak areas and work on shortcomings accordingly. Sometimes in the test you may get questions where the answer is a fraction. These can range from easy to where you just have to simplify the numbers provided to complex where you have to do multiple calculations to arrive at final answer. Problems can also be in either text or tabular format, so be sure to recognise which format you struggle with the most if this is an area of concern. Here are a few tips to help with calculating fractions in the UCAT:

- **Adding and Subtracting fractions mentally without using a least common multiple:** This is a good method to save time in the exam because you are able to shorten the number of steps involved when adding fractions.

$$\frac{3}{4} \times \frac{1}{6} = \frac{18+4}{24} = \frac{22}{24} = \frac{11}{12}$$

Step 1. Multiply the denominators in order to calculate the denominators.

Step 2. Multiply the numerator of the first fraction with the denominator of the second fraction, and then multiply the numerator of the second fraction with the denominator of the first fraction.

Step 3. Add these two solutions together to calculate the numerator
3 x6 =18, 1 x4 =4 and 18+4 = 22 (this will be the numerator).

Step 4. Reduce the final answer.

- **Dividing Fractions by flipping one fraction and multiplying them together:** This tip makes dividing fractions much easier. You simply create a reciprocal of one fraction and multiply it to the other fraction. For example: $\frac{3}{4} \div \frac{5}{7}$, can be calculated as $\frac{3}{4} x \frac{7}{5} = \frac{21}{20}$.

- **Memorize decimal and percentage equivalents of common fractions:** We know our times tables and understand how much time they save when doing calculations. In the same way by memorizing this list of fractions can be a real time saver and help you with fractions, percentages and decimals. I provide a comprehensive list of fractions to decimal equivalent in strategy #141.

#149. Fraction, Ratio & Proportion: Currency Conversions

When dealing with exchange rates and foreign currency problems in the UCAT, many times it helps to set up as a proportion problem when converting from one currency into another. For example, how many euros would Daniel have to spend to get £85, at the exchange rate of £0.89? We can solve this using ratio and proportion:

Since 1 euro = £0.89

We can express this a ratio **1: 0.89**

in order to find out how much Daniel's £85 is worth we can set up a ratio where x is the amount in euros:

x:100

Using the exchange rate ratio x = 85 x 0.89 = £75.65

#150. Fraction, Ratio & Proportion: Scaling Ratios

Some questions in the quantitative reasoning may include a scale factor as part of the problem. A **scale factor** is a ratio which scales or multiples a quantity. They are used to create maps and other scale diagrams

Example: The floor plan of a flat shows a rectangular bathroom 2 cm by 3.5 cm. The scale of the map is 1:20,000. 1 hectare = $10,000m^2$. What is the area of the bathroom in hectares?

A. 2.8

B. 28

C. 280

D. 2800

Solution

First thing you should have noticed is that the conversion scale is in metres not cm, so we have to do a conversion at some point. You may be tempted to convert 2cm and 3.5 cm to metres straightaway but that's will give you two decimals to work with which is little more difficult to compute mentally. It's easier to convert them later after you have scaled them up so you don't have to deal with decimals. See below:

Area (cm^2) = (2 x 20,000) x (3.5 x 20,000) = 40,000cm x 70,000cm (now it's easier to convert to metres without having to compute with decimals)

Area (m^2) = 400m x 700m = 280,000 m^2

Since 1 hectare = 10,000 m^2 (i.e. 1:10,000)

Using proportion: 280,000 m^2 = 28 hectares.

(expect the examiners to include options such as 2.8 hectares and 280 hectares to catch students out – if you were to use decimals during computation, you risk misplacing the decimal point and picking one of these wrong answers)

Expect smiliar reasoning in geometry questions where you may be asked to work out the volume.

#151. Fraction, Ratio & Proportion: Direct and Inverse Proportion

If two quantities are dependent up on each other, then a change in one of the quantities makes a corresponding change in the other quantity. Here one quantity varies as the other or the quantities are in proportion.

Direct Proportion

One quantity X is said to be in vary directly as another quantity Y. If the two quantities depends up on each other, in such a manner that if Y is increased (or decreased) in a certain ratio, X also increases (or decreases) in the same ratio.

It is expressed as X $\propto$ Y (X varies directly as Y or X is directly proportional to Y)

If X $\propto$ Y, then X = kY, where k is the proportionality constant => k = X/Y.

If both the quantities X and Y have two sets of parameters such as x_1 corresponding to y_1 and x_2 corresponding to y_2, then their direct proportionality can be expressed in the following way:

$x_1/x_2 = y_1/y_2$ OR $x_1/y_1 = x_2/y_2$

Illustrated example:

Cost of 15 books $\rightarrow$ £ 75.

Therefore;

351

Cost of 10 books $\rightarrow$ £ 50

Here number of books (P) is directly vary with the total cost (C).

P $\propto$ C, i.e.

$P_1/P_2 = C_1/C_2 \rightarrow 15/10 = 75/50$

Inverse Proportion

A quantity X is said to be vary inversely as another quantity Y, if the two quantities depends up on each other, in such a manner that if Y is increased (or decreased) in a certain ratio, then X will decrease (or increase) in the same ratio.

More simply;

If X increases $\rightarrow$ Y decreases.

If X decreases $\rightarrow$ Y increases.

It is expressed as X $\propto$ 1/Y (X varies inversely as Y or X is inversely proportional to Y).

i.e. X = k/Y, where k is proportionality constant, and k = XY.

Then, $x_1/x_2 \neq y_1/y_2$ but $x_1/x_2 = y_2/y_1$
ie. $x_1 * y_1 = x_2 * y_2$

Example: *If a car travels at a rate of 30 kmph, then it will take 4 hours to cover a certain distance. How long the car will take to cover the same distance at a constant rate of 40 kmph?*

A.   *4 hours*

B.   *3.5 hours*

C.   *3 hours*

D.   *2.75 hours*

Solution:

There basically two quantities: speed and time. You may be tempted to use the formula covered in strategy #144 to find the distance then solve the time at the higher speed (40 kmph) – this is fine but it's quicker to use proportionality, since the distance is constant. Therefore, speed and time are dependent on each other. It is clear that if the speed is increasing then the time taken for journey should reduce.

Therefore,

$S_1 / S_2 = T_2 / T_1 \rightarrow 30/40 = T_2/4 \rightarrow T_2 \rightarrow = (30 * 4)/40 = 3$ hours

Always try to spot constants and the type of relationship between variables (direct or inverse) when solving problems in the exam and apply the above techniques to save time.

#152.   Times   &   Schedules   (Trip Schedules & Time Zones)

Questions based on trip schedules or difference in time zones fall under this category. Learning how to read timetables and interpret schedules builds on basic numeracy. The challenge with these questions isn't so much the level of maths required but figuring out **what the times given mean** and being comfortable **converting in-and-out of minutes and hours** to solve a problem. Time-consuming questions may present scenarios where you have to perform multiple calculations to **compare given trips or time zones.** Also expect examiners to include questions where you have to apply **speed, distance and time concepts** (strategy #144).

Example: The table below is part of a train timetable for six high speed trains from Manchester to London

Train	A	B	C	D	E	F
Manchester	06:35	07:00	07:15	07:30	07:45	08:00
London	08:09	08:39	08:48	09:04	09:59	09:39

Question 1: *Which train takes more than two hours to go from Manchester to London?*

A.   Train A

B.   Train B

C.   Train C

D.   Train E

Solution:

Using eyeballing (strategy #105) and guesstimation (strategy #142) we can deduce that Train E takes longer than 2 hours.

Question 2: *Patrick has a meeting at 9 am in London, what is the latest train he can take considering that he wants to arrive 5 mins early and the time it takes for him to get to his office from the London station takes 10 minutes?*

A.   Train A

B.   Train B

C.   Train C

D.   Train D

Solution:

We can automatically eliminate option C and option D, since he will get to the office late. Using eyeballing and guesstimation we can select Train B.

Question 3: *Trains C and F are the newly introduced TS2015 model. The distance from Manchester to London is 336 km. What is the approximate speed of the new TS2015 model?*

A.   84 m/s

B.   72 m/s

C.   58 m/s

D.   *43 m/s*

Solution:

Tip: *Under exam conditions I would personally guess, flag and move on as I would have recognised this problem will take up some time. My approach would be as follows:*

I would eyeball the table to work out the average time: **1.5 hours** then divide 336 km by 1.5 to get the average speed $\approx$ 224 Km/hr.

Then converted it to m/s using strategy #145 $\rightarrow$ 224.27 x $\dfrac{5}{18}$ = 62.2

Guessimated answer $\approx$ 62.2 m/s, I would therefore would pick the option C as it's within the same ball park.

More Precise Solution :

Speed of C (km/hr) = 336/1.55 = 216.8

Speed of F (Km/hr) = 336/1.65 = 203.6

Average speed of C and F = 210.2 km/hr

Convert 210.2 km/hr to m/s = 58.4 m/s

Question 4: *One of the trains to London was held at a red signal for 40 minutes and turned up 10 minutes before the next train from Manchester. Which train was delayed?*

A.   *Train A*

B.   *Train B*

C.   *Train C*

D.   *Train E*

From eyeballing the data we can deduce it is Train A

Here are common skills required for dealing with time & schedule problems in the exam, use it as a rough guide to identify areas you may need to improve:

355

- Draw out the required information to solve a problem

- Convert from minutes to hours and vice versa

- Make comparisons when required and

- Apply speed, distance and time calculations when required

Here are a few tips to help with solving time and schedule problem in the UCAT:

- **Expose yourself to different time zones and schedule problems:** Practice loads of time schedules maths questions (e.g. train, bus, flights) so that you become quicker at interpreting and drawing out information in the exam. Do problems that include a single schedule (e.g. schedule time for one train) and multiple schedules (e.g. schedule times for more than one train).

- **Expose yourself to time zone problems:** These can feel complicated but are not necessarily harder. Questions on flight times and international calls tend to be common themes in the UCAT. Practice loads of questions on these so you become quicker at drawing out information on test day.

- **Have an approach that allows you work through calculation quickly and accurately:** it's common to get a little confused when attempting these types of problem. During practice develop a method that is quick and applicable in a given scenario.

- **Don't be intimidated by complex schedules:** Expect examiners to include large schedules with multiple times for more than one train, bus or flight). Most of the data will be irrelevant so don't panic!

- **Pay close attention to format of arrival times, departure times and other events that might influence answers:** Examiners might try to trick you by providing times in different formats as well different modes of transports that might influence answer.

- **Expect Speed, Distance and time calculations:** Time schedule or time zone problems where distance travelled provided tends to include a speed type problem as one of the questions. It's good to prime yourself when you spot this so you can draw information quicker in the exam.

#153. Conversion Shortcut for Metres, Litres and Grams

Converting from one unit to another is one of the most applied skills in the exam as it is usually a common sub-step when solving problems in the exam. It is important that you practice converting from one unit to another quickly and accurately. If this is an area of weakness, try using this trick when converting units. The trick uses a mnemonic device for the six most commonly used prefixes from kilo to milli:

King Henry Died Unexpectedly Drinking Chocolate Milk

Where,

King – Kilo
Henry – Hecta
Died – Deka
Unexpectedly – Unit (which can be metre (m), gram (g) or lites (l))
Drinking – Deci
Chocolate – Centi
Milk - Milli

The benefit of using this mnemonic is that **it helps with remembering how many places to move decimal points when doing a calculation and in what direction**. Let's look at some examples:

Convert 4.44 mm to cm: 4.44 mm to cm = 0.444 cm

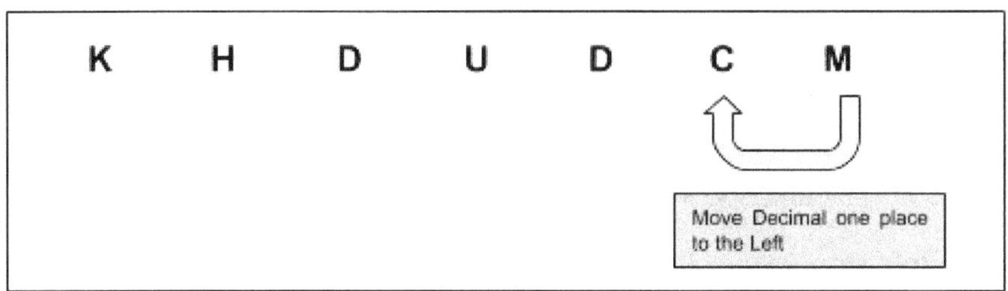

Convert 6.73 m to mm: 6.73 m to mm = 6730 mm

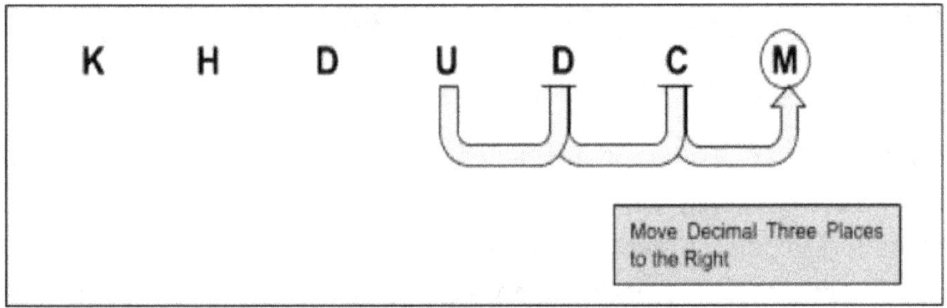

Remember: Unit (U) can be metre, gram or litre

Convert 5.75 kg to mg: 5.75kg to mg = 5,750,000 mg

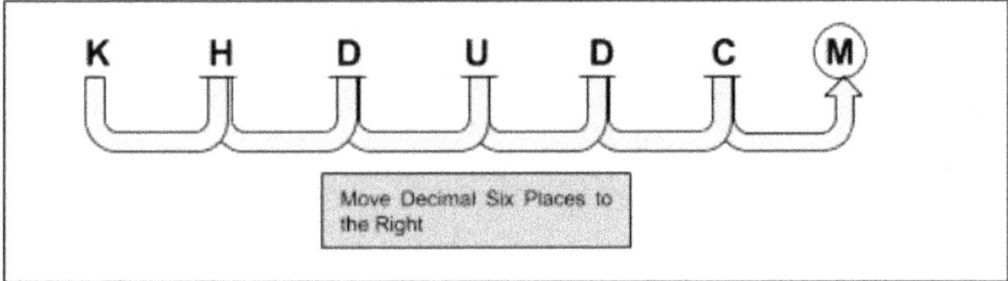

Convert 6,762 ml to l: 6,762 ml to l = 6.72

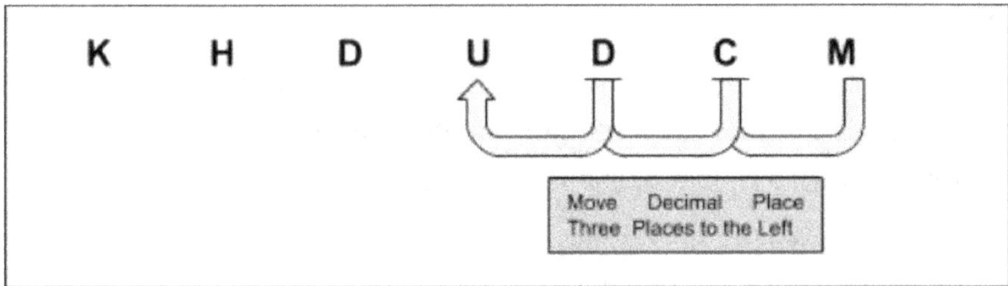

As you can see the acronym can be particularly helpful when moving the decimal point. Practice using it until you become comfortable eough and don't need to write it out. Here are some helpful tips to improve your accuracy and speed at converting units

- **Avoid converting in multiple steps**: Say you wanted to convert 3.43 mm to cm, it's a waste of time to convert 3.43 mm to metres then to cm. Using the above trick, you can do this in one step by moving the decimal one step to the right (0.343 cm).

- **Understand the meaning of prefixes**: Understanding the meaning of each prefix lets you comprehend how big or small numbers are in relation to each other.

- **Practice converting numbers:** practice more GCSE style conversion questions so that you get good enough that you don't need to write out the mnemonic every time you need to convert.

- **Practice difficult Conversion problems**: UCAT style conversion problems are not straightforward, they usually include multiple steps where doing a unit conversion is a sub-step. Practice difficult problems so you get into the habit of adopting the mnemonic when solving complex problems.

#154. Converting Seconds, Minutes and Hours

There are two numbers you need to know when converting time - **60** and **3600**. When combined with the mental maths tricks covered earlier in this guide (strategy #134 - #140), you should be able to convert from one measurement to another pretty quickly.

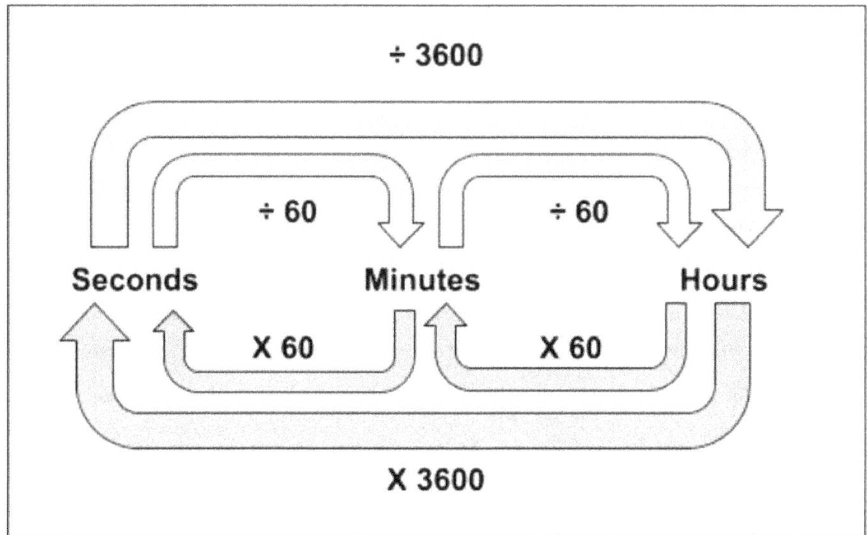

When converting seconds, minutes and hours, there are three steps involved. First, think about whether the new number you are trying to solve

359

is bigger or smaller. For example, if you were converting 5.4 hours to minutes, you will expect your answer to be bigger right? Same goes for if you were converting 6.3 minutes to seconds. Here are more examples, try to think if the expected answer will be bigger or smaller:

- 6.3 seconds to hours
- 4.45 minutes to seconds
- 3.78 hours to minutes
- 9.5 seconds to minutes
- 10.4 hours to seconds
- 34.3 minutes to hours

Secondly, recognise the type of operation to perform. As a rule of thumb, if **the expected number is bigger you multiply and if it is lower you divide**. For example:

- 6.3 seconds to hours → answer expected to be smaller (**divide**)
- 4.45 minutes to seconds → answer expected to be bigger (**multiply**)
- 3.78 hours to minutes → answer expected to be bigger (**multiply**)
- 9.5 seconds to minutes → answer expected to be smaller (**divide**)
- 10.4 hours to seconds → answer expected to be bigger (**multiply**)
- 34.3 minutes to hours → answer expected to be smaller (**divide**)

Thirdly, recognise how much big of an increase or decrease the new number is going to be. As a rule of thumb, **use 60 if it's one level above or below the base measurement, use 3600 if it's two levels above or below the base measurement**. For example, moving from seconds to minutes is one level, whilst moving from hours to seconds is two. Consider the example where we will convert 6.3 seconds to hours, we expect the answer to be lower, and since we are moving two levels (seconds to hours) we will **divide by 3600.**

- 6.3 seconds to hours → divide by 3600
- 4.45 minutes to seconds → multiply by 60
- 3.78 hours to minutes → multiply by 60

- 9.5 seconds to minutes → divide by 60

- 10.4 hours to seconds → multiply by 3600

- 34.3 minutes to hours → divide by 60

Practice converting more seconds, minutes and hours until this method becomes second nature. Also incorporate mental maths tricks such as 2-by-2 multiplication and 2-by-1 division to save more time.

#155. Memorise Decimal Equivalents when working with Time

When solving time problems, you can save a ton of time by memorising the decimal equivalents of common seconds and minutes. For example, 7 hours 30 mins is 7.5 hours, 4 minutes 15 seconds is 4.25 minutes. By memorising common decimal equivalents, you save time during calculations, thus increasing speed.

seconds / minutes	Decimal equivalent
15	0.25
30	0.50
45	0.75
60	1

However, in the UCAT time conversions tend not to be straightforward but odd instead. For example, converting 5 hours 23 minutes to decimals or 8 hours 21 minutes to decimals. There are a couple tricks you can adopt to help you convert quicker.

Method 1 - Rounding one minute/second to 0.02

The decimal equivalent of 1 second/minute is 0.017. However, this is harder to compute mentally, so rounding it to two decimal places to derive **0.02** can make life easier as it is simpler to work with mentally. Note that by rounding up the decimal value there will be a slight error margin, so your answer option in the exam will be slightly off the answer you derive.

Example: an employee at Google worked for 4 hours 23 minutes at a rate of £13.50. How much did they earn?

Solution:

Step 1 - Convert 23 mins to decimals by multiplying 0.02 x 23 $\approx$ 0.46 (solved mentally – double number and move two decimals to the left)

Step 2 - Salary earned = 4.46 x 13.5 = 60.21 (input in onscreen calculator)

The exact answer is £59.17. That's an error margin of under 2%, that's pretty good! That's close enough to eliminate and pick a correct answer option.

Method 2 - Spotting multiples of three (in minutes/seconds) and Five (in decimals)

When you look at a time conversion chart, there is something interesting going on with minutes/seconds that are multiples of three: **when converted to decimal they increase in multiples of 5**. For example, 3 minutes is 0.05, 6 minutes is 0.10, 9 minutes is 0.15, 12 minutes is 0.20 and so on.

Minutes	Decimal Hours	Minutes	Decimal Hours	Minutes	Decimal Hours
1	.02	21	.35	41	.68
2	.03	22	.37	42	.70
3	.05	23	.38	43	.72
4	.07	24	.40	44	.73
5	.08	25	.42	45	.75
6	.10	26	.43	46	.77
7	.12	27	.45	47	.78
8	.13	28	.47	48	.80
9	.15	29	.48	49	.82
10	.17	30	.50	50	.83
11	.18	31	.52	51	.85
12	.20	32	.53	52	.87
13	.22	33	.55	53	.88
14	.23	34	.57	54	.90
15	.25	35	.58	55	.92
16	.27	36	.60	56	.93
17	.28	37	.62	57	.95
18	.30	38	.63	58	.97
19	.32	39	.65	59	.98
20	.33	40	.67	60	1.0

This can help save a ton of time in the exam when converting from one to the other. For example, 8 hours 33 minutes is simply 8.55 in decimals! Since 33 is multiple of 3 (3 x 11), then we can find the equivalent in decimals by multiplying the **factor** (11) by 5 (which is 55). Let's look at another one, what is 4 minutes 48 seconds in decimals? Since 48 is a multiple of 3 (3 x 16), then we can find the decimals equivalent easily by multiplying 16 x 5 = 80. The final answer is 4.8 minutes. Here are a few more for you to solve mentally:

- Convert *8 minutes 30 seconds* to decimal
- Convert *5 hours 54 minutes* to decimal
- Convert *4 hours 24 minutes* to decimal
- Convert *3 minutes 45 seconds* to decimal
- Convert *1 minute 33 seconds* to decimal

You can work in reverse when converting from decimal to actual time. For example, convert 3.4 minutes to seconds. It is important to realise that 3.4 is the same as 3.40 where 40 is a multiple of 5 (5 x 8). So, 0.40 in seconds will be 3 x 8 = 24 seconds. So the final answer will be 3 minutes 24 seconds = **204 seconds**. Let's put this skill into action, a train leaves the Edinburgh station at 10:15 and takes 3.6 hours to get to Manchester. What time will it arrive in Manchester?

Step 1 – simplify 3.6 hours by converting 0.6 to minutes.

0.6 – since 60 is a multiple of 5 (5 x 12) then the equivalent in minutes will be (3 x 12) = 36 minutes

Step 2 – time of arrival will be 10:15 + 3 hours 36 minutes = 1:51 pm

When you are converting from decimals to minutes/second: **find the factor of 5 then multiply it by 3** and when you are converting from minutes/seconds (time) to decimal: **find the factor of 3 then multiply by 5.** Keep practising until it becomes second nature. I would recommend when finding the decimal equivalents of time to use method 2 when seconds/minutes are multiples of three, and method 1 for method for seconds/minutes that are not multiples of three.

#156. Mixtures and Composition

These types of problems build on fraction, ratio and proportion (strategy #147 -#151) as well as your ability to work with percentages. The subject matter varies, but you are typically presented with the composition of an object in terms of the percentage or ratio of its constituents. They can be either word or tabular problems where items or quantities of different values are mixed together and you have to determine some quantity (percentage, price, weight...) of the resulting object or mixture.

Example: *a farmer mixes 20kg of type A wheat, which costs £0.60/kg, with 60kg of type B wheat, which costs £0.80/kg, what is the price per kg of the resulting mixture?*

20 kg. of type A wheat costs 20 x 0.6 = £12
60 kg. of type B wheat costs 50 x 0.8 = £48
The resulting mixture is: 80 Kg of wheat with a price of £60
Each kg costs: 60/80 = **£0.75**

More difficult mixture and composition problems might require you to create an algebraic equation to solve them. For example, a seed farmer mixes some pumpkin seeds that sell for £2.50/lb with sunflower seeds that sell for £5/lb to make a 12-pound mixture worth $3/lb. How many pounds of pumpkin seeds were in the mixture?

Amount of Pumpkin + Amount of Sunflower = total Amount of Mixture
$2.50x + 5(12 - x) = (3 \times 12)$
Where x is the quantity of pumpkin seeds in lb
$2.5x + 60-5x = 36$
$60-36 = 5x - 2.5x$
$24 = 2.5x$
$x = 9.6$
There were 9.6 pounds of pumpkin seeds.

Let's look at another problem:

Example: *100g of silver which is 90% pure is mixed with an amount of silver which is 75% pure. The purity of the resultant mixture is 85%. What quantity of the silver with 75% purity was added?*

If the purity of the first silver is 90% then it contains 90g of pure silver.

Silver in 90% pure + Silver in 75% pure = Silver in 85% pure

$90 + 0.75x = 0.85 (100 + x)$

$90 + 0.75x = 85 + 0.85x$

$5 = 0.1x$

$X = 50$ (therefore 50 g of the 75% pure was added)

It never gets more complicated than this in the UCAT. Practice as many mixture and composition problems as possible if this is an area of weakness, you may be asked to find one of the following the exam:

- Total quantity (percentage, price, weight, etc.) of the mix when given the quantity of an item.
- The quantity (percentage, price, weight, etc.) of an item given the quantity of another.
- The quantity of an item when given the total quantity
- The ratio or percentage composition of two items in the mix

#157. Currency Conversion and Commissions

This is another type of problem that builds on ratio where you have to work with exchange rates (provided in text or tabular format) to convert from one currency into another. For example, the exchange rate for converting US dollars to Chinese yuan is 6.11. How much is 600 US dollars' worth in China? (answer: 600 x 6.11 = 3666). Unfortunately, questions in the exam will not be as straightforward, instead you'll be given scenarios where converting currencies is one of many steps to derive final answer. Usually, you are provided with currency exchange data in tabular form then given a scenario and have to use the table to solve it. Complicated questions will introduce commissions to throw you off, as long as you understand how it fits into the conversion then you should be fine. For example, John is going to Portugal on holiday and changes £200 to euros. The bank where he is exchanging the money charges a 5% commission. The exchange rate is £1 = 1.60 euros. How many euros does he get after paying the commission?

Step 1: how much John gets in euro – 200 x 1.6 = 380 euros
Step 2: deduct commission – 0.95 x 380 = 361 euros

Let's look at more challenging question, this is more in line with what you can expect in the UCAT:

How much pounds would John have to spend to get 500 euros, if the commission charged reduced to 2.5%?

Amount in pounds X exchange rate = amount in euros
Amount in pounds X exchange rate = 500
1.6x = 500
x = £312.50

However, there's is a 2.5% commission charge. So, £312.50 will not be enough. Therefore, we have to add the 2.5% commission price.

1.025 x 312.50 = £320.31

It rarely gets more complicated than that in the UCAT. The only other scenario is when you have to do similar calculations gathering data presented in tabular form. Here are a few tips to improve both accuracy and speed when dealing with currency conversion problems:

- **Learn basic formulas** - this will help reduce confusion when dealing with direct and reverse conversion problems.

- **Practice problems that involve commissions** – practice multi-step problems where converting currencies is one of many steps. During practice work on improving your speed.

- **Practice interpreting different types of currency exchange tables** – practice reading currency exchange tables. Learn to interpret both simple and complex tables, so if it comes up you can work through them quicker.

- **Always determine which currency is stronger** – when analysing conversion rates always determine which currency is stronger. For example, 1 USD = 0.7155 EUR. The EUR is stronger than the USD. When compared to 1 USD its value is lower than 1. Applying this pattern you can switch between any two currencies as well as using additional third currency as a converting factor.

- **Always have a reference point when reading tables** – To avoid confusion, make sure to use the left-most column in currency exchange tables as the reference point. Choosing a currency from that left-column, means you are now comparing the value of one unit of that currency to other currencies within that row.

Symbol	USD	EUR	GBP	AUD
USD	1	0.7582	0.6292	0.9728
EUR	1.3192	1	0.8299	1.2829
GBP	1.5896	1.2049	1	1.5459
AUD	1.0283	0.7794	0.6468	1

If we look at USD in the left-most column, and then compare it to currencies within the first row, we are actually comparing the value of 1 USD to other currencies including USD. In this case, USD is weaker than all other currencies as one unit of it is worth less than 1 of any other currency, with

GBP being the strongest: 1USD = 0.6292GBP. Moving on to row 3 in the left-most column, we see that 1 GBP is worth 1.5896 USD, which is the inverse 0.6292GBP.

#158. Geometry and Measure

Standard Geometry questions usually draw on basic understanding of perimeter, area or volume during calculations. For example, when dealing with scaling ratio problem (strategy #150), a calculation may require you to find the area of a rectangular kitchen floor plan, where you have to apply the area formula. More difficult problems might give you a 3-D shape where you have to apply understanding of surface area and volumes to solve them, e.g. finding the surface area of a conical tent. Cases where you have to use the π in the exam will provide the formula, so don't get caught up in memorising the area and volumes of sphere, cones etc. Here is a rough checklist of skills to go over during revision:

- Calculating Perimeter and Circumference
- Calculating Area
- Calculating the length of a missing side with given side or area (some problems can be solved with algebra)
- Calculating volume and surface area (when dealing with 3D shapes: cylinder, cone, sphere, etc.)
- Calculating how many objects of a specific size fits into a larger space
- Dealing with Geometry in Scale problems
- Making comparisons*

*Making Comparison: This is where you are given a shape and asked to compare to another one. For example, *a farmer has a square field, A, with an area greater than $1600m^2$. He decides to fit in a new barn, so increases the fields length by 20m and decreases width by 20m to give a rectangular field, B. What is the difference in perimeter and area?*

#159. Averages: Mean, Median and Mode

Mean, median, and mode are three kinds of "averages". There are many "averages" in statistics, but these are, I think, the three most common, and are certainly the three you are most likely to encounter in the UCAT.

The "mean" is the "average", where you add up all the numbers and then divide by the number of numbers. The "median" is the "middle" value in the list of numbers. To find the median, your numbers have to be listed in numerical order from smallest to largest, so you may have to rewrite your list before you can find the median. The "mode" is the value that occurs most often. If no number in the list is repeated, then there is no mode for the list. The "range" is another term where it is the difference between the largest and smallest values within a list of numbers.

Unfortunately, in the UCAT, you won't be given a list of numbers to work with, instead **you will be given a graph or table and be required to deduce the values you need to calculate the mean, median or mode**. The difficulty with these questions isn't the calculations but knowing which values to compute. During revision, practice calculating mean, median and mode **from tabular and graphical data**.

#160. Mental Rephrasing Technique

This strategy works well when dealing with questions that seem too complex – i.e. text, tabular or graphical questions with loads of information. The idea is that you **break down the problem by rephrasing it in your own words in a way that makes sense to you**. Try getting into the habit of doing this before attempting a question and always keep your "version" as simple as possible. This might seem basic, but it makes such a huge difference in the exam especially when dealing with unfamiliar data. For example, a question could ask *"What is the approximate cube foot of water needed to fill swimming pool A"*, this could be mentally rephrased as *"what is the volume of cuboid A"*, seems less complicated right? Another way to adopt this technique is where you rephrase the question based on how you intend to solve it. For example, *"What percentage of people that voted for party A in May voted for the same party in October?" This could be rephrased as "Total people that voted both months divided by Total May voters times 100"*.

#161. Have a Guessing Strategy

Guessing requires strategy for a test like the UCAT, and there are a number of strategies you can employ to help increase your chances of guessing the correct answer. Never resort to blind guessing too because the exam isn't negatively marked, you may not lose points but you'll be selling yourself short.

Strategy #1. Approximate

This is the art of Guesstimation where you approximate and estimate the numbers used in calculations to solve a problem more easily. Your derived answer will be off with a slight error margin which you can use to eliminate options that are not within the same ballpark. This is great when answer options have huge difference.

Strategy #2. Eyeball

This builds on strategy #105 and it is great for tabular and graphical questions, where you can use a bit of common sense to pick the right answer without doing any calculations. These kinds of questions come up more than you might think in the exam, so always keep an eye out for them.

Strategy #3. Odd-Even Rules

This builds on strategy #109 where you pick final option based on the rules governing odd and even numbers. For example, if you had a problem where you the final step required multiplying 259 + 24, you could save time by guessing and eliminating the answer options that are odd.

Strategy #4. Elimination

This is a helpful skill to master for the QR subtest, involves using a bit of logic to eliminate answer options that seem too extreme to be correct. When combined with the PIN method (strategy #X) you can work in reverse and save time in the test.

Strategy #5: half-calculations

Sometimes you do not have to finish calculations, you can get half way and make an educated guess. I encourage you to practice this during prep. When faced with multiple step calculations, try to do 1 or 2 steps then use a bit of common sense to guess final answer

#162. Master the Art of Elimination

Eliminate wrong options using a bit of logic and common sense to shortlist potential answers. When evaluating options, try to think which ones seem too extreme (either too high or too low) to be correct. Then work with the remaining options either by doing half-calculations (strategy #161), eyeballing (strategy #105), PIN method (strategy #108) or Guesstimation (strategy #142). If you can eliminate one wrong answer, your chances of picking the correct answer jumps to 33%. If you can eliminate two, those chances jump even higher, to 50%. This means that even if you can't definitively identify the correct answer, eliminating wrong answers will be a huge help.

#163. Build confidence in Deploying triage

Again, you are going to have to fight the urge of doing QR questions in order. Examiners intentionally include *time waster*s. In some cases, questions tend to be simple but have a lot of irrelevant information that may throw you off. Other times, they are three or more step calculations that take ages to solve. Whatever the case may be, build confidence in deploying triage. This will help increase your chances of finishing the subtest on time. Here are some example of QR triage strategies, use them as a rough guide in designing your own:

Strategy #1: Skip and come back to text, graphical or tabular questions that seem too long or complex.

Strategy #2: Skip and come back to a specific type of question-type identified during preparation as threats and weakness

Strategy #3: Skip and come back to questions you can't solve in 30 seconds.

Strategy #4: Skip and come back to questions that you have categorised as hard.

#164. Practice using Basic Onscreen Calculator Functions

In the image below, I've labeled each of the non-numerical functions of the UCAT calculator. I'll go through all of the functions below.

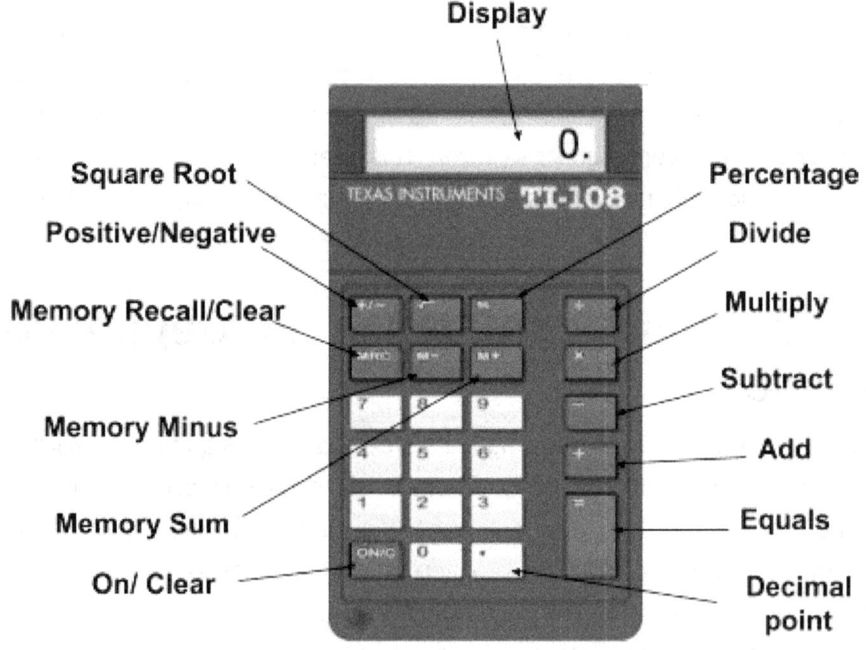

Percentage: Use this function for calculating percentages (see strategy #123)

Divide: Use this function for division of one number by the other.

Multiply: Use this function for multiplication of two numbers

Subtract: Use this function for subtraction of one number by the other.

Add: Use this function to add two numbers together.

Equals: Use this button to get a result of a function (addition, subtraction, multiplication, division, and so on). The equals sign is also useful for getting around the calculator's order of operations.

Decimal Point: Use this button to delineate decimals, like 3.45 or 2.3.

Square Root: Use this button to take the square root of a number. You must first enter in the number you want to take the square root of, then click then "root" sign.

Positive/Negative: Use this button to toggle back and forth between positive or negative for a number.

Memory Recall/Clear: Has two function - to recall a stored answer, hit MRC. You can do this to begin a calculation (e.g. MRC – 8) or at the end of a calculation (e.g. 86/MRC). Second function is to clear the stored answer by pressing M- then MRC, you'll know it was successful when the "M" disappears from the left-hand side of the display (see strategy #124).

Memory Minus: Use this to store the negative of an answer for later use in calculations. An M will appear to the left of the display to show that an answer's been stored.

Memory Sum: Use this to store an answer for later use in calculations, hit "M+". An M will appear to the left of the display to show that an answer's been stored (see strategy #124).

On/Clear: Use this to switch on calculator or clear the display. For example, let's say you wanted to divide 161 by 4, but accidentally put in "5" instead of 4, pressing the ON/Clear button would get rid of the entire operation so you could start over.

Tips for using the onscreen calculator:

- **Don't rely too heavily on calculator balance with mental maths:** Don't use the UCAT calculator for simple maths that would be quicker to solve mentally. Not only is it simpler to solve things like (4 x 8) or (2400/3) without going through the calculator, but it also cuts down on key strokes thus reduces the likelihood of error.

- **Use the Computer Keyboard When Possible:** Use the keyboard of the computer, rather than clicking each number/function, to save time. You should be able to use numbers on the keyboard to enter in numbers to the calculator. Similarly, you may be able to use other common shortcuts like *, -, /, +, =, and the return/enter key instead of having to click the functions on the calculator individually (and go back and forth between keyboard and mouse). The one limitation is that you can't use the backspace, delete, or C on the keyboard to clear the calculator display.

- **Be Careful of Order of Operations:** Keep order of operations straight by using the equal sign. If all else fails, you can solve for one part of an equation at a time. Write what that answer is on the white board provided in the exam, solve for the next part, write that down, and so on. But using the "equals" function speeds up the process tremendously.

#165. Save time with the Onscreen Calculator

This strategy assumes you are familiar with the contents in strategy #164.

Using calculator for multi-step percentage problems:

The percentage function is great for calculating percentages for problems where you have multiple steps.

Example: The population of Venezuelan refugees has risen in neighbouring countries due to the economic crisis in Venezuela. The refugee population in country A is 43% higher than the refugee population in Country B. The population of refugees in country C is 50% of that in Country B. If number of refugees in country C is 127,000, what is the population of Venezuelan refugees in Country A?

A.   *296,965*

B.   *363,219*

C.   *410,564*

D.   *310,549*

Solution:

This problem can be solved with 11 keystrokes:

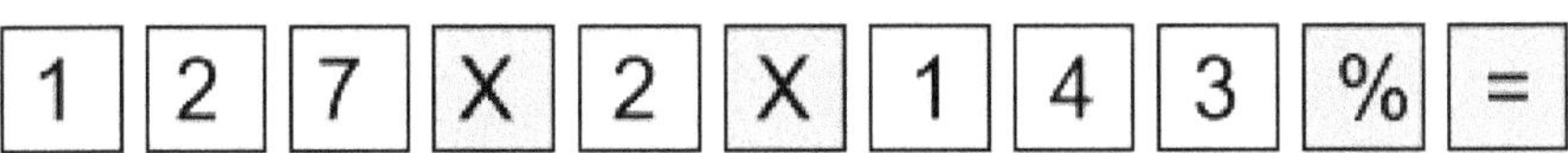

Answer on display screen: 363.219999 (Option B)

Using calculator for Compound interest (or exponential problems)

The memory recall function is great for solving exponential problems like compound interest. The trick is **to store the multiplier** (e.g interest rate) in the memory.

Example: *Amy bought a one bedroom flat in London for £93,450. In the three years that followed it's value appreciates by 8%. How much is the flat worth after three years?*

A. £97,765

B. £100,285

C. £102,395

D. £117,720

Solution

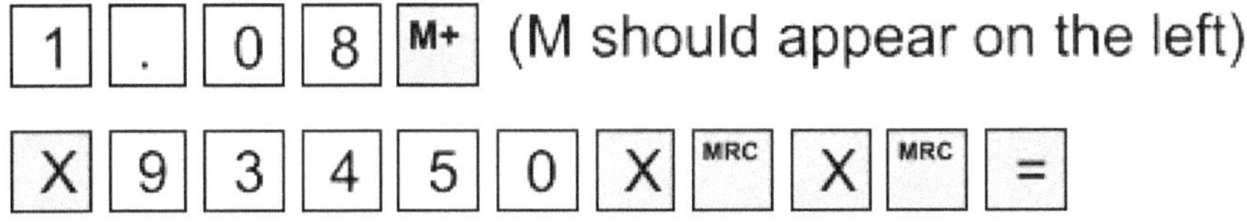

Answer on display screen: 117720.086 (option D)

Additional Strategies

Have a Timing contingency plan (see Strategy #48)

Have a Question Triage Strategy (See Strategy #47)

Have a Flagging Strategy (See Strategy #41)

Use Keyboard Shortcuts (See Strategy #42)

ABSTRACT REASONING

TIPS, TACTICS AND STRATEGIES TO IMPROVE YOUR UCAT ABSTRACT REASONING SCORE

#166. Decoding Rules – SCANS Method (Basics)

A great starting point for decoding rules in the AR subtest is to use the SCANS method. It is an acronym and mnemonic device to help structure your approach to finding rules and patterns within a set. It stands for:

S – Shape: What shapes are present? Are all the elements the same or different shape? (Refer to strategy #171)

C – Colour: Is there a consistent or relevant colour theme? Does any shape or element have a particular colour? (Refer to strategy #172)

A – Angle/Arrangement: How are the different shapes arranged in the box and in relation to each other? If faced with patterns like lines or arrows consider the ANGLE, i.e. obtuse or acute. (Refer to strategy #173)

N – Number: How many shapes, sides, intersections, right angles etc (refer to strategy #174)

S – Size: How does the size of each shape differ between boxes. Does it relate to colour, arrangement, number or a conditional feature, such as the existence of another shape or the total number of sides in the box? (refer to strategy #175)

Practice using the SCANS method during preparation, there is a tendency at the beginning of prep for students to get flustered, but it's just a case of training your brain through practice. You'll start to pick up speed over a week or two. Other similar mnemonics include SPONC or NSPCC, to find out more visit the blog at www.themedicblog.co.uk/abstract-mnemonics.

#167. Decoding Rules – SAMSSPEOE Method (Advanced)

The SAMSSMPEOE method is more relevant for decoding rules in the exam. It stands for:

Should All Medical Students Study Physics English or Economics

Where,

Should – **Shape**

All – **Adjacent**

Medical – **Mirror image**

Students – **Shading**

Study – **Symmetry**

Physics – **Position**

English – **Enclosure** (

Or – **Opposite**

Economics – **Equivalence**

The SAMSSPEOE method is more detailed than the mnemonics in strategy #166. With enough practice, it will become easy to remember when working through questions in the abstract reasoning subtest.

#168 Decoding Rules – The Three R's

For difficult problems where you cannot seem to spot the pattern, it is worth considering the three R's, they include: Reflection, Rotation and Ratio.

Reflection – Are the shapes or elements in a box a reflection?

Rotation - Do the shapes or elements follow a rotational pattern?

Ratio – Does the number of one shape to another a ratio? E.g. the number of triangles to circles is in the ration of 3:1.

#169 Decoding Rules – Beware of Conditional Patterns

Conditional patterns are where a characteristic of one object in a box dictates a characteristic of another item in the same box. This a popular scenario in difficult questions posed by examiners. For example, a pattern where each box contains a triangle and a circle, where if the circle is shaded it is positioned to the right of the triangle, if the circle is not shaded it is positioned to the left of the triangle. Conditional patterns are not that common so only really look for them if you can't find any relationships straightaway.

#170. Decoding Rules – Beware of Distractors

Distractors are shapes that have no relationships with other features in the box. You may find your yourself paying attention to certain elements that have no bearing on the relationship between objects. These tend to catch out candidates that overthink the entire pattern finding process. Just remember, if your hypothesis is correct, you will find no exceptions to the commonality rule despite the difference between the elements in the boxes. Always remember this: if a rule applies to a majority of the boxes in set but there is maybe one box that doesn't fit the rule, you've most likely fallen for a distractor. Recognise this immediately and switch hypothesis. There is likely something more complex or simpler going on.

#171. Things to Consider: Shape

- Are all the elements the same type of shape (e.g. square, circle, etc.)?
- Are the elements symmetrical or asymmetrical?
- Do the elements have curved or straight edges?
- Do the elements have right or acute angles?
- Is there an object which consistently appears in each box?
- Are shapes concave or convex?
- Are the shapes solid or dotted?

#172. Things to Consider: Colour or Shading

- Are some elements always a particular colour?
- Does each box have a certain number of colours?
- Does the colour of elements influence the counting of some of the key features (e.g. black shapes have even number of sides; white shapes have odd number of sides)?
- Are some elements always a particular colour?
- Does each box have a certain number of colours?

#173. Things to Consider: Position

* Does each element have certain shapes arranged relatively to each
* other?
* Does each box have rotated shapes?
* Does each box have elements arranged by features (colour, size, number of sides, etc.)?
* Are some shapes always in the same place?
* Are some objects inside others?
* Do some objects point in a particular direction?
* Are some components arranged along the x-axis or y -axis (i.e. 'stand' vertically or 'lie down' horizontally)?
* Do shapes overlap or intersect?
* Are some shapes parallel or at tangent to each other?
* Do some shapes mirror each other?
* Does each box have an object pointing to a particular direction? (e.g. a triangle always pointing to a black box)

#174. Things to Consider: Numbers

* Does each box have an odd or even number of shapes?
* Is the number of components or a particular shape the same in each box?
* Is the number of one type of shape the same?
* Is there a relative relationship between two different types of shapes (e.g. the number of black objects = number of white objects + 2)?
* Is the number of one type linked to a feature of another object (e.g. the number of dots in a box is equal to the number of sides of another object within the box)?
* Is the total number of edges of smaller shapes equal to the number of edges of the bigger shape (e.g. a box that has 2 small squares and 1 large octagon)?

#175. Things to Consider: Size

* Are some objects the same size or are they all different sizes?

- Is a particular object small or big in each box?
- Is there a relative relationship between the shapes of two different objects? (e.g. when triangle is small the circle is big and vice versa)

#176. Type 1 – Start with Simplest Box

This approach involves starting with the simplest box in either set A or set B to find the rule in a set. This is a good approach as the simplest boxes contain the fewest distractors, and thus will help you identify the true pattern. If the simplest box contains only one shape, your job becomes more straightforward. For example, if a box contains a single shaded circle in the corner of the box, you now have a clue that the pattern is either about circles, shaded shape or about arrangement in the corner. By checking other boxes in the set for these characteristics you will find the commonality quickly.

#177. Type 1 – Reverse Rule and Test

Once you have identified the pattern with a set, say set A, it is worth reversing the rule to see if it follows for the other set. For example, if the rule for Set A is *shaded circles on the top right corner of a box*, when reviewing set B consider the reverse which may be non-shaded circles on the bottom left corner of a box. Sometimes, Set A and set B tend to be opposites, so it's worth reversing the rules to find the pattern for the other set and seeing if it follows.

#178. Type 1 – Always look for at least two patterns

Always look for more than one pattern, sometimes this may include a set which has more than one rule. Even when you've found a rule, double check that no other rule exists. Get into the habit of doing this when working through sets in type 1 problems.

#179. Type 1 – Practice Focussed and Diffused thinking

When trying to figure out patterns that do not come to you immediately, try changing your perspective by moving closer and away from the computer screen. When you are close to the screen, you are using focussed thinking, which takes advantage of your prefrontal cortex to focus on one specific set of data and concentrates on it, but it doesn't let the rest of your brain become activated. Thus, other patterns are more difficult to spot this way, a helpful trick is using diffused thinking where you move further away from the screen to change perspective.

#180. Type 1 – Avoid Matching

It can be tempting when you cannot figure out the pattern straight away to look at the test shape and find a similar looking box in a shape. This should be **avoided at all cost**. Always seek to find relationships in a set, you are better off finding partial relationships than matching boxes.

#181. Type 1 – Never start with the Test Shape

I strongly recommend to start looking at the patterns in each set before looking at the test shape. The test shape may not even have the pattern for either set, so you waste time if you start with it. Also, you run the risk of matching test shapes to a similar looking box in one of the sets. If you can't find a pattern straightaway, go with your gut, flag and move on to the next set of questions.

#182. Type 1 – Two Box Comparison Technique

The comparison technique works by comparing the simplest box (strategy #176) to another box within the set. Compare the boxes, looking for any similarity with regards to the shapes, patterns, shading etc. Also checking if rules apply to the rest of the boxes in that set. During practice, start by

383

comparing two boxes at a time. As it becomes more natural begin comparing three boxes at a time.

#183. Type 1 - 40 seconds Rule

If you get stuck on a pattern for more than 40 seconds, go with your gut, FLAG IT and move on. Most patterns you spot will jump out at you within the first 40 seconds, and it is much more important to answer each pattern than get stuck for 3 minutes trying to answer one of the more complicated ones. You'll be surprised how easily you spot the pattern when you come back to it, this is usually because by answering more questions your eyes become more trained.

#184. Type 2 – Focus on one item at a time

It can be tempting to look at everything going on within a box in an effort to figure out what's going on. However, this is a common mistake that students make. Focus on one item at a time, see how it compares to the adjacent box. Focus on differences and changes of each item from one box to the next. Things to consider - position, shading, direction, rotation and size.

#185. Type 2 – Start by Only Assessing Box 1 and Box 2

Start by only focusing on the changes of each item in boxes 1 and 2, break the boxes into individual items that exist in both boxes and come up with a 'thesis' on how each items changes from one box to the next. Check thesis by validating it with boxes 3 and 4 (see strategy #186).

#186. Type 2 – Anticipate Box 3 and Box 4 before assessing in-depth

As you assess boxes 1 to 2, try to anticipate box 3 and 4 before looking at them in-depth. Validate thesis developed in strategy #185 by anticipating the components in box 3 and 4. For difficult problems where assessing box

1 and 2 is not enough, consider box 3 as well and anticipate patterns in box 4.

#187. Type 2 – Eliminate as-you-go Technique

As you identify the rule for each component eliminate answer options that do not fit the next anticipated change for an item. Many of the times you can narrow down the correct answer without defining all the rules covering each component.

#188. Type 2 – Beware of Alternate Patterns

These are situations where patterns work in an alternate fashion. For example, a series where certain a shape only appears in some boxes – like a black square in every other box (say box 1 and box 3 but not in box 3 and 4).

#189. Type 2 – 30 seconds Rule

If you get stuck on a type 2 problem for more than 30 seconds, go with your gut, FLAG IT and move on. Try coming back to it if time permits.

#190. Type 2 – Recognise the scenarios that you struggle to spot

Always remind yourself that there are a limited number of ways an item can move or change from one box to the next. During revision identify which common changes take you long to spot, there is always a pattern. Try to set a plan or technique in place to ensure you spot them quickly on exam day.

#191. Type 3 – Focus on one component at a time

Focus on one item at a time, see how it compares to the adjacent box. Focus on similarities, differences and changes of each to form your 'thesis'.

#192. Type 3 - Asses what components hasn't changed

Though not mandatory, I would recommend to start looking for similarities between boxes, i.e. items or elements that are static or DO NOT change. This may allow you to apply the same rule to the test box and eliminate answer options that do not contain the static item.

#193. Type 3 – Assess components that have changed

Identify changes in each item and come up with a 'thesis' to apply to the test box. Common components that change in the exam include colours, position and rotation.

#194. Type 3 – Predict Before looking at Answer options

Avoid looking at the answer options right way. Once you have formed your thesis, try to picture what changes in the test box would look like before assessing the answer options in-depth.

#195. Type 3 – Eliminate as-you-go

As you identify the rule for each component, eliminate answer options which do not fit the next anticipated change for an item.

#196. Type 3 – 20 seconds Rule

If you get stuck on a type 2 problem for more than 20 seconds, go with your gut, FLAG IT and move on. Try coming back to it if time permits.

#197. Type 4 – Same Strategies as Type 1

The strategies and techniques for type 4 questions are the same for Type 1 questions. See strategies #176 - #183.

SITUATIONAL JUDGEMENT

TIPS, TACTICS AND STRATEGIES TO IMPROVE YOUR UCAT SITUATIONAL JUDGEMENT SCORE

#198. Always Read the Scenario First

Always read the scenario thoroughly before answering questions. The good news is that they tend to be about one paragraph and do not take too long to read, so make sure you fully understand what is stated before attempting the accompanying questions.

#199. Identify Character and Respond Accordingly

The first thing you need to pay attention to in every scenario is the character or profession of the person involved (e.g. junior doctor, consultant, nurse etc.). This is particularly important for when considering what is expected from a medical student compared to a fully trained doctors. Even though both must display the same competencies, generally, medical students might not be as knowledgeable, so depending on the scenario you might have to take that into account that reporting to a higher authority might be appropriate thing to do. Typically, scenarios that compromise patient safety, confidentiality and data handling must be reported to higher authority.

#200. Make Independent Judgements

The responses provided for each scenario should be judged independently from one another. In other words, only base answer on the response option you're presented with not the answer picked from an earlier question (i.e. responses option) from the same scenario. Remember to **never make an assumption** and to always pick an option based on **what is expected from you not what you would do**.

#201. Understand the meaning of Answer options for Appropriateness

Appropriateness questions require you to rate how appropriate a response is in the context of the scenario. You have four answer options to choose from:

- A very appropriate thing to do

- Approprate, but not ideal
- Inappropriate, but not awful
- A very inappropriate thing to do

Some students can find it difficult to choose between the various options because they do not fully understand the definition of each one, make sure that you do, they are as follows:

- *A very appropriate thing to do*: it addresses at least one aspect (not necessarily all aspects) of the scenario.
- *Appropriate, but not ideal:* it could be done but not necessarily the best thing to do.
- *Inappropriate, but not awful:* it should not really be done, but would not be terrible.
- *A very inappropriate thing to do:* it should definitely not be done and would potentially make things worse.

#202. Appropriateness Questions – Categorise Your Reaction

When reading a scenario and determining how appropriate a response, it's a good strategy to categorise whether you think it is positive or negative. This can help with eliminating answer options:

- A very appropriate thing to do – positive (feels right)
- Appropriate, but not ideal - uncertain but positive overall
- Inappropriate, but not awful – uncertain but negative overall
- A very inappropriate thing to do – ngative (feels wrong)

When deciding which principles need further reading (strategy #206), it's a good idea to consider areas where you thought the response was positive but it's actually negative and vice versa.

#203. Appropriateness Questions – Options can be picked more than once

With each scenario you will be presented with 2 to 4 accompanying questions. It is important to realise that just because you rate an earlier response as 'A very appropriate thing to do', this doesn't mean that later responses cannot have the same rating. When you are rating a response, remember that an answer option can be picked more than once. For example, all responses provided <u>can be different but still all be a very appropriate thing</u> <u>to do</u>.

#204. Understand the meaning of Answer options for Importance

Importance questions require you to rate how important you think a response is, in the context of the scenario. You will have four options to choose from:

- Very Important
- Important
- Of minor importance
- Not important at all

The following are definitions of each term:

Very Important: response is vital and <u>must</u> be taken into account

Important: response <u>should</u> be taken into account (although not essential)

Of minor importance: response <u>could</u> be taken into account (but equally acceptable if it was not taken into account)

Not important at all: response is irrelevant or negative and <u>should not</u> be taken into account

#205. Importance Questions – Pay close attention to tone and wording

The wording and tone of the response can help you decide whether the provided response is important or not. The use of a positive words (e.g. support, propose, listen, etc.) tend to indicate overall positive response and the use of a negative tone (e.g. words like blame, ignore accuse, etc.) tend to indicate a negative response. Use a bit of common sense and pay close attention to the wording especially in cases where you are presented with a difficult scenario. Sometimes it helps to also consider how appropriate a response is in addition to overall tone/wording to help guide you on the degree of importance.

#206. Recognise Principles that need Further Reading

When reviewing incorrect answers during practice, try to recognise the underlying principles being tested and spend additional time reading up on them (see strategy #207). I strongly recommend prioritising the areas based on the following criteria:

Level of Priority	Explanation
Top Priority	Areas where you thought the response was positive/negative but was the opposite. E.g. picking 'appropriate' when response is 'inappropriate'
Mid Priority	Areas where you correctly identified whether it is negative or positive but were not able to recognise to what degree. E.g. picking 'important' when answer is 'very important'
Low Priority	Areas where you understand and can answer correctly.

Scenarios in the situational judgement can come in any form but test certain core principles, they are as follows:

- Integrity
- Teamwork
- Adaptability
- Resilience
- Managing difficult situations from multiple perspectives

You do not need any prior knowledge for the STJ subtest but I strongly recommend you recognise areas where you may misunderstand and need further reading to understand concept.

#207. Review the Good Medical Practice Guide

The *Good Medical Practice (UK or Australian)* are great blueprints that give detailed advice on how doctors should behave. Many of the principles and themes of the situational judgement test are derived from these document so I strongly recommend reading them beforehand. Make sure to take notes along the way. Here are some of the key lessons from the guide:

- Always be honest, open and act with integrity
- Patient's health and safety always comes first. The care of patient must be your first concern in any given scenario.
- Always respect patient privacy and right to confidentiality
- All actions must justify patients trust in you and the public's trust in the profession.
- Patient should always have informed consent
- Support a patient's wishes regarding treatment. Respect the patients' right to seek a second opinion.
- Address any issues immediately. Always speak with people involved before escalating it with a senior.
- Never apologise on behalf of a colleague.
- Seeking advice from a senior is almost always an appropriate thing to do.
- Respect the skills and contributions of your colleague. Never undermine them even if they are wrong. Support colleagues when appropriate.
- Work with colleagues in the ways that best serve patients' interests.
- Illegal acts and lying are totally inappropriate
- Always report inappropriate behaviour directly. Do not confront the person involved.

#208. Review the official Practice tests and Question Banks Multiple times

Attempt the official situational judgement question banks and practice test questions as many times as possible. I strongly recommend attempting them at the beginning of your preparation and keep a record of your performance, once sufficient time passes (say 2 weeks or so) go over them again and compare your performance. During review try to recognise the underlying principle being tested and do further reading to fully grasp concept. Once you are able to improve accuracy then focus on improving your speed (refer to step 4 and 5 in the preparation guide).

#209. Consider Answer Options irrelevant of Time frame

It is important to realise that the response options provided are not meant to represent all possible outcomes nor are subject to time. A response may still be right even though it might not be done immediately. When you think about it the other way round its easy to get your head around – an option that is wrong will never be an appropriate or an important thing to do regardless of time frame.

#210. Never Consider Response as the only course of action

Sometimes in the exam you may be given a scenario that you are familiar with and may know the "most appropriate" thing to do. However, the response provided is completely different. It common for students to pick the wrong answer say "appropriate" instead of "very appropriate" because they are subconsciously comparing their 'made up' response to the response provided in the question. Avoid this by understanding that the responses provided are not the only course of action.If it addresses at least one of conflicting issues in the scenario then it is right.

BEST FROM THE BLOG

10 MOST READ ARTICLES FROM THE MEDIC BLOG

How I Achieved a UCAT Score in the 90th Percentile

I took the UCAT, formerly known as the United Kingdom Clinical Aptitude Test (UKCAT), back in 2015. In this article, I dive into how I achieved a UCAT score in the 90th percentile. We will look at the TEN most helpful tips that were a game changer for me.

In case you don't know already, my name is Michael, I'm one of the guys behind the MEDIC BLOG. If you are reading this then you have probably clicked on a tweet, Facebook post or link on my blog and want to find out how exactly I smashed the UCAT! To be completely honest, the UCAT was one of the most challenging things I've ever had to overcome. I failed to get into medical school TWICE before finally succeeding on my third attempt and scoring one of the highest scores in 2015. However, it wasn't easy! I made so many mistakes when I initially prepared for the exam and noticed so many students offering bad advice on **The Student Room** that I had to share my preparation tips. The following TEN tips were a game changer for me, and I highly recommend you incorporate them into your preparation plan, they are as follows:

1. Set A Target Score

Obviously, you want to achieve the highest UCAT score possible. However, I highly recommend setting a goal, typically this would be the minimum UCAT score needed to be invited for an interview. However, universities assess the UCAT differently, some have a total cut-off, others use a percentile cut-off, whilst others do not have a cut-off at all. You need to find out how your choices assess the exam and set yourself an ideal and minimum target score based on your findings. When I took the UCAT the third time I came to the conclusion after researching all my choices that I needed to achieve an average score of 700 in each section and a minimum of 650. This was the benchmark I set myself during my preparation. If I achieved below 650 in a mock exam, I would consider it a fail. My entire preparation was based on beating this mark.

2. Identify Your Weakness first

Before buying any practice book or enlisting on any course, identify which areas of the UCAT you find difficult. The UCAT is made up of 5 subtests, they include Verbal reasoning, Abstract reasoning, Decision Making, Abstract Reasoning and Situational Judgement. The most reliable way to find out your weakness is by attempting the **official practice tests** on the UCAT website. It is updated each year to reflect the same level of difficulty candidates can expect in the exam. I recommend you attempt the tests at the beginning of your preparation, it will help you identify which areas you need to work on the most. I remember when I took the UCAT, I quickly discovered that the verbal reasoning subtest was my weakest section, I did not perform well in the official verbal practice tests so I spent a majority of my preparation time learning and adopting new strategies to improve my verbal score. In addition, I took things further by recognising that the inference and mostly likely verbal question-types were the questions I struggled with the most and thus, worked on those areas the most.

3. Prioritise Smartly

A common mistake candidates make is that they can at times find themselves feeding their ego, where they spend the majority of their time on sections of the exam they enjoy the most. This can be a waste of time, think about it, if you find the Abstract reasoning section easier than verbal reasoning. It doesn't make sense to practice more abstract questions than verbal. Studies show that honing your strongest section only boosts your overall UCAT score by 10-15%, but focusing on your weakest section can boost your overall score by 20-30%. That is double the results! Give priority to your weakest section and spend most of your preparation improving it. I spent 45% of my preparation time practising verbal questions (weakest section) and about 10% of my time practising my strongest section, which was the abstract section.

4. Practice Question-types not just Sections

I realised that the second time I took the UCAT my average score didn't improve by much despite practising thousands of questions. This is because practising questions only familiarizes you with the exam, it doesn't significantly improve your reasoning skills. In order to really smash the UCAT, you need to dig deeper! Try to understand which type of question in each subtest you struggle with the most. For instance, in the Abstract reasoning section there are four types of questions that examiners include, you might find one type of question difficult and another easy. It makes sense to focus your efforts on improving on the one question-type you find most difficult instead of the entire abstract section. Use this to your advantage by adopting strategies to fix the problem or a triage approach that levels your strengths and weaknesses.

5. Evaluate Your Progress

Another mistake to avoid is just practising questions after questions with no strategy. You must evaluate your progress throughout the duration of your preparation. A good way to evaluate your progress is by attempting a mock exam every week until your big day. After each mock exam compare your results with the previous one. This will help identify areas for improvement and ensure you are working effectively to boost your weakest skills. I remember when I took the exam I did a total of 5 mock exams before my big day. I noticed by the end of week 3 I had significantly improved my verbal reasoning score but my quantitative score hadn't improved much. Consequently, I spent a majority of the remaining weeks working on my quantitative skills.

6. Learn Exam Strategies To Boost Reasoning Skills

It is virtually impossible to significantly improve your cognitive skills in a short amount of time. For example, if you are a slow reader, you won't be able to increase your reading speed in 2 weeks or a month. However, you can learn exam strategies and tactics to improve your ability to read and comprehend information presented in the verbal section. I'm really slow at working out maths in my head, but I learned a few mental maths tricks to combat this so I can save time in the quantitative section.

7. Practice with an Online Course

The UCAT is a computer-based test, you need to practice questions under the same exam conditions as the real test. Pick an online course that closely mimics the testing experience and allows you to familiarize yourself with the onscreen format of the exam. The best online courses contain answer items at the same equivalent standard as UCAT and allow you review your responses against answer rationales. Online courses are also a great way to hone your exam strategies and techniques. There are loads of companies offering online courses so be sure to read reviews and customer feedbacks before choosing one.

8. Improve skill don't Just Practice

Practising questions only increases your familiarity with the exam. You need to also identify which elements or skills you struggle with and work on improving it. For instance, if you find the verbal section difficult, this might be due to a number of things, you might have poor comprehension skills or poor critical thinking skills, perhaps you are a slow reader? Try to identify what element you struggle with and try to improve it. I'm a naturally slow reader, in order to combat this I spent a month before the test reading everything online with *Spreeder* and adopting strategies to comprehend information in the verbal section quicker.

9. Do A Mock Exam Every Week

There is no other better way to assess yourself than attempting mock exams. Treat them like the real test. Do an entire 2-hour test with no breaks and no distractions. I recommend attempting your mocks on an online course to mimic the testing environment.

10. Be Confident

My last tip, do not let your nerves get the better of you, with practice you'll become more confident. However, the combination of applying and sitting the UCAT can be stressful but try to stay calm during your preparation – not only do you feel better, but also perform better.

Best time to take the UCAT

As a former UCAT candidate that took the exam three times I know a thing or two about the best time to take the exam.

If you plan on taking the UCAT (formerly known as UKCAT), you should already be aware that you are free to take the test anytime between July to October, but when is the best time to take the UCAT?

The Short answer: It depends

Most students take the UCAT at the end of the summer, in either August or September. This is probably due to the fact that summer is a busy time. Many students will either be working or enjoying a break from their studies. Some students might be travelling for part or all of the summer. Depending on your personal plans, there are any number of factors that could impact your decision on when to sit the UCAT. You can select any date from July 1st to October 5th to take the test, depending on availability at your preferred test centre. Thus, the choice is really up to you.

My advice is to consider factors that might affect your preparation or performance on the test day, and schedule your test appointment appropriately. Since you can choose any available test appointment, there is no reason not to choose the appointment that will give you the greatest advantage.

Factors To Consider Before Booking Your Test

The following are factors to consider before booking your UCAT test

1. Will you be working in the summer?

If you are working or volunteering, then you might need longer time to prepare for the exam. I recommend setting up study schedule, to ensure that you will have sufficient time to revise and practise before your test. Depending on your working hours, you might want to schedule your test for later in the summer

2. Will you be travelling, whether for a week or two or even longer?

If you have travelling plans, how realistic is it for you prepare for the UCAT? You might find it challenging to get a bit of space and quiet to revise and practise for the UCAT whilst on holiday. Taking a practice test in one sitting (and being able to concentrate, even for a bit of quick practice) could be very difficult indeed. If a vacation is on the cards, then you might want to consider delaying your UCAT preparation until after the holiday. Depending how long you are away for you could consider getting up to speed by attending a UCAT seminar upon your return, with your test appointment to follow 2 to 4 weeks later

3. Are You Taking the BMAT or GAMSAT?

If you are planning on taking the BMAT (in November) or GAMSAT (in September) then you might want to schedule your test early in the summer to give you time to prepare for the other exams.

4. How Prepared Are You?

I recommend booking your test depending on how easy you find the official UCAT practice tests. If you score well and find it easy I reckon 4 – 8 weeks is enough preparation. However, if you achieve a low score I recommend giving yourself longer.

5. How much time do you need To Prepare?

I personally do not think you need longer than 2 months to prepare for the exam. Typically students take between 2 weeks to a month to prepare for the UCAT. Attempt the official UCAT practice tests first then set a date depending on how easy you find it.

6. What's the best time of day for your test appointment?

The options to take the UCAT range from early morning – as early as 8am – to late in the afternoon – as late as 3 or 4pm, depending on the test centre. I strongly advise you consider past experiences taking tests, when are you the sharpest? A study recently published concluded that students are at the height of their cognitive abilities in the morning and perform better at exams. Remember, the UCAT will be a very intense 2 hours of staring at a monitor, while working incredibly quickly through a wide range of question types and completing over 200 questions, without a break, so you want to be at your best.

How I Would Prepare for the UCAT if I had to Re-take it Again

Last year, I got asked by a student 'how would I prepare for the UCAT if I had to re-take it?'. I thought it would be a good idea to share this with you.

Step #1 - Get Familiar with the Overall Interface and Format of the UCAT

I would visit the official UCAT website and go through all the free tutorials, these include the: question tutorial, tour tutorial and official guide. The goal here is to become familiar with the UCAT interface and gain familiarity with the different questions I can expect in the exam.

Step #2 - Become Familiar with the content and feel of the UCAT

I would begin to go through the official question bank for each subtest. I'll make note of areas that I struggled with and create an actionable list to go through later. I would also take note of anything that took me ages to solve or I guessed on.

Step #3 - Pinpoint Weaknesses

Once I feel generally oriented to the test, I'll want to figure out what areas I'm weak at and set a baseline. The best way to do this is by completing the Official UCAT practice tests under exam conditions. I would attempt at least 2 of them to accurately gauge my weak areas. I would use the UCAT conversion to calculate my score out of 3600 and identify my baseline score. The subtest I do the best in is clearly my strongest, but I'll try to get more granular than that. I would look back through the test to see which questions I missed and note down any patterns.

Step #4 - Set a target score

Once I have an idea of my baseline, I would set a target score! Ideally I would want it to be something I can realistically accomplish in the time frame I have for preparing for the UCAT. Realistically, from my experience I would say the following is realistic:

0-50 point improvement: 10 hours

60-80 point improvement: 20 hours

90-110 point improvement: 40 hours

120-200 point improvement: 80 hours

200+ point improvement: 90+ hours

Please Note: A 100-point improvement from your baseline in a month is definitely doable; a 300-point improvement in that time frame is much less so. And remember that the more you want to improve your score, the more time you'll have to put into it!

Step #5 - Create a Study Schedule

Based on my target score and how much time I scored in the practice test, I would make a study schedule for myself. I would aim to spend a consistent amount of time every week studying until test day. For example, if I thought I needed to study 40 hours to hit my target score, and the test is in 4 weeks, I would study about 10 hours a week for 4 weeks.

Step #6 - Review Important Content

Once I have my goal and schedule, I'll start reviewing content. I will learn any material I need for the test that I didn't know yet, and review what I already know. Mainly targeting the areas, I know I'm weak at, but not neglecting anything.

Step #7 - Learn Test Strategies

An important part of preparing for the UCAT is learning the best strategies to approach the test. I would learn as much as possible including how to best eliminate answers, guess when I need to, manage my time, and additional section-specific tips.

Step #8 - Practice

Practicing for the UCAT has two facets. The first facet is targeted practice of the skills I'll need to hone for the test. I would do this through practicing specific question types, topics, or entire sections that I need more work on. When I get questions wrong, I'll make sure to really work through them to understand where I went astray. Also, I'll engage in a couple of complete test practice runs. For these, I'll take practice tests under the same conditions as on test day.

Five Free Ways to Prepare for the UCAT in your Spare time

You do not have to wait until your exam is around the corner before you start preparing for the UCAT. There are some things you can do in your spare time to prepare for the UCAT and improve the reasoning skills needed for the exam.

In this article I'll share some of the best ways to prepare for the UCAT that take no longer than 5 -10 minutes. You can do this in your spare time and improve the skills needed in the exam.

#1. Use the Official UCAT Mobile App

This is a very helpful app to prepare for the UCAT. I recommend adjusting the settings so that you are prompted to attempt one question a day. You can choose to pick a specific subtest or a random section. I recommend downloading the app straightway! You can start preparing for the UCAT months ahead.

#2. Brain Training Apps

I recommend downloading apps such as Elevate or Luminosity to help improve speed reading and cognitive skills. These apps have free versions that will help boost memory, mental maths, vocabulary and comprehensive skills. Do daily exercises which usually last 5 minutes to complete.

#3. Read Newspaper articles and summarise from memory

Start reading articles more regularly, I recommend summarising articles once you've read them to improve recall and retention, which are useful for the UCAT.

#4. YouTube Videos

It is worth having a look at YouTube videos by previous applicants, offering helpful tips, reviews and more on preparing for the UCAT. You could watch one video per week to get more insight into preparing for the exam, learn from their experience and prepare more effectively for the exam.

#5. Read Articles from Blogs

Not to toot our own horn, but toot. My team and I provide comprehensive and detailed advice on how to prepare for the UCAT. From preparation tactics to exam strategies to adopt on test day, the MEDIC BLOG has you covered. Search the blog for specific tips and advice.

How to Use these Resources During Revision

While the above resources won't replace the majority of your regular, unglamorous studying, they can supplement it in a few key ways.

#1: To Target Specific Skills/Concepts

They can be helpful in **targeting specific skills or concepts that you have trouble with.** For type 2 questions in the abstract reasoning session, try reading an article or watching a YouTube video to learn or reinforce a strategy to help improve error rate.

#2: Keep Material Fresh Between Study Sessions

A quick UCAT mobile app session can be a good way to **keep things fresh between dedicated preparation sessions.** A few questions on official UCAT will help keep your "problem-solving brain" fresh when you go a day or two without any serious prep time.

#3: As Warm-ups, Breaks, and Rewards

These are also a great way to **warm up your brain at the beginning of a study session,** and a good way to re-energize yourself during a quick break. Watching a YouTube video on the UCAT from an influencer you like for a few minutes before you take a practice test will help turn on your brain and get the gears moving before the main event.

Achieved a low UCAT Score? Here is What to DO!

Let me start by saying that achieving a low UCAT score isn't the end of the world. It just means you might have fewer options available. Universities with a high cut-off mark are obviously not an option to apply. However, a UCAT score below the cut-off of one medical or dental school may be good enough for admittance to another. The following six things I recommend you do if you achieve a low UKCAT score:

1. Find Out Your Decile/Percentile Rank

The UCAT exam board uses a statistical approach called deciles to report the overall performance of candidates each year. A decile is any of nine values that divide data into ten equal parts so that each part represents 10% of the sample population. This statistical approach is descriptive and gives the exam board a good overview of the overall test performance each year. I recommend finding out where your overall score ranks before applying. It could be that the year you take the UCAT it is difficult and most students find it hard as well. This could potentially put you in a higher decile. You ideally want to be in the 6th decile and above. Applicants below the 4th decile are normally rejected before the interview stage.

2. Consider Universities that use a Point-based System

If you score a low UCAT score I recommend you research all the universities and find out how they each assess the UCAT. You want to shortlist universities that do not have a cut-off mark or have a cut off below your achieved score. Shortlist universities that also use a point-based system when picking applicants to interview and lay more emphasis on the entire application when shortlisting applicants i.e. predicted grades, work experience, reference, personal statement etc. Once you have shortlisted the universities, I recommend giving their admissions team a call, I cover this in detail in the next step.

3. Call Admission Tutors for More Information

Let's assume you've found seven universities that do not have a cut-off or use a point-based system. You want to get an idea on how heavily they rely on the UCAT. The best way to find out is by calling their admissions team. Here are a few questions you could ask:

- How heavily do you rely on the UCAT?
- How are applicants shortlisted for interview?
- What was the average UCAT score for applicants you interviewed last year?
- What was the lowest UKCAT score from last year's interview pool?

- What do you consider a good UCAT score? The admissions team's answer to these questions will give you a rough indication on how much they rely on the exam and the likelihood of you being invited for an interview. You want to shortlist four universities that will most likely invite you for an interview.

4. Strengthen Other Parts of Application

To give yourself the best possible chance of being invited for an interview you need to strengthen other parts of your application. There are a few things you could do to give you a bit of an edge:

- Show individual marks to modules on your UCAS application, show the marks of your highest scoring modules, GSCE subjects, etc.
- Personal Statement – highlight your commitment to a career in medicine and what you've learned from work experience. Try to stand out in whatever way you can.
- Provide a reference from someone in a medical or dental profession.
- Review your letter of recommendation – make sure all the attributes the university is looking for is highlighted by your referee. Ask your referee to also include an example of when you've demonstrated these skills in the letter.

5. Consider BMAT or GAMSAT Universities

There are many medical and dental programmes that do not require the UCAT as part of their application process. I would recommend taking the time to also research these options, they might actually be a more suitable or an easier route for you to study medicine or dentistry.

6. Consider Alternative Routes

There is more than one route to medicine or dentistry, for instance – you could consider graduate medicine or dentistry with a foundation year. There are alternative routes to both courses. One of my friends actually studied nursing at university before getting into medicine and I have another mate that did Biomedical Sciences before getting a place on the dental programme at King's College. These routes might be longer but will strengthen your application if you've achieved a high grade or degree class.

Achieved Target UCAT Score? READ THIS!

Let me first start by saying WELL DONE on achieving your target UCAT score! If you are anything like me you probably did the Carlton dance at some point to celebrate.

With one huge hurdle out the way there are still a few more you need to cross before reaching the finish line. In this article I share 5 key things to ensure you do before submitting your application.

1. Find out Your Decile/Percentile

I recommend finding out where your overall score ranks before applying. It could be that the year you take the UCAT is easier and most students scored highly as well. This could potentially put you in a lower decile or percentile.

2. Research Your Choices (Again!)

It is important to understand how universities use the UCAT before submitting your application. You can make more informed decisions after taking the exam. Use your results to shortlist universities based on the outcome of your results, I strongly advise to speak with the respective admission teams if you have any further questions or would like more information on how they assess the exam.

3. Strengthen Other parts of your application

Further increase your chances of being invited for an interview by strengthening other parts of your application.

4. Pick Final four choices Strategically

It is tempting to apply to all your ideal choices when you have a high UCAT score. However, it is important to tread with caution because Medicine and Dentistry are so competitive. I recommend after the test research all the medical or dental schools that use the UCAT. Split them into three groups:

- First Group – Rely zero to little on UCAT results
- Second Group – Do not rely too heavily on UCAT results
- Third Group – Rely heavily on UCAT results

Also look at their application:place ratio, this is a measure of how competitive a course is based on how many students apply versus the number of places on the course. You can find out the number of places and number of applicants by visiting the respective university website or calling their admissions office. A dental school with 380 places and 3000 applicants per year will have an application:place ratio of 7.9, which means about 8 people were applying for every place. The lower the application ratio the higher your chances, use both information to make a more calculated decision on where to apply to increase your chances of getting a place. You may want to pick a couple universities in the 1st or 2nd group that have a low application:place ratio if your first and second choices are really competitive.

5. Have a Back-up Plan

I think it is important to have a well thought out back up before applying, this could be anything from picking your 5th choice to studying abroad or taking a gap year. It is important to have this all planned out in case things do not go as planned. Take into consideration the following factors when constructing your back-up plan.

- What would you do if you do not get an offer?
- What else are you good at?
- What else do you enjoy?
- Will you take a gap year?
- Will you consider alternative routes?

Five Big Mistakes I Made When I Applied to Medicine

I want to share 5 Mistakes to avoid when picking your medical or dental school. These are some of the mistakes I initially made when I applied to Medicine the first time and was left with 4 rejections and no university place.

1. Research all medical schools

I appreciate you probably have 4 medical or dental schools picked out at this point. However, you need to keep an open mind when applying to these competitive courses. I remember when I first applied I only really looked into London medical schools because I wanted to live in London so badly, I didn't take the time to look into ALL the medical school programmes in the UK. I recommend researching into all the schools that offer your desired programme, find out their entry requirements, understand their selection process and how they assess the UCAT. This will help you make a more informed decision when shortlisting your choices.

2. Not Fully Understanding Their Selection Process

It is not enough to just understand what the entry requirements are, look into the selection process of these course, i.e. take the time to find out how they shortlist applicants to invite for interview. Do they put more emphasis on academics or the UCAT? Do they use a UCAT cut-off? Finding this out helps you know how realistic your chances are of being invited for an interview. You can make smarter decisions with regards to the final 4 courses you decide to shortlist. Just a quick tip, do not settle for just the information provided on university website. Get more details by calling their admissions office and asking more direct questions like "what was the minimum UCAT score for students you invited for interview last year" etc.

3. Only practising questions for the UCAT

The UCAT is a tough exam in my opinion, however, you can smash it if you prepare smartly. Just attempting questions with no real strategy isn't enough, you'll only end up familiarising yourself with the exam, not actually improving your reasoning skills. I recommend having a strategy for your preparation and developing an attack plan for each section of the exam.

4. Not focusing on "what I've learned" on my Personal Statement

I might as well just put it out there now, admission tutors care more about what you've learned from an experience. You can have 6 weeks placement at your local GP, but if you do not mention what you've learned you are no different from the thousands of applicants that apply to their course. Be reflective on everything you mention on your personal statement. This makes a huge difference.

5. Not Keeping Your Referee up to date

This is overlooked by many students, keep your referee in the loop about everything you are doing to get into medicine or dentistry! Tell them about your volunteer experience, what you've learned, what you hate, etc! Basically, treat them like a HUMAN DIARY and meet with them regularly either biweekly or monthly. I guarantee you they'll write a more compelling reference, backed up with examples of why they think you should be accepted into your desired course.

How to Pick Your Medical or Dental School

You probably have your ideal choices in mind but make sure to take the following factors into account before submitting your final application.

When I first applied to medicine I only looked into entry requirements - I was predicted to achieve 3 A's. I was naive to think I would get at least an interview based on my predicted grades. I laugh at myself every time I look back because the year I applied there were 80,000 applicants for medicine, which meant that there were 1-in-10 applicants per place. Medicine and Dentistry are so competitive, choosing a course largely based on thinking you will hit the entry requirements is not enough! The following are some of the KEY factors I took into account when I began narrowing down my choices the third time I applied:

1. Course Structure & Teaching: This is the most important factor when picking your medical or dental school. I recommend you choose a university largely based on course structure and its teaching style.

2. UCAT Assessment & Selection Process: Every university uses the UCAT differently, some have cut-off marks, whilst others use a scoring or point based system where they look at different components of one's application before deciding who to invite for interview. It is by understanding this process you can have a rough idea on how good your chances are of getting an interview. I actually cover this step-by-step in my UCAT Study Guide, I explain how to use this understanding to set a target score during practice. In fact, I would go as far as to say do not shortlist your choices until you have taken the UCAT. I remember I shortlisted 12 universities when I applied, I had my 4 ideal choices if I did well in the test. Another 4 if I did OK and a final 4 if I didn't perform so well.

3. Application to Places Ratio: The third time I applied I went a little 'crazy'. I looked into how many places against the number of students that applied to get a rough idea of the competition. For example, let's say that 2000 students applied to Queen Mary, which has 250 places. Then the Application:Places ratio would be 8 i.e. 8 students were applying to every place. I don't recommend using this as the main criteria to shortlist but could be worth using if you have to decide between two universities that are equal in comparison.

I took all THREE factors into account when shortlisting my choices and ended up with 4 medical school interviews. It is worth taking the time to think tactically about where to apply, don't just look at entry requirements.

Developing a SOLID Backup Plan

I think it is important to develop a backup plan before applying to medical or dental school because they are highly competitive courses. UCAS requires all medical school applicants to pick a fifth choice that is an alternative degree. For some this might be alternative routes to medical school or dental school, for others it could be a completely different career path but I recommend considering the following to help develop your medical school backup plan.

1. What Am I Good At?

I know loads of students that went into Biomedical Sciences hoping they will get into graduate medicine later down the road. Make sure you are picking your fifth choice based on what you are good at, look into core modules, teaching styles and course structure. I remember when I was at the University of Manchester there were students that struggled with the chemistry modules of the course.

They just couldn't get their heads round the core chemistry principles they needed to apply to key Pharmaceutical concepts. I actually dated a girl on my course who hated chemistry and struggled with the chemistry concepts, but was very good with the physiology modules. She would have probably found it a lot easier if she stuck solely with her passion and studied physiology instead. Take the time to really think about what you are good at, do not pick a fifth choice solely because it could potentially get you a place into graduate medicine or dentistry later down the road.

2. What Do I enjoy?

In my opinion, this is the most important question you must ask yourself. Pick a fifth choice that you enjoy. You have to imagine that if a career in medicine or dentistry doesn't work out what would you rather do? What would you dedicate the next 4 years studying? Or maybe what other career would you consider? For some this might still be in the health sector, for others it could be something completely different. I have a mate I studied with in Pharmacology that now runs a mobile app company that helps enhance cognitive function – combining both his passion in neuroscience and technology. Remember that whatever you decide will take 3-4 years, that's a really long time if you are not passionate.

3. What Are the Entry Requirements, Course Structure and Teaching Style?

Another consideration that makes a significant difference from one university to another is how you are taught and assessed. There are three main approaches: traditional, integrated and problem-based learning. Check out which approach your preferred choices use and consider if this suits the way you enjoy learning.

4. Should I take A Gap Year?

Taking a gap year can be tremendously beneficial to one's personal growth, whether one decides on enrolling in a structured gap year program, spend time volunteering abroad or simply traveling the world. Regardless, taking a gap year gives you the chance to think things through, do not rush into university if you aren't sure. I took a gap year and it was probably one of the smartest things I've ever done despite getting pressured from family to get into university. You can use the time to reflect on your achieved grades or get relevant work experience to enhance your application.

5. How Can I Make My Application Stronger?

This last point is really for those who are determined to get in medical or dental school if they do not make it the first time applying. I recommend you consider how you can make your application stronger the next time you reapply. For instance, if you did not achieve the grades, you'll need to work hard enough to get a strong degree class in your backup choice.

UCAT CHECKLIST

USE AS GUIDANCE TO COVER ALL BASES

Preparation Checklist

Tick Once Completed

Understand test format, question-types and timing	
Practise using the exam interface and tools (keyboard shortcuts, calculator and flagging)	
Understand UCAT marking	
Understand how choices use the UCAT	
Set minimum and ideal target scores	
Identify and rank subtests according to strengths	
Achieve target score in at least 2 mocks	

Verbal Reasoning Checklist

Tick Once Completed

Identify and rank question-types according to strengths	
Reading strategy and Approach for long passages with "True,False and Can't Tell" questions.	
Reading strategy for short passages with "True, False and Can't Tell" questions.	
Reading strategy and Approach for long passages for each type of multiple-choice question type.	
Reading strategy and Approach for short passages for each type of multiple-choice question type.	
Approach for dealing with weakest areas and most difficult question-types	
Test and develop Triage Strategy	
Test and develop Guessing Strategy	
If necessary, develop flagging strategy	

Consistently complete 44 questions in 21 minutes with a low error rate	
Have a timing contingency plan	

Decision Making Checklist

Tick Once Completed

Identify and rank question-types according to strengths	
Approach for solving logical puzzles	
Approach for drawing conclusions	
Approach for interpreting questions	
Approach for evaluating arguments	
Approach for solving venn problems	
Approach for solving probability problems	
Approach for dealing with weakest areas and most difficult question-types	
Test and develop Triage Strategy	
Test and develop Guessing Strategy	
If necessary, develop flagging strategy	
Consistently complete 29 questions in 31 minutes with a low error rate	
Have a timing contingency plan	

Quantitative Reasoning Checklist

Tick Once Completed

Identify and rank question-types according to strengths	

Recognise and practice weak and rusty maths concepts	
Recognise whether a question is easy, medium or hard before attempting it	
Approach for short text problems	
Approach for long text problems	
Approach for simple tabular problems	
Approach for complex or unfamiliar tabular problems	
Approach for simple graphical problems	
Approach for complex or unfamiliar graphical problems	
Learn formulas and shortcuts for most common concepts (e.g. percentage change, speed, etc.)	
Learn mental maths tricks to save time	
Use onscreen calculator to save time	
Approach for dealing with weakest areas and most difficult question-types	
Test and develop Triage Strategy	
Test and develop Guessing Strategy	
If necessary, develop flagging strategy	
Consistently complete 36 questions in 24 minutes with a low error rate	
Have a timing contingency plan	

Abstract Reasoning Checklist

Tick Once Completed

Identify and rank question-types according to strengths	
Approach for Type 1 questions	

Approach for Type 2 questions	
Approach for Type 3 questions	
Approach for Type 4 questions	
Approach for dealing with weakest areas and most difficult question-types	
Approach for spotting distractors	
Approach for spotting conditional patterns	
Approach for spotting alternate patterns (Type 2)	
Test and develop Triage Strategy	
Test and develop Guessing Strategy	
If necessary, develop flagging strategy	
Consistently complete 55 questions in 13 minutes with a low error rate	
Have a timing contingency plan	

Situational Judgement Checklist

Tick Once Completed

Identify and rank question-types according to strengths	
Approach for Appropriateness questions	
Approach for Importance questions	
Review official question banks and practice tests to compile list of concepts tested in exam (e.g integrity, teamwork, resilience, etc)	
Read Good Medical Practice booklet and tomorrow's doctor's guide to understand qualities and key medical principles	
Further reading for most commonly tested principles: Integrity, teamwork, resilience and Adaptability	

Approach for dealing with weakest areas and most difficult question-types	
Test and develop Triage Strategy	
Test and develop Guessing Strategy	
If necessary, develop flagging strategy	
Consistently complete 69 questions in 26 minutes with a low error rate	
Have a timing contingency plan	

Index

A

B

C

D

K

L

M

N

O

P

W

CPSIA information can be obtained
at www.ICGtesting.com
Printed in the USA
BVHW040712100621
609205BV00020B/61